BIOACTIVE ANALYTES, Including CNS Drugs, Peptides, and Enantiomers

METHODOLOGICAL SURVEYS IN BIOCHEMISTRY AND ANALYSIS

Series Editor: Eric Reid

Guildford Academic Associates
72 The Chase
Guildford GU2 5UL, United Kingdom

The series is divided into Subseries A: Analysis, and B: Biochemistry
Enquiries concerning Volumes 1–11 should be sent to the above address.

Volumes 1–10 edited by Eric Reid

Volume 1 (B): Separations with Zonal Rotors

Volume 2 (B): Preparative Techniques

Volume 3 (B): Advances with Zonal Rotors

Volume 4 (B): Subcellular Studies

Volume 5 (A): Assay of Drugs and Other Trace Compounds in Biological Fluids

Volume 6 (B): Membranous Elements and Movement of Molecules

Volume 7 (A): Blood Drugs and Other Analytical Challenges

Volume 8 (B): Cell Populations

Volume 9 (B): Plant Organelles

Volume 10 (A): Trace-Organic Sample Handling

Volume 11 (B): Cancer-Cell Organelles
Edited by Eric Reid, G. M. W. Cook, and D. J. Morré

Volume 12 (A): Drug Metabolite Isolation and Determination
Edited by Eric Reid and J. P. Leppard
(includes a cumulative compound-type index)

Volume 13 (B): Investigation of Membrane-Located Receptors
Edited by Eric Reid, G. M. W. Cook, and D. J. Morré

Volume 14 (A): Drug Determination in Therapeutic and Forensic Contexts
Edited by Eric Reid and Ian D. Wilson

Volume 15 (B): Investigation and Exploitation of Antibody Combining Sites
Edited by Eric Reid, G. M. W. Cook, and D. J. Morré

Volume 16 (A): Bioactive Analytes, Including CNS Drugs, Peptides, and Enantiomers
Edited by Eric Reid, Bryan Scales, and Ian D. Wilson

BIOACTIVE ANALYTES, Including CNS Drugs, Peptides, and Enantiomers

Edited by

Eric Reid
Guildford Academic Associates
Guildford, United Kingdom

Bryan Scales

and

Ian D. Wilson
ICI Pharmaceuticals Division
Alderley Park, United Kingdom

PLENUM PRESS • NEW YORK AND LONDON

Library of Congress Cataloging in Publication Data

International Bioanalytical Forum (6th: 1985: University of Surrey)
    Bioactive analytes.

    (Methodological surveys in biochemistry and analysis; v. 16.)
    "Based on the Sixth International Bioanalytical Forum, held September 10–13,
1985, at the University of Surrey, Surrey, Guildford, United Kingdom"—T.p. verso.
    Includes bibliographies and indexes.
    1. Psychotropic drugs—Analysis—Congresses. 2. Drugs—Analysis—Congresses. 3.
Neuropeptides—Analysis—Congresses. 4. Central nervous system—Congresses. I.
Reid, Eric, 1922–   . II. Scales, Bryan. III. Wilson, Ian D. IV. Title. V. Series.
[DNLM: 1. Central Nervous Systems Agents—analysis congresses. 2. Peptides—
analysis—congresses. W1 ME9612NT v. 16 / QU 68 I583 1985b]
RM315.I538   1985   615'.78   86-21204
ISBN 0-306-42400-2

Based on the Sixth International Bioanalytical Forum, held September 10–13, 1985,
at the University of Surrey, Guildford, United Kingdom

© 1986 Plenum Press, New York
A Division of Plenum Publishing Corporation
233 Spring Street, New York, N.Y. 10013

Printed in the United States of America

Senior Editor's Preface

The bibliographic usefulness of what many readers may not recognize to be a book *series* has again encouraged the customary thorough editing and indexing, in the interests of clarity, integration and effectiveness of retrieval. Repeated allusions in the present book to articles in past volumes testify to the continuity of the biennial Forum series that gives rise to successive volumes; the present one arose from the 6th International Bioanalytical Forum held* in Guildford, U.K., in September 1985.

The continuity has been **coupled** with evolution. There are striking trends, apparent from this book, in the analytical area concerned with determining drug levels in body samples. HPLC, usually without elaborate sample preparation, has pushed aside traditional GC, although not capillary GC. Solvent-extraction lore remains invaluable; but the solid-phase approach now dominates sample preparation. It is now hardly esoteric in HPLC to use electrochemical (EC) detection ('ECD' is a *banned term* unless electron-capture detection is meant!). Proton NMR offers promise, but not in connection with the ever-increasing demand for high sensitivity, especially for pharmacokinetic or bioavailability studies on low-dose drugs (maybe administered with little appreciation of the analytical skills needed to supply requisite blood-level data). Largely in this connection, there is a vogue for ligand methods, sometimes preceded by HPLC (thereby minimizing specificity problems). This sensitivity need is especially great in two areas - CNS-active drugs, and peptides - which, along with chiral separations, warranted special attention at the Forum and in these pages. For drug determinations in general, HPLC and other analytical literature has become dominated by humdrum recipes which seldom match a 'Forum philosophy' - that the rationale of method development should be presented, with consideration of unsatisfactory as well as adopted procedures.

Fortunately, many knowledgeable and critical analytical investigators participated enthusiastically in the Forum. Moreover, almost all of them 'made time', promptly or eventually, to furnish a publication text, albeit varying in quality of presentation. The Co-Editor who first looked at the MSs. was prompted by one MS. to compose a pseudo-Shakespearean playlet which opened with his coming on-stage amid "Alarums and wailing". The second Co-Editor's contribution to the playlet alluded to the anticipated reaction of the Senior Editor - who, with a "wicked smile", exclaims "Steady-on, my children: there's much more to come!" as he makes his exit, thinking "This is Heaven!". The help from Co-Editors to which this thought refers

*with valued support from U.K. pharmaceutical companies - Beechams, Glaxo, ICI and SK&F (Smithkline Beckman) - and from Bachem (U.K.).

was in fact a boon. Both are blameless for any editorial idiosyncrasy that a book reader may notice. Their initial editing was in turn edited, e.g. with reprieval of "quantitate" where a Co-Editor preferred "quantify". — The Senior Editor felt that each author's preference should usually be respected, but confesses to his own idiosyncrasies, e.g. abhorrence of "extremely" where "very" would convey the meaning, and partiality to "due to", arguably a solecism, and to hyphenation as a visual aid within multi-adjectival phrases.

Achievement of readable, terse and unambiguous presentation whilst not violating each author's style was, then, the aim of the editing, which earned commendation from some authors even where 'tidying-up' was drastic. There was a gratifying response from one author when discrepancies between a Table and the text in assay sensitivities were pointed out.- "The problem appeared because of an interpretation of the terms sensitivity, detection limit, lower limit of measurement and reliability within the people in our laboratory. We have corrected the problem and thank the Editors for pointing this problem out." (Vol. 10 is especially pertinent to this 'grey area'.)   Editorial effort has also been devoted to the aim of a true, integrated book as distinct from a 'Conference Proceedings' patchwork. This, coupled with the calibre of the material, should benefit analysts working in a challenging but treacherous field.

'Permissions': the publishers, especially Elsevier, were generous.

Abbreviations.- Standard terms, undefined, include: ACTH, MSH, TSH; GC, HPLC ('LC' is disfavoured), TLC, UV [absorbance]; GC detection: (A)FID, NPD ($\equiv$ AFID), ECD (*see above*; EC = electrochemical); also statistical terms (e.g. C.V.) and column features (e.g. inside diameter, i.d.; HETP). Temperatures (°) are always Celsius. In the articles concerned, some well-known terms are usually redefined:-

Ab, antibody (M, monoclonal)   MS, mass spectrometer (CI, chemical
RIA, radioimmunoassay   ionization; EI, electron impact;
RRA, radioreceptor assay   FAB, fast atom bombardment)
IMA, immunometric assay (cf. p. 95) CSP, chiral stationary phase
BSA, bovine serum albumin   NP/RP, normal/reverse phase (HPLC);
IE, ion exchange   C-18 and ODS are synonymous.

PG (= peptidoglycan in #A-1) usually = prostaglandin; see #NC(A)-3, for LT, TX also. For peptides (GF = growth factor; see p. 128 for opioid types) there are text listings, notably on pp. 17, 65 and 75.

Analyte Index.- Following past practice, compounds are grouped according to chemical features that could guide method development, especially solvent extraction, derivatization, GC response, ion-pairing.

Guildford Academic Associates   ERIC REID
72 The Chase, Guildford,
Surrey, GU2 5UL, U.K.   *20 May, 1986*

Contents

The 'NOTES & COMMENTS' ('NC' items') at the end of each section
include comments (with initial sub-index) made at the Forum on
which the book is based, along with some supplementary material.

Senior Editor's Preface, with an abbreviations list   v

List of Authors   xi

#A   **PEPTIDES AND OTHER ENDOGENOUS-TYPE ANALYTES**   1

#A-1   Assays of peptidoglycans and specific antibodies in
biological samples - JELKA TOMAŠIĆ   3

#A-2   Cyclic decapeptides in kidney - IAN R. TEBBETT   13

#A-3   Analysis of protein growth factors and optimization
of their separation by HPLC - JOHN A. SMITH &
MICHAEL J. O'HARE   17

#A-4   HPLC-EC measurement of neuropeptides in biological
samples - G.W. BENNETT, J.V. JOHNSON & C.A. MARSDEN   37

#A-5   Determination of substance P and neurokinins by a
combined HPLC/RIA procedure - J.M. CONLON & C.F. DEACON ..   45

#A-6   Methods and problems in the assay of CSF for
β-endorphin and other endogenous peptides -
RICHARD F. VENN, STEPHEN J. CAPPER, JOHN S. MORLEY &
JOHN B. MILES   55

#A-7   The importance of defined tracers in RIA -
K.G. McFARTHING, M.R. HARRIS, A. SMITH, R.J. PITHER,
D. SILVER, A.L. HAMILTON, D.G. SMYTH & R.H. JACKSON   65

#A-8   The use of radioimmunoassays for cryptic regions
of peptide precursors, in the study of biosynthetic
mechanisms - R. DIMALINE, H. DESMOND, A-C. JONSSON,
S. PAUWELS, H. RAYBOULD, A. VARRO, L. VOWLES &
G.J. DOCKRAY   75

#A-9   Clinical assay of somatomedins by RIA - J.D. TEALE
& V. MARKS   87

#A-10   Immunometric approach to peptide hormone analysis
- J.G. RATCLIFFE, A. WHITE, S. DOBSON, A.D. SWIFT &
S. BRUCE   95

#NC(A)   **NOTES and COMMENTS relating to the foregoing topics**   107
including Notes on:

#NC(A)-1   Endogenous molecules in relation to drugs: comments
prompted by the focus on peptides - STEPHEN H. CURRY ..   109

#NC(A)-2   Determination of 2-pyrrolidone in plasma -
D. DELL, G. WENDT, F. BUCHELI & K-H. TRAUTMANN   113

#NC(A)-3   Determination of prostaglandins, prostaglandin
           analogues and leukotrienes in biological samples
           - M.V. DOIG & J.A. SALMON 117

#NC(A)-4   Dynorphin-(1-9) and enkephalin studies with
           vas deferens - MICHAEL J. RANCE, LYNNE MILLER,
           JOHN S. SHAW & JOHN R. TRAYNOR 121

#B   CNS-ACTIVE DRUGS AND THEIR METABOLITES 131

#B-1   Thirty years of antipsychotic drug analysis -
           STEPHEN H. CURRY 133

#B-2   Determination of benzodiazepines: the present-day
           scene - M. DANHOF, J. DINGEMANSE & D.D. BREIMER 141

#B-3   Analytical pitfalls with tricyclic and newer anti-
           depressants in biological samples - C. LINDSAY DEVANE 149

#B-4   Determination of phenothiazines: the present-day
           scene - G. McKAY, S.F. COOPER & K.K. MIDHA 159

#B-5   Analysis of thioxanthenes by HPTLC, HPLC, capillary
           GC, and RIA - A. JØRGENSEN, K. FREDRICSON OVERØ,
           T. AAES-JØRGENSEN & J.V. CHRISTENSEN 173

#B-6   HPLC-EC determination of physostigmine in biological
           samples - ROBIN WHELPTON & PETER HURST 181

#B-7   HPLC-UV determination of substituted benzamides in
           biological fluids for their pharmacokinetic
           study - F. BRESSOLLE, J. BRES & M. SNOUSSI 189

#NC(B)   NOTES and COMMENTS relating to the foregoing topics .. 199
           including Notes on:

#NC(B)-1   Applicability of disposable extraction columns to
           CNS-drug analysis - J.P. DESAGER 201

#NC(B)-2   Isomerism of the ring-sulphoxides of thioridazine
           and of some other phenothiazine drugs -
           A.S. PAPADOPOULOS & J.L. CRAMMER 207

#NC(B)-3   Relevance of metabolism to methods for determining
           nomifensine in biological samples - M. UIHLEIN,
           W. HEPTNER & I. HORNKE 211

#NC(B)-4   HPLC determination of diclofensine and metabolites in
           plasma -J.A.F. DE SILVA & N. STROJNY 213

#C   SEPARATION TECHNOLOGY APPLICABLE TO VARIOUS DRUGS
           AND TO ENANTIOMERS 219

#C-1   Novel capillary gas-chromatographic phases applicable
           to drugs - B. CADDY & W.M.L. CHOW 221

#C-2   Liquid-solid sample preparation - R.D. McDOWALL,
        J.C. PEARCE, G.S. MURKITT & R.M. LEE 235

#C-3   Applicability of HPLC chiral stationary phases to
        pharmacokinetic and disposition studies on
        enantiomeric drugs - IRVING W. WAINER 243

#C-4   Attempts to obtain separations of chiral anti-
        cholinergic drugs - KARLA G. FEITSMA, BEN F.H. DRENTH,
        KOR H. KOOI, JAN BOSMAN & ROKUS A. DE ZEEUW 259

#NC(C) NOTES and COMMENTS relating to the foregoing topics 271
        including Notes on:

#NC(C)-1 Separation of fenfluramine and norfenfluramine
          enantiomers by derivatization and GC-ECD -
          R.P. RICHARDS, S. CACCIA, A. JORI, M. BALLABIO,
          P. DE PONTE & S. GARRATINI 273

#NC(C)-2 Towards chiral TLC plates: some preliminary
          studies - IAN D. WILSON 277

#NC(C)-3 RP-HPLC separation, as diastereoisomers, of acebutolol
          and related compounds - A.A. GULAID, O.R.W. LEWELLEN
          & A.R. BOOBIS 283

#NC(C)-4 Separation of chiral drugs and metabolites by
          capillary gas chromatography - H. FRANK 285

#NC(C)-5 Preparation, properties and use of capillary GC
          columns for drug analysis - H. FRANK 289

#NC(C)-6 GC analysis with a dedicated automated derivatizer
          - H. FRANK, G.J. NICHOLSON & J. GERHARDT 291

#NC(C)-7 Robotics in drug analysis - J.C. PEARCE,
          M.P. ALLAN & R.D. McDOWALL 293

#NC(C)-8 Fluorimetric assay of an antihypertensive drug with
          automated sample processing and HPLC - P.R.J. CEELEN,
          H.M. RUIJTEN & H. DE BREE 297

#NC(C)-9 HPLC separation of maloprim-related analytes,
          exemplifying computer-guided optimization -
          C.R. JONES & B.C. WEATHERLEY 299

#NC(C)-10 Bulky ion-pair reversed-phase HPLC: some applications
          in biomedical research - HERMANN-JOSEF EGGER &
          GUY FISCHER 303

#D   APPROACHES TO ANALYTE DETECTION, IDENTIFICATION
        AND MEASUREMENT 319

#D-1   The application of high resolution proton NMR
        spectroscopy to the detection of drug metabolites
        in biological samples - J.K. NICHOLSON, P.J. SADLER,
        K. TULIP & J.A. TIMBRELL 321

#D-2   Detection, identification and quantitative analysis
          of drugs by ^{1}H NMR - ISMAIL M. ISMAIL & IAN D. WILSON .. 337

#D-3   Pre-column (HPLC) fluorescence labelling of
          glucuronides - H. LINGEMAN, G.W.M. MEUSSEN,
          C. VAN DER ZOUWEN, W.J.M. UNDERBERG & A. HULSHOFF 343

#D-4   Photodiode array HPLC detectors in metabolic profiling
          and other analytical screening techniques -
          ROKUS A. DE ZEEUW 355

#D-5   A rotating filter disc alternative to photodiode
          array detection systems - PETER C. WHITE 373

#NC(D)   NOTES and COMMENTS relating to the foregoing topics 383
          including Notes on:

#NC(D)-1 Metabolic study of two unlabelled drugs using HPLC
          with UV-Vis diode array detection - M.P. VAN BERKEL,
          B.J. DE JONG, H. DE BREE, E. KOORN & W.R. VINCENT 385

#NC(D)-2 Determination of the glucuronide(s) of the anti-
          neoplastic agent etoposide - J.J.M. HOLTHUIS,
          W.J. VAN OORT & A. HULSHOFF 389

#NC(D)-3 Recent developments in post-column reactors for
          HPLC - U.A.Th. BRINKMAN 395

#NC(D)-4 HPLC with on-line electron-capture detection -
          U.A.Th. BRINKMAN 397

#NC(D)-5 Liquid chromatography— mass spectrometry (LC-MS) -
          L.E. MARTIN, M.S. LANT & JANET OXFORD 399

ANALYTE INDEX 409

GENERAL INDEX 415

List of Authors

Primary author

Co-authors, with relevant name to be consulted in left column

G.W. Bennett - pp. 37-43
Queen's Med. Centre, Nottingham

J. Bres - pp. 189-197
Univ. of Montpellier, France

U.A.Th. Brinkman -
pp. (i) 395-396, (ii) 397-398
Free Univ., Amsterdam

B. Caddy - pp. 221-234
Univ. of Strathclyde, Glasgow

J.M. Conlon - pp. 45-54
Max-Planck-Gesellschaft,
Göttingen, W. Germany

S.H. Curry -
pp. (i) 109-112, (ii) 133-140
Univ. of Florida, Gainesville

M. Danhof - pp. 141-148
Univ. of Leiden

H. de Bree - pp. (i) 297-298,
(ii) 385-388
Duphar, Weesp, The Netherlands

D. Dell - pp. 113-116
Hoffmann-La Roche, Basel

J.P. Desager - pp. 201-206
UCL, Brussels

J.A.F. de Silva - pp. 213-214
S. Orange, NJ, U.S.A.

C.L. DeVane - pp. 149-157
Univ. of Florida, Gainesville

R.A. de Zeeuw -
pp. (i) 259-269, (ii) 355-372
State Univ., Groningen

R. Dimaline - pp. 75-86
Univ. of Liverpool

M.V. Doig - pp. 117-120
Wellcome Res. Labs., Beckenham

T. Aaes-Jørgensen - Jørgensen
M.P. Allan - Pearce

M. Ballabio - Richards
A.R. Boobis - Gulaid
J. Bosman - de Zeeuw (i)
D.D. Breimer - Danhof
F. Bressolle - Bres
S. Bruce - Ratcliffe
F. Bucheli - Dell

S. Caccia - Richards
S.J. Capper - Venn
P.R.J. Ceelen - de Bree (i)
W.M.L. Chow - Caddy
J.V. Christensen - Jørgensen
S.F. Cooper - Midha
J.L. Crammer - Papadopoulos

C.F. Deacon - Conlon
B.J. de Jong - de Bree (ii)
P. De Ponte - Richards
H. Desmond - Dimaline
J. Dingemanse - Danhof
S. Dobson - Ratcliffe
G.J. Dockray - Dimaline
B.F.H. Drenth - de Zeeuw (i)

Primary author

Co-authors, with relevant name to be consulted in left column

H-J. Egger - pp. 303-307
Hoffmann-La Roche, Basel

K.G. Feitsma - as for de Zeeuw
(i)

H. Frank - pp. (i) 285-287,
(ii) 289-290, (iii) 291-292
Inst. f. Toxikol., Tübingen

A.A. Gulaid - pp. 283-284
May & Baker, Dagenham

J.J.M. Holthuis - pp. 389-393
State Univ., Utrecht

A. Hulshoff - pp. 343-353
(& as for Holthuis)
State Univ., Utrecht

C.R. Jones - pp. 299-301
Wellcome Res. Labs., Beckenham

A. Jørgensen - pp. 173-180
Lundbeck A/S, Copenhagen

R.D. McDowall - pp. 235-242
& as for Pearce
SK&F, Welwyn

K.G. McFarthing - pp. 65-74
Amersham Internat., Amersham

L.E. Martin - pp. 399-402
Glaxo Group Res., Ware

K.K. Midha - pp. 159-171
Univ. of Saskatchewan, Canada

J.K. Nicholson - pp. 321-335
Birkbeck Coll., London

A.S. Papadopoulos - pp. 207-210
Inst. of Psychiatry, London

J.C. Pearce - pp. 293-296
(& as for McDowall)

M.J. Rance - pp. 121-122
ICI Pharm., Alderley Edge

J.G. Ratcliffe - pp. 95-106
Univ. of Manchester

R.P. Richards - pp. 273-276
Servier R&D, Fulmer, Slough

G. Fischer - Egger
S. Garratini - Richards
J. Gerhardt - Frank (iii)

A.L. Hamilton - McFarthing
M.R. Harris - McFarthing
W. Heptner - Uihlein
I. Hornke - Uihlein
P. Hurst - Whelpton

I.M. Ismail - Wilson (ii)
R.H. Jackson - McFarthing
J.V. Johnson - Bennett
A-C. Jonsson - Dimaline
A. Jori - Richards
K.H. Kooi - de Zeeuw (i)
E. Koorn - de Bree (ii)

M.S. Lant - Martin
R.M. Lee - McDowall
O.R.W. Lewellen - Gulaid
H. Lingeman - Hulshoff

G. McKay - Midha
V. Marks - Teale
C.A. Marsden - Bennett
G.W.M. Meussen - Hulshoff
J.B. Miles - Venn
L. Miller - Rance
J.S. Morley - Venn
G.S. Murkitt - McDowall

G.J. Nicholson - Frank (iii)
M.J. O'Hare - Smith
K.F. Overø - Jørgensen
J. Oxford - Martin

R.J. Pither - McFarthing
S. Pauwels - Dimaline
H. Raybould - Dimaline
H.M. Ruijten - de Bree (i)

P.J. Sadler - Nicholson
J.A. Salmon - Doig
J.S. Shaw - Rance
D. Silver - McFarthing
A. Smith - McFarthing
D.G. Smyth - McFarthing
M. Snoussi - Bres
N. Strojny - de Silva
A.D. Swift - Ratcliffe

Primary author	*Co-authors, with relevant name to be consulted in left column*
J.A. Smith - pp. 17-36 Ludwig Inst., Sutton, London	J.A. Timbrell - Nicholson
J.D. Teale - pp. 87-93 St. Luke's Hosp., Guildford	K-H. Trautmann - Dell J.R. Traynor - Rance K. Tulip - Nicholson
I.R. Tebbett - pp. 13-16 Univ. of Strathclyde, Glasgow	W.J.M. Underberg - Hulshoff
J. Tomašić - pp. 3-12 Inst. of Immunology, Zagreb	M.P. van Berkel - de Bree (ii)
M. Uihlein - pp. 211-212 Hoechst Pharm., Frankfurt	C. van der Zouwen - Hulshoff W.J. van Oort - Holthuis A. Varro - Dimaline
R.F. Venn - pp. 55-63 Pain Relief Foundn., Liverpool	W.R. Vincent - de Bree (ii) L. Vowles - Dimaline
I.W. Wainer - pp. 243-257 FDA, Washington DC	B.C. Weatherley - Jones
R. Whelpton - pp. 181-187 London Hosp. Med. Coll.	G. Wendt - Dell A. White - Ratcliffe
P.C. White - pp. 373-382 Met. Police Forensic Science Lab., London	
I.D. Wilson - pp. (i) 277-281, (ii) 337-342 Hoechst Pharm., Milton Keynes	

Section #A

PEPTIDES AND OTHER ENDOGENOUS-TYPE ANALYTES

#A-1

ASSAYS OF PEPTIDOGLYCANS AND SPECIFIC ANTIBODIES IN BIOLOGICAL SAMPLES

Jelka Tomašić

Institute of Immunology
P.O.B. 266, 41000 Zagreb, Yugoslavia

The presence of bacterial peptidoglycan fragments in mammals is apparently due to enzymic action on cell walls, yielding peptidoglycans (PG's) differing in size and chemical composition. The fragments can be manifested in the host by immunomodulating activity and an influence on sleep regulation. Antibodies (Ab's) can be raised to soluble fragments of higher mol. wt., and have been detected in serum from patients with bacterial infections, particularly staphylococcal. Several sensitive immunoassays are now available for detecting soluble PG's or specific Ab's, to distinguish patients with the most serious infections and to complement other diagnostic methods. Consideration is given to methods for isolating, purifying and characterizing PG's of low mol. wt., including HPLC and fast atom bombardment mass spectrometry (FAB-MS).

This article aims to review the recent advances in the area of peptidoglycan (PG) assay. PG's have received increasing attention in the last 10 years due to their remarkable biological activities, particularly as potent immunomodulators and very recently as sleep factors affecting slow-wave sleep. The term peptidoglycans covers the PG molecules of high mol. wt. and rather complex structure, besides the fragments of low mol. wt. and well defined structure. Several types of assays for various PG molecules have been described in the last few years, as considered below together with detection of the specific Ab's that complex high-mol. wt. PG's induce in mammals.

STRUCTURE AND BIOLOGICAL ACTIVITY OF PEPTIDOGLYCANS

Bacterial cell walls are formed of a number of polymeric components, each possessing immunological and biological activities. In gram-positive bacteria PG is a major component and in gram-negative organisms PG is present in the form of a unimolecular rigid layer. PG's consist of a glycan backbone with alternating residues of *N*-acetylglucosamine and of muramic acid - which is a unique molecule, present only in bacteria and blue-green algae and found nowhere else in nature. It is usually N-acetylated, but in some species is in N-glycolylated form.

Short peptide chains consisting of alternating L- and D-amino acids, are linked to muramic acid residues (by an amide bond at the carboxyl group). The first amino acid linked directly to muramic acid is always L-alanine, and the second is D-glutamic acid in free or amidated form; the third is usually L-lysine or diaminopimelic acid, and the fourth is D-alanine. Peptide chains are cross-linked either through peptide bridges or directly through D-alanyl-diamino-pimelate linkages. Thus, in streptococci the cross-linking bridge consists of two L-alanine units and in staphylococci of five glycines. Not all the peptide chains in PG molecules need be cross-linked; in bacteria lacking D,D-carboxypeptidase some chains are not cross-linked (up to 20% of the peptide content in the PG molecule). Primary structures of PG's were discussed recently in a review by Schleifer & Kandler [1]. A method for obtaining PG monomer units (fragments without cross-linking) was outlined in Vol. 12 of this series by Tomašić, in connection with 'PGM' adjuvant use, and an investigation of its metabolic fate when adminstered to mice was described.

Naturally occurring PG's are large molecules which are also substrates for several bacteriolytic enzymes, e.g. lysozyme (murami-dase), *N*-acetylglucosaminidase, *N*-acetylmuramyl-L-alanine amidase and specific peptidases [2]. Bacteriolytic enzymes have also been found in mammalian sera [3-5]. A possible physiological function of these enzymes might be their action on bacterial residues in mammalian organisms, resulting in release of PG fragments varying in size and structure and also of different biological activities.

Structure-activity relationships in various PG molecules have been thoroughly investigated and well documented [6, 7]. Molecules of higher mol. wt. exhibit marked biological activity, mainly affecting the immune system, but are also toxic to the host. Some PG's of low mol. wt. and well defined chemical structure also possess immunomodu-lating and anti-tumour properties and affect slow-wave sleep [8, 9]. When present in a host organism, PG's affect its vital functions. Elevated levels of soluble PG fragments or related specific Ab's in a host might be an indication of pathological conditions or altered immune status. It has, therefore, been of importance to develop reliable and sensitive assays for detecting PG molecules of various types and also specific Ab's.

ASSAY OF MURAMIC ACID (MA)

MA is the unique internal marker for PG material. Measurement of this specific component could serve for an indirect estimation of bacterial biomass. The procedures for determining individual components in a complex molecule involve several steps such as extraction, hydrolysis, derivatization, chromatographic separation and final detection and characterization. Assay of MA in various samples, including mammalian tissues, could be carried out mainly in two ways: on large complex PG molecules and on fragments extractable from tissues respectively.

MA determination in large PG molecules.- Samples should first be submitted to hydrolysis in order to release MA from PG molecules under conditions that should not affect the molecular structure of the amino sugar. Fox et al. [10] described a method for detecting MA in various mammalian tissues where the localization and persistence of toxic, immunogenic bacterial cell-wall fragments was suspected. Relevant tissues were first homogenized and dialyzed, then hydrolyzed with 1 M H_2SO_4. Extraction with organic solvents removed some impurities, and MA present in the aqueous layer was partially purified by TLC. It was further converted to alditol with sodium borohydride and then acetylated in order to get volatile alditol acetates. The derivatives were subjected to GC-FID (3% SP 2430 on 100/200 mesh Supelcoport) or to GC-MS with selected ion monitoring (SIM) for characterization.

A modified and improved procedure also based on GC-MS of volatile alditol acetate was reported recently [11]. Instead of extraction with organic solvents, solid extraction using disposable Bond-Elut and Chem-Elut columns, before and after derivatization, was performed. Sodium acetate-catalyzed derivatization was also improved, and only a single ion was monitored, resulting in sensitive and selective analysis of MA (ng quantities per mg of wet tissue).

Mimura & Romano [12] measured MA as an indicator of bacterial biomass in marine samples (surface micro-layer, sediment, and the water in between). Following hydrolysis of freeze-dried samples with 6 M HCl, reaction with o-phthaldialdehyde was carried out to give a fluorescent derivative for HPLC separation as described previously (6 μm Ultrasphere ODS column)[13, 14]. MA was accurately assayed in μg quantities.

MA determination in PG fragments from tissues.- Sen & Karnovsky [15] reported the extraction and assay of MA as a component of small extractable muramyl peptides from rat tissues. Homogenates were extracted with 8% trichloroacetic acid. Dried extracts were hydrolyzed with 6 M HCl, and the released amino sugars and MA were recovered and separated on three different cation-exchange columns. Partially purified MA was reacted with fluorescamine and characterized by TLC by co-chromatography with standard preparations, and by chemical methods applied to the isolated fluorescamine derivative. It was oxidized with sodium periodate, and formaldehyde originating from C-6 of the muramate ring was detected fluorimetrically. Alternatively, D-lactate was released by base treatment (β-elimination) and assayed by reaction with NAD$^+$ and D-lactic dehydrogenase leading to NADH formation. Thereby MA was detected in rat brain, liver and kidney in pmol amounts per g of tissue.

STUDIES ON PEPTIDOGLYCAN PRIMARY STRUCTURES

PG's confer rigidity on the bacterial cell wall and thus guarantee the integrity of the microorganism. The integral PG molecule present in a bacterial cell wall in the form of sacculi is too large to permit of direct analysis. Following isolation from bacterial cells, sacculi should be treated with enzymes in order to obtain smaller fragments.

Most of the numerous studies on PG composition and primary structure have entailed methods such as enzymic hydrolysis and amino acid analysis [6, 16]. Only a few recent studies using HPLC will be cited here. RP-HPLC applied to PG's from *E. coli* [17], *Caulobacter crescentus* [18] and *Neisseria gonorrhoeae* [19] revealed much greater heterogeneity in PG structure than previously thought. Novel types of cross-bridges were found and average chain lengths estimated. Prior to HPLC, PG sacculi were prepared from the respective bacterial cells by treatment with detergents and digestion with amylase and pronase, and submitted to hydrolysis with muramidase which cleaves glycan backbones. PG fragments thus obtained were subsequently reduced with sodium borohydride to prevent anomerization of muramic acid residues. Particular aspects of these studies warrant mention.

Fractionation of material originating from *E. coli* [17] by RP-HPLC yielded ~60 well separated peaks, detected at 202 nm; the column (Hibar, Lichrosorb RP18) was equilibrated with phosphate buffer and eluted with this buffer plus methanol. Amino acid analysis was performed on the peaks after partial enzymic hydrolysis. In the other studies cited above, on muramidase digests, HPLC under similar conditions helped elucidate the structure of murein [18] and, with ODS-Hypersil and a linear gradient (15% methanol in phosphate buffer), disclosed 13 major species of muropeptides comprising ~70% of total PG and ~45 minor peaks [19]. The latter study also included structural investigations with [^{3}H]glucosamine-labelled PG, entailing TLC to give muropeptide classes based on cross-linkage and O-acetylation or passage through G-50 and G-25 Sephadex columns in series to give 4 main peaks which were desalted and then separately studied by HPLC.

STUDIES ON METABOLISM OF PEPTIDOGLYCANS

Data are needed on metabolic fate; but studies so far have been confined to the mouse with low mol. wt. PG's, radiolabelled.

In studying muramyl di-, tri- and penta-peptide metabolites in body samples, Yapo et al. [20] used anion exchange and high-voltage paper electrophoresis for partial purification. For radiolabelled muramyl and nor-muramyl dipeptide metabolites, Ambler & Hudson [21] performed solid-phase extraction on ODS-Porasil and then HPLC with Partisil ODS-2 (phosphate buffer for elution). Studies in our laboratory (with B. Ladešić, Z. Valinger and I. Hršak; cited in Vol. 12 of this series, and submitted for publication) have concerned metabolites of PG monomer. Separations were by gel and ion-exchange chromatography and then TLC.

The above-mentioned experimental procedures had shortcomings and achieved only partial purification and characterization of radioactive products. The need for reliable methods in such investigations of metabolites in biological material might be met by RP-HPLC combined with FAB-MS, as described below for 'sleep factors'; but such an approach needs costly special instruments that are not widely available.

INVESTIGATION OF 'SLEEP FACTORS'

The role of PG's as modulators of various processes in mammals has been reinforced by the recent discovery that the composition of sleep-promoting factors isolated from CSF, urine and brain is closely related to that of bacterial PG's. New sensitive methods were developed and applied for isolating and characterizing endogenous substances that promote natural sleep. Even pmol amounts of these sleep factors given intraventricularly to rabbits were reported to significantly increase slow-wave sleep [9].

A sleep-promoting agent, Factor S, was isolated from animal brains by a combination of relatively simple procedures involving extraction, ion-exchange chromatography, gel filtration, partition chromatography and electrophoresis [22]. Such material was sufficiently purified to allow use for physiological experimentation.

Factor S was isolated from human urine [22] in 0.5-300 l batches extracted initially with CM-Sephadex. Purification entailed chromatographic steps (gel filtration; ion-exchange; paper) with final amino acid analysis; sleep-promoting activity was monitored throughout. Methods such as HPLC and high-voltage paper electrophoresis were unsatisfactory for Factor S isolation, causing serious inactivation. However, HPLC was found indispensable in final purification steps prior to MS structural analysis of Factor S, isolated from urine and further purified by DEAE-resin chromatography [22]. HPLC was carried out on a Waters Bondapack C-18 column with acetonitrile (in water containing trifluoroacetic acid) rising linearly to 10%. Thereby structurally closely related compounds were resolved, e.g. PG α- and β-anomers, and compounds containing muramic acid or anhydro-muramic acid (lacking a free reducing end).

For sleep-promoting factors from human urine, Martin et al. [23] ascertained by FAB-MS that the main component was *N*-acetylglucosaminyl-*N*-acetylmuramylalanylglutamyldiaminopimelyl-alanine (MH^+ at m/z 922) accompanied by two additional minor components. The advantage of FAB-MS in this work was that it allows thermally labile and high mol. wt. compounds to be detected without derivatization. Protonated molecular ions are formed in the process in the presence of glycerol and acetic acid. The technique also permits the detection of compounds in a complex mixture. Conclusive evidence for the structure of sleep-promoting factor was derived from the FAB mass spectra of the reference compounds, PG monomer from *Brevibacterium divaricatum* [24] and muramyl pentapeptide [20].

DETECTION OF SOLUBLE PEPTIDOGLYCANS IN BIOLOGICAL FLUIDS

The occurrence of soluble PG's (SPG's) in mammalian serum or urine is supposedly the consequence of release from indigenous bacteria. Cross-linking of PG molecules is inhibited by penicillin, and hence elevated amounts of SPG's could be expected in hosts treated with penicillin.

Park et al. [25] described recently the unique enzyme-linked immunosorbent assay (ELISA) for detecting SPG in human serum and urine. The assay exploits the specificity and affinity of vancomycin for the PG precursor sequence found in SPG's (D-Ala-D-Ala sequence). Ab's raised in rabbits against the synthetic pentapeptide immunogen Ala-γ-D-Glu-Lys-D-Ala-D-Ala were used in the assay after purification by affinity chromatography. The ELISA steps were incubations as follows: (1) of polyvinyl wells with vancomycin; (2) with samples containing SPG; with (3) rabbit anti-SPG and biotinylated anti-rabbit IgG and (4) avidin-biotin-horseradish peroxidase complex; (5) with added substrate, *o*-phenylenediamine and H_2O_2. The detection limit in serum was 500 pg/ml and in urine 50 pg/ml.

The essential difference between customarily used ELISA tests and the assay described above is in the use of the antibiotic vancomycin instead of specific Ab's for coating of the plastic wells on microtitre plates. This unique feature renders the assay more specific, since it is highly unlikely that any other peptide sequence would be detected in such an ELISA. The ability of vancomycin to form a stable complex with peptide constituents of bacterial PG's [26] could also be used for affinity purification of PG's on vancomycin-Sepharose [27].

MEASUREMENT OF ANTIBODY LEVELS TO PG IN HUMAN SERA

Large PG structures are immunogenic, inducing the formation of specific Ab's in the host. Mammalian organisms are continuously exposed to bacteria, and accordingly anti-PG Ab's are constantly detectable in serum. With higher amounts of bacterial material in the organism the titre of specific Ab's will rise too. PG fragments

could occur abundantly at, for example, various inflammation sites and
also in serum or urine as a consequence of bacterial cell-wall degradation and processing by macrophages and bacteriolytic enzymes.
Such a situation is conceivable and probable in all bacterial infections. Several attempts have therefore been made to develop sensitive
methods for measuring anti-PG Ab's and to use such assays in diagnostic
procedures connected with serious bacterial infections.

PG molecules reveal five antigenic epitopes, viz. the glycan
moiety, N- and C-terminal sequences of the inter-peptide bridges,
tetrapeptide subunits and non-crosslinked pentapeptide subunits [28].
The pentapeptide subunits appear to be the predominant antigenic
determinants in PG molecules, with carboxy-terminal D-Ala-D-Ala as
the immunodominant site. A major portion of the humoral immune
response to PG was found to be directed against the pentapeptide subunits.

Radioimmunoassay (RIA)

Heymer et al. [29] applied RIA for measuring Ab response to
the pentapeptide determinant of PG, using ^{125}I-labelled synthetic
pentapeptide hapten, L-Ala-γ-D-Glu-L-Lys-D-Ala-D-Ala. The labelling
was performed by the active ester method of Bolton & Hunter [30].
Radioiodinated active ester was presumably attached to the free
amino group of L-Ala. The labelled hapten was incubated with respective sera to be tested, followed by precipitation of antigen-Ab
complex with ammonium sulphate. Binding curves for the labelled
hapten exhibited a large linear range, permitting Ab measurement
from 50 to 500 µg/ml serum. The binding specificity in tested sera
was apparently directed against the PG precursor pentapeptide sequence,
as shown by inhibition studies with various PG's and synthetic oligo-
peptides.

A possible relationship among the PG-binding capacities of
patients' sera and gram-positive infections was studied by Zeiger et
al. [31], besides the effects of treatment with β-lactam antibiotics
on the PG-binding activity. They showed that patients with staphylococcal endocarditis and bacteraemia have elevated levels of PG-binding
titres (expressed as % binding of radiolabelled antigen). Synthetic
antigen, $(D-Glu^{60}-D-Ala^{40})_n(Ala-\gamma-D-Glu-Lys-D-Ala-D-Ala)$, was first
tyrosylated and then radioiodinated using the chloramine T procedure.
Precipitation of the antigen-Ab complex was done with ammonium sulphate
or with anti-human Ig. Non-specific binding using a double-Ab method
was lower and therefore conducive to reliability. The isolation
of binding factor from positive sera was also described [31]. Affinity
chromatography of such sera was carried out with Sepharose to which
the pentapeptide Ala-γ-D-Glu-Lys-D-Ala-D-Ala was covalently attached.
Ab's eluted from the column were shown to be primarily of the IgG
class, with a smaller amount of IgM and a trace of IgA.

Solid—phase RIA (SPRIA)

Measurement of anti—PG Ab's by SPRIA was used to complement serological methods for diagnosing staphylococcal infections ([32] and B. Christensson, unpublished). These infections are difficult to diagnose by common bacteriological and clinical methods. The method of Christensson et al. [32] proved particularly sensitive and useful for diagnosing *S. aureus* endocarditis, provided that the PG preparation used as antigen was appropriate. It was isolated from a trichloro-acetic extract of whole bacteria; the solubilized PG obtained by tryp-sinization and then sonication was coated onto the polystyrene tubes. Patient's and control sera (diluted 1:10) were then incubated, and finally ^{125}I-labelled Protein A was added, being stated to bind to IgG Ab's of subclasses 1, 2 and 4.

Wheat et al. [33] developed a RIA for IgM and IgG Ab's to PG. The PG for coating plastic wells was prepared by disrupting *S. aureus* cells, digesting with DNase, RNase and trypsin, and extracting with trichloroacetic acid. Solubilization was achieved by sonication or by lysozyme digestion – the respective products being equally satis-factory for the assay. After coating the solid phase with PG, incuba-tion was carried out with highly diluted control and patient's sera, to avoid the pro-zones seen with more concentrated sera. The class-specific response was measured using ^{125}I-labelled goat IgG Ab's specific for the Fc fragment of either human IgM or IgG, the results being expressed as ng anti-IgG or -IgM bound per serum sample. High levels of IgG or IgM Ab to staphylococci were demonstrated in sera of patients with various staphylococcal infections, but levels of both IgG and IgM were significantly elevated only in patients with endo-carditis or complicated bacteraemia caused by *S. aureus*.

ELISA

ELISA proved invaluable in the serological diagnosis of serious staphylococcal infections through very sensitive measurement of Ab response to *S. aureus* PG [34]. PG extracted as above [32] was solubilized by lysostaphyne treatment, or by lysozyme treatment or by sonication and the three products tried in an ELISA for detecting and quantita-ting IgG Ab's to PG. After coating the plastic wells and incubating with sera, a final incubation with anti-human IgG-alkaline phosphat-ase conjugate was performed. ELISA was found to be more reprodu-cible than SPRIA for detecting the Ab's.

Franken et al. [35] showed human sera to contain anti-PG Ab's of the IgA class, for which the ELISA was tailored with binding specifi-city for the terminal R-D-Ala-D-Ala sequence of the PG peptide subunit.[⊗] Synthetic antigen, albumin-$(D-Ala_3)_9$, was used for coating of poly-styrene tubes. After incubation with serum, IgA Ab's were selectively detected by anti-human IgA conjugated with horseradish peroxidase.

⊗ R denotes peptidyl residue

Synthetic antigen linked to random polymer was used by Zeiger et al. [31] in ELISA for detecting IgG Ab's to the D-Ala-D-Ala moiety of PG.   Antigen-coated   polystyrene   test   cups   were   first   incubated with test and control sera and then with alkaline phosphatase-conjugated anti-human IgG. Elevated Ab levels were demonstrated in patients with ankylosing spondylitis and Reiter's syndrome [36].

COMMENTS

The sensitivity and general performance characteristics of immunoassays for measurement of anti-PG Ab's depend mainly on the type of PG preparation or synthetic PG used in the reaction.   Bacterial PG is a very complex molecule which could give rise to different mixtures of immunogenic or non-immunogenic fragments of both protein and carbohydrate origin depending on the procedures used for isolation and solubilization. In several RIA, SPRIA and ELISA tests, different antigen or hapten preparations were used and, therefore, it is virtually impossible to compare the respective results. Various authors also recommend different serum dilutions varying from 1:10 to 1:3000. Evidently, if immunoassays for measuring anti-PG Ab's are to be used in routine serological diagnosis of bacterial infections, methodological aspects of these assays should be standardized.

References

1. Schleifer, K.H. & Kandler, O. (1983) in *The Target of Penicillin* (Hackenbeck, R., Höltje, J-V. & Labischinkski, H., eds.), Walter de Gruyter, Berlin, pp. 11-17.
2. Strominger, J.L. & Ghuysen, J-M. (1967) *Science 156*, 213-221.
3. Selsted, M.E. & Martinez, R.J. (1978) *Infect. Immun.* 20, 782-791.
4. Calvo, P., Revilla, M.G. & Cabezas, J.A. (1978) *Comp. Biochem. Physiol. 61B*, 581-585.
5. Valinger, Z., Ladešić, B. & Tomašić, J. (1982) *Biochim. Biophys. Acta 701*, 63-71.
6. Schleifer, K.H. (1975) *Z. Immun.-Forsch. 149*, 104-117.
7. Chedid, L. & Lederer, E. (1978) *Biochem. Pharmacol. 27*, 2183-2186.
8. Adam, A. & Lederer, E. (1984) *Med. Res. Rev. 4*, 111-152.
9. Krueger, J.M., Karnovsky, M.L., Martin, S.A., Pappenheimer, J.R., Walter, J. & Biemann, K. (1984) *J. Biol. Chem. 259*, 12659-12662.
10. Fox, A., Schwab, J.H. & Cochran, T. (1980) *Infect. Immun.   29*, 526-531.
11. Whiton, R.S., Lau, P., Morgan, S.L., Gilbart, J. & Fox, A. (1985) *J. Chromatog. 347*, 109-120.
12. Mimura, T. & Romano, J-C. (1985) *Appl. Environ. Microbiol. 50*, 229-237.
13. Lindroth, P. & Mopper, K. (1979) *Anal. Chem. 51*, 1338-1345.
14. Mimura, T. & Delmas, D. (1983) *J. Chromatog. 280*, 91-98.

15. Sen, Z. & Karnovsky, M.L. (1984) *Infect. Immun.* *43*, 937-941.
16. Petit, J.F., Wietzewrbin, J., Das, B.C. & Lederer, E. (1975) *Z. Immun.-Forsch. 149*, 118-125.
17. Glauner, B. & Schwartz, U. (1983) *as for* 1., pp. 29-34.
18. Markiewicz, Z., Glauner, B. & Schwartz, U. (1983) *J. Bacteriol. 156*, 649-655.
19. Dougherty, T.J. (1985) *J. Bacteriol. 163*, 69-74.
20. Yapo, A., Petit, J.F., Lederer, E., Parant, M., Parant, F. & Chedie, L. (1982) *Int. J. Immunopharmacol. 4*, 143-149.
21. Ambler, L. & Hudson, A.M. (1984) *Int. J. Immunopharmacol. 6*, 133-139.
22. Krueger, J.M., Pappenheimer, J.R. & Karnovsky, J.L. (1978) *Proc. Nat. Acad. Sci. 75*, 5235-5238, & (1982) *J. Biol. Chem. 257*, 1664-1669.
23. Martin, S.A., Karnovsky, M.L., Krueger, J., Pappenheimer, J.R. & Biemann, K. (1984) *J. Biol. Chem. 259*, 12652-12658.
24. Keglević, D., Ladešić, B., Tomašić, J., Valinger, Z. & Naumski, R. (1979) *Biochim. Biophys. Acta 585*, 273-281.
25. Park, H., Zeiger, A.R. & Schumacher, R. (1984) *Infect. Immun. 43*, 139-142.
26. Harris, C.M., Kopecka, H. & Harris, T.M. (1985) *J. Antibiotics 38*, 51-57.
27. DePedro, M.A. & Schwartz, U. (1980) *FEMS Microbiol. Lett. 9*, 215-217.
28. Seidl, P.H., Franken, N. & Schleifer, K.H. (1983) *as for* 1., pp. 299-304.
29. Heymer, B., Bernstein, D., Schleifer, K.H. & Krause, R. (1975) *J. Immun. 114*, 1191-1196.
30. Bolton, A.E. & Hunter, W.M. (1973) *Biochem. J. 133*, 529-539.
31. Zeiger, A.R., Tuazon, C.U. & Sheagren, J.N. (1981) *Infect. Immun. 33*, 795-800.
32. Christensson, B., Espersen, F., Hedström, S.A. & Kronvall, G. (1983) *Acta Path. Microbiol. Immunol. Scand. 91B*, 401-406.
33. Wheat, L.J., Wilkinson, B.J., Kohler, R.B. & White, A.C. (1983) *J. Infect. Dis. 147*, 16-22.
34. Christensson, B., Espersen, F., Hedström, S.A. & Kronvall, G. (1984) *J. Clin. Microbiol. 19*, 680-686.
35. Franken, N., Seidl, P.H., Kuchenbauer, T., Kolb, H.J., Schleifer, K.H., Weiss, L. & Tympner, K-D. (1984) *Infect. Immun. 44*, 182-187.
36. Park, H., Schumacher, H.R., Zeiger, A.R. & Rosenbaum, J.T. (1984) *Ann. Rheum. Dis. 43*, 725-728.

#A-2

CYCLIC DECAPEPTIDES IN KIDNEY

Ian R. Tebbett

Forensic Science Unit
University of Strathclyde
204 George Steet, Glasgow Gl lXW, U.K.

The Cortinarius genus of mushrooms contains a number of species that have caused poisonings throughout Europe. Cortinarins A and B have been isolated from these fungi and ascertained to be cyclic polypeptides; they have been shown in laboratory animals to cause nephrotoxicity characteristic of Cortinarius mushroom poisoning. HPLC systems, besides TLC, have been developed to examine methanolic extracts of kidney tissue from poisoned animals for these compounds, and for cortinarin C which is non-toxic. The toxicity of the mushrooms seems to entail a metabolic process, possibly explaining the genetic and sex-linked differences in susceptibility observed among individual humans and animals.

In 1979 two men and a woman were poisoned in the North of Scotland after eating a meal of the fungus *Cortinarius speciosissimus*. Apparently they had mistaken this mushroom for *Cantharellus cibarius*, an edible Chantrelle [1]. The toxic symptoms associated with Cortinarius poisoning only become apparent after an unusual latent period, 3-20 days after ingestion. Symptoms include an intense thirst together with gastric disturbances, vomiting and persistent headaches. Some subjects also experience a constant sensation of coldness. In severe cases renal function may be impaired and oliguria and sometimes anuria may be observed [2]. In the Scottish episode all three subjects were hospitalized suffering from renal failure. The two males subsequently required kidney transplants whereas the female regained renal function. Similar toxic reactions have been reported following the ingestion of *Cortinarius speciosissimus* and *C. gentilis* in Scandinavia [2], of *C. splendens* in France and Switzerland [3] and of *C. orellanus* throughout Central Europe. In fact there have been over 500 cases of Cortinarius poisoning in Europe during the last 10 years.

Three major components of *C. speciosissimus* were isolated from methanolic extracts of the fungi and identified as cyclic decapeptides in our laboratories [4]. Cortinarins A and B (which show a brown fluorescence under UV light) were found, in laboratory animals, to cause nephrotoxicity characteristic of Cortinarius mushroom poisoning. Cortinarin C which is non-fluorescent was found to be non-toxic. The structures of these compounds were confirmed by mass spectrometry of the linear peptides after derivatization by permethylation and acetylation [4].

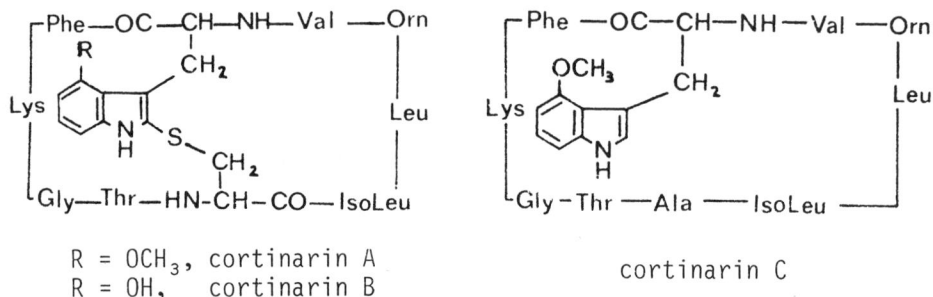

R = OCH$_3$, cortinarin A
R = OH, cortinarin B

cortinarin C

Having determined the structures of the major components of *C. speciosissimus*, other members of the genus were screened for the presence of cortinarins A, B and C. The material was air-dried, Sohxlet-extracted with methanol, and the extractives were examined by TLC and HPLC [5]. For preparative TLC, on silica gel G, cyclohexane/ethyl acetate (3:1 by vol.) was a suitable developing solvent for A and B, and butanol/acetic acid/water (0.4:1:1) for B. HPLC was performed as stated in the legend to Fig. 1, with UV detection; recourse to fluorescence detection was unnecessary as sensitivity was adequate (100 ng or, for B, 200 ng was detectable). Cortinarins A, B and C were well separated (Fig. 1).

The following results, as % of mushroom dry wt., are representative; cortinarin B was found only in the first three species.-
C. speciosissimus: 0.47% A, 0.60% B (& 0.20% C); *C. orellanus*: 0.42% A, 0.52% B (& 0.24% C); *C. orellanoides*: 0.45% A, 0.47% B (& 0.20% C); *C. pinicola*: 0.19% A (& 0.03% C); *C. callisteus*: 0.20% A (& 0.19% C); *C. turmalis*: 0.32% A (& 0.05% C); *C. mucifluus*: 0.05% A (& 0.07% C); *C. betuletorum*: 0.28% A (& 0.05% C); *C. trivialis*: 0.10% A (& 0.06% C); *C. torvus*: 0.01% A (& 0.12% C). Besides cortinarin B, the first three species also contained relatively high concentrations of A; they have been reported to be the three most toxic species within the genus Cortinarius. *C. callisteus* which contains only A was also found to be toxic to mice if sufficiently high doses were given. *C. splendens* which contains high concentrations of A but no B has been reported as causing a number of poisonings. These results suggested that the toxicity of Cortinarius species is

Fig. 1.   Mixture of cortinarins
A, B and C: RP-HPLC separation.
Column: 5 μm ODS-silica, 25 cm ×
4.5 mm i.d. Mobile phase: aceto-
nitrile/water, 1:3 by vol.; 1.5 ml
/min. Injection: 20 μl.
Detection at 220 nm.

From [5], courtesy of Elsevier.

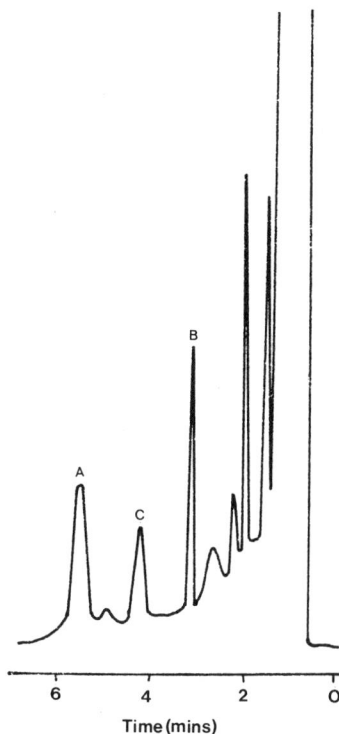

Time (mins)

proportional to the sum of the concentrations of cortinarins A and
B.   Whilst A was found to some extent in the majority of the species
examined, in most it was present only in low concentrations. However,
tests with laboratory animals indicated that this toxin may accumulate
in the kidney, and it is suggested that all species of Cortinarius
be considered as being potentially toxic.

INVESTIGATIONS ON MOUSE KIDNEY

Toxicity was investigated by administering the toxins i.p.
(A or B) [4]. Renal damage was apparent 3 days after a 1 mg dose: the
kidneys were enlarged and showed a blue fluorescence in the cortex
under UV light.   The blue fluorescent compound was isolated from
the kidneys by methanol extraction after homogenization, and examined
by UV, TLC and HPLC. The chromatographic and spectral data obtained for
this compound were identical with those for a sulphoxide metabolite
of cortinarin B, readily separable from B by HPLC with no tissue
interferences (Fig. 2). This metabolite is also found in the kidneys
of mice poisoned with cortinarin A, which is presumably converted
to B followed by S-oxidation to produce the sulphoxide metabolite.
This metabolite was produced semi-synthetically and given to mice to
determine its toxicity relative to that of the cortinarins themselves.
Severe damage to the kidneys was observed less than 24 h after its
administration – although the actual fungi and the isolated toxins take
at least 3-4 days before any effects are observed.

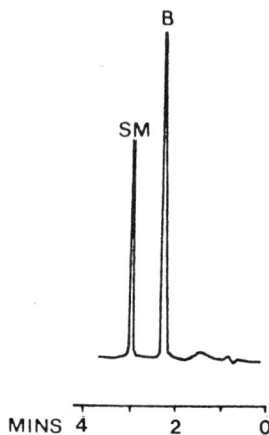

Fig. 2. RP-HPLC analysis of a methanolic extract, spiked with cortinarin B, from mouse kidney. HPLC conditions as for Fig. 1. SM = sulphoxide metabolite of cortinarin B.

It would seem, then, that the compounds present in the fungus are are metabolized to an active metabolite which causes the toxic effect. This would explain why some animals are apparently more susceptible than others to the toxins [6]. Those which form the active metabolite rapidly are greatly affected, whilst others which lack this ability are resistant. Females may not be as efficient as males in producing it, as evidenced by the fact that female mice are more resistant to the toxins than males. In the Scottish case of Cortinarius poisoning it was the female who recovered renal function despite having consumed more of the fungus than the males.

References

1. Short, A.I.K., Watling, R., MacDonald, M.K. & Robson, J.S. (1980) *Lancet ii*, 942-943.
2. Grzymala, S. (1957) *Z. Pilzk. 23*, 139-142.
3. Colon, S., Deteix, P., Bervard, M., Gerault, A., Finaz, A., Zech, P. & Traeger, J. (1982) *Kidney International 21*, 121.
4. Tebbett, I.R. & Caddy, B. (1984) *Experientia 40*, 441-446.
5. Tebbett, I.R. & Caddy, B. (1984) *J. Chromatog. 283*, 417-420.
6. Hulmi, S.P., Siddonen, P., Forström, J. & Vilska, J. (1974) *Duodecim. 90*, 1044-1055.

#A-3

ANALYSIS OF PROTEIN GROWTH FACTORS AND OPTIMIZATION OF THEIR SEPARATION BY HPLC

John A. Smith and Michael J. O'Hare

Ludwig Institute for Cancer Research
London Branch, Royal Marsden Hospital
Sutton, Surrey SM2 5PX, U.K.

For polypeptide and protein GF's*, which may occur in very small amounts and whose bioassay may lack specificity, chromatographic systems are needed which give high resolution and recovery and preserve biological activity. Resolving power in RP-HPLC depends on the nature of the stationary phase, on the pH and ionic strength of the primary solvent, and on the organic modifier used. Hydrophobic ion-pairing agents, anionic or cationic, can enhance selectivity. Protein recovery depends on solubility in the eluent, which must not irreversibly disrupt secondary structure and so cause inactivation.

Milder conditions are possible using 'hydrophobic interaction' HPLC - with packings still to be fully tested - or ion-exchange HPLC as in conventional operation but with enhanced speed and resolution, extendable by use of hydrophobic ion-pairing agents. Size-exclusion HPLC resolves no better than conventional operation.

HPLC techniques are now widely used for polypeptides and proteins, both for rapid isolation and for ascertaining homogeneity prior to amino acid analysis and sequence determination, at levels below 1 nM - even 50 pM - in conjunction with the new generation of gas-phase sequencers. This technology has put within the scope of the analyst a whole range of highly active GF's found in normal tissues, and related compounds in tumour cells (e.g. transforming GF's), the characterization of which has become a major goal of tumour-cell biology.

---

* GF, growth factor (EGF, epidermal; FGF, fibroblast). RP, reversed-phase; HFBA, heptafluorobutyric acid; PDFOA, pentadecafluorooctanoic acid; SDS, sodium dodecyl sulphate; TEA, triethylamine; TFA, trifluoroacetic acid.

Correct identification and accurate measurement of such factors calls for separation systems that give maximum resolution and recovery and preferably full retention of biological activity. Unfortunately there may be some mutual incompatibility of these goals. The precise choice of chromatographic conditions can, therefore, be crucial. In a recent example from our Institute, the composition and complete amino acid sequence of rat EGF has been established for the first time [1, 2], using only HPLC techniques in various modes as considered below. In the past the choice of both stationary and mobile phases in the HPLC of polypeptides and proteins often seems to have been dictated by availability and precedent, rather than through systematic optimization.

In this brief overview we attempt to identify some of the parameters which we have found to be especially important, particularly with regard to optimizing resolution of closely related protein GF's. While some of these compounds have individual characteristics, as a whole they epitomize the problems likely to be encountered with any group of small soluble proteins. The approaches described should therefore have some general applicability in analyzing other mixtures.

RP-HPLC

It may seem perverse to start with the so-called reversed-phase techniques for protein analysis as these bear the least resemblance to conventional techniques based on size or charge. It is, however, separations based on the intrinsic hydrophobicity that give the greatest resolution of complex mixtures of closely related proteins. A protein's hydrophobicity dependent on amino acid composition affords an essentially novel dimension for separation. However, the complex (and heterogeneous) natures of the stationary phases created by chemically bonding alkyl moieties of various chain lengths to microparticulate (3-10 μm), meso-porous (10-35 nm) silicas (Fig. 1) creates opportunities for various forms of essentially uncontrolled 'mixed-mode' chromatography that can interfere with effective separations.

On the other hand, controlled forms of mixed-mode chromatography can be created by the use of various mobile-phase additives, which can significantly enhance separations. Our efforts to optimize protein RP-HPLC have therefore concentrated on devising conditions in which reproducibility is ensured by minimizing unwanted stationary phase-dependent effects, and maximizing resolution by manipulating the mobile phase.

Basic mechanism of RP-HPLC of proteins

In order to understand the factors controlling resolution, recovery and activity of proteins in RP-HPLC runs, it has to be appreciated that their behaviour is quite unlike that encountered with small-molecular solutes. Firstly, the interaction of a protein with a

Fig. 1. Schematic representation
of the stationary phase created by
bonding a long-chain alkylsilane
to silica - exemplified by the
octyldimethylsilyl (ODMS) groups -
and then 'capping' most residual
accessible silanol groups with
trimethylsilyl (TMS) residues.
Residual mono-, di- and tri-hydroxy
residues are depicted that can
undergo cation exchange even
in the pH range 2-6, and some
weakly hydrophobic siloxane
groups (see Unger [3]).

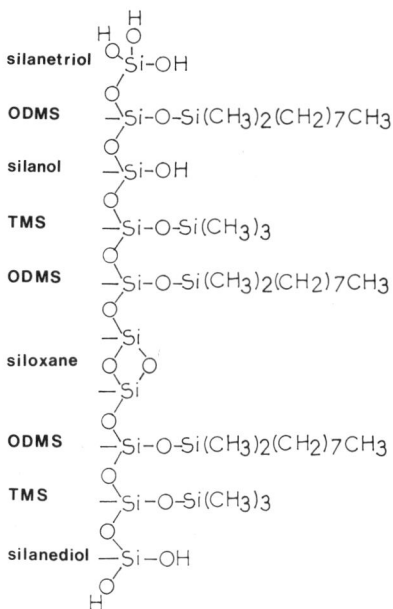

typical alkyl-bonded stationary phase is so strong that an organic
modifier is required to elute it. Secondly, the range of concentrations of organic modifier over which true (i.e. interactive) chromatography of the protein takes place is extremely narrow (Fig. 2).
In general, the larger the polypeptide, the more closely does the
relationship between organic modifier concentration and elution volume
approach a rectilinear form (e.g. compare ref. [4] with Fig. 2).
At its extreme, therefore, RP-HPLC of proteins with organic modifier
elution comes to resemble a form of frontal displacement; the distinction is basically between tenacious binding to the stationary phase
below a certain modifier concentration and total loss of binding or
interaction above it. Most protein RP-HPLC systems therefore employ
some form of organic modifier gradient (Fig. 3), each protein eluting
at a characteristic and individual organic modifier concentration.

The extremely narrow concentration range over which true chromatographic interaction occurs (Fig. 2) has several consequences. (1) It
ensures, under gradient conditions, a highly reproducible elution time
(±0.2 min) for a given protein, provided that the gradient is formed
accurately. This feature can greatly aid in the identification
of closely related analytes. Such reproducibility is very difficult to
achieve under isocratic conditions as any deficiencies or imbalance
in pump performance are amplified; even when using a single pump it
is very difficult to guarantee the organic modifier content of mixtures
prepared manually within ±0.1%. (2) Many of the procedures used to
enhance separation of small-molecular solutes in RP-HPLC, e.g. increasing the column's efficiency (plate no.) or length, have little effect

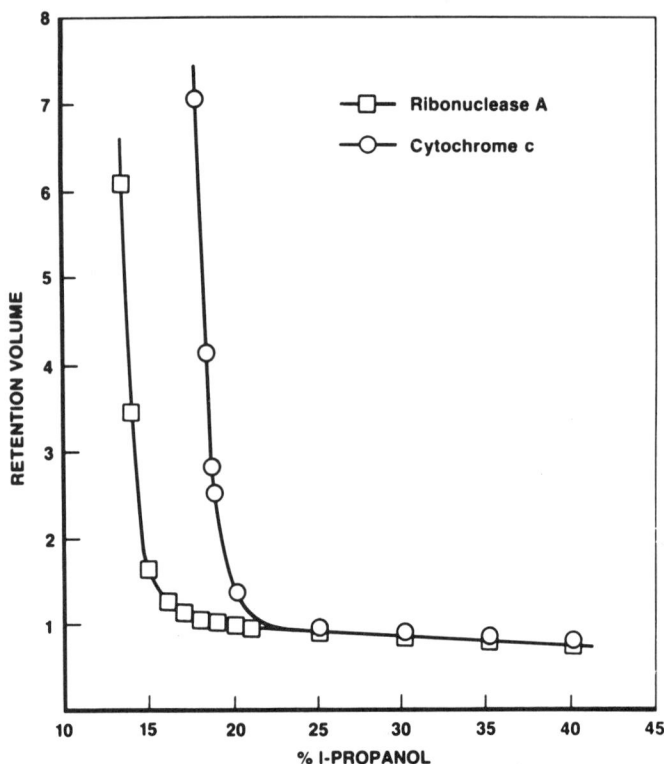

Fig. 2. Effect of organic modifier concentration on elution volume of cytochrome **c** and ribonuclease A. Separations were carried out isocratically at ambient temperature with 10 mM TFA as primary and and propan-1-ol as secondary solvent. Data from Archer & Cooke *(see Acknowledgements)*.

on proteins because the true chromatographic time for each compound is so short (1-2 min). Thus, short, fat columns give virtually identical separations to long, thin ones, with in the former case the advantage of enhanced capacity. (3) The solubility limit of a protein, particularly if late-eluting, may have been exceeded by the gradient before all the protein has had time to detach from the stationary phase. Incomplete recovery ensues, with the likelihood that 'ghost' peaks will recur in the same position on subsequent chromatograms; stringent control of column use and frequent 'blank' runs are therefore necessary.

What is actually happening to the protein, especially its 3-D structure, during this critical phase has been the subject of much surmise. The density of alkyl moieties is very high (up to 5 $\mu mol/m^2$) on well-covered RP packings, due to reaction with the majority of accessible hydroxyls (occupancy 8 $\mu mol/m^2$ on underivatized silica)[3]. The effect of this seems to be that most, if not all, hydrophobic amino acid residues come into contact with the stationary phase, as inferred from the fact that retention orders of most proteins are directly correlated with overall hydrophobic amino acid content [4, 5]. As a corollary it must be assumed that much of the tertiary structure is lost, resulting in a form of *in situ* denaturation, to which the modifier may itself contribute once the protein has been eluted. Although retentions can be predicted to some extent on the basis of known composition [4], the predictions differ significantly with different mobile phases [6, 7].

In endeavours by ourselves and others to optimize protein RP-HPLC, the effects of varying both stationary-phase and mobile-phase composition have been examined, besides extrinsic factors such as temperature, flow rates and gradient profiles.

Stationary-phase effects

Most early work on polypeptide and protein HPLC was carried out with C-18 bonded packings [4, 8], mainly b cause these were the only high-efficiency columns available at the time and because they were widely used for small molecules. With increased availability of alkyl-bonded packings of different chain lengths it became possible to compare the effect of chain-lengths from C-1 to C-18 on protein resolution and recovery [5]. Initial results, mostly based on packings from different manufacturers, showed virtually no specific selective effects attributable to the chain lengths of individual packings, and very little change in absolute retention times. Recoveries of the more hydrophobic test substances did, however, vary, with an optimum at C-3 chain length [5] and a marked reduction in 'ghost' peaks (see above).

All these early studies were done with silicas of 10 nm pore size, having nominal exclusion limits of ~70 kD. To eliminate unwanted exclusion effects and to improve mass transfer, similar short-chain RP (RPSC) packings were prepared with silica having 30 nm pore size by the Beckman-Altex group. Similar packings have now been marketed by several companies. In comparison with end-capped packings (cf. Fig. 1) uncapped short-chain packings gave less retention and lower recoveries of proteins [9], particularly with acetonitrile as the organic modifier – which illustrates the danger of making comparisons between packings from different sources: differences are as likely to be due to unknown (and possibly uncontrolled) variations in coverage as to other more specified parameters. Changes in stationary phase coverage can also occur during prolonged use of columns. A solvent system which minimizes such variations and counteracts the effects of exposed silanol groups is therefore desirable.

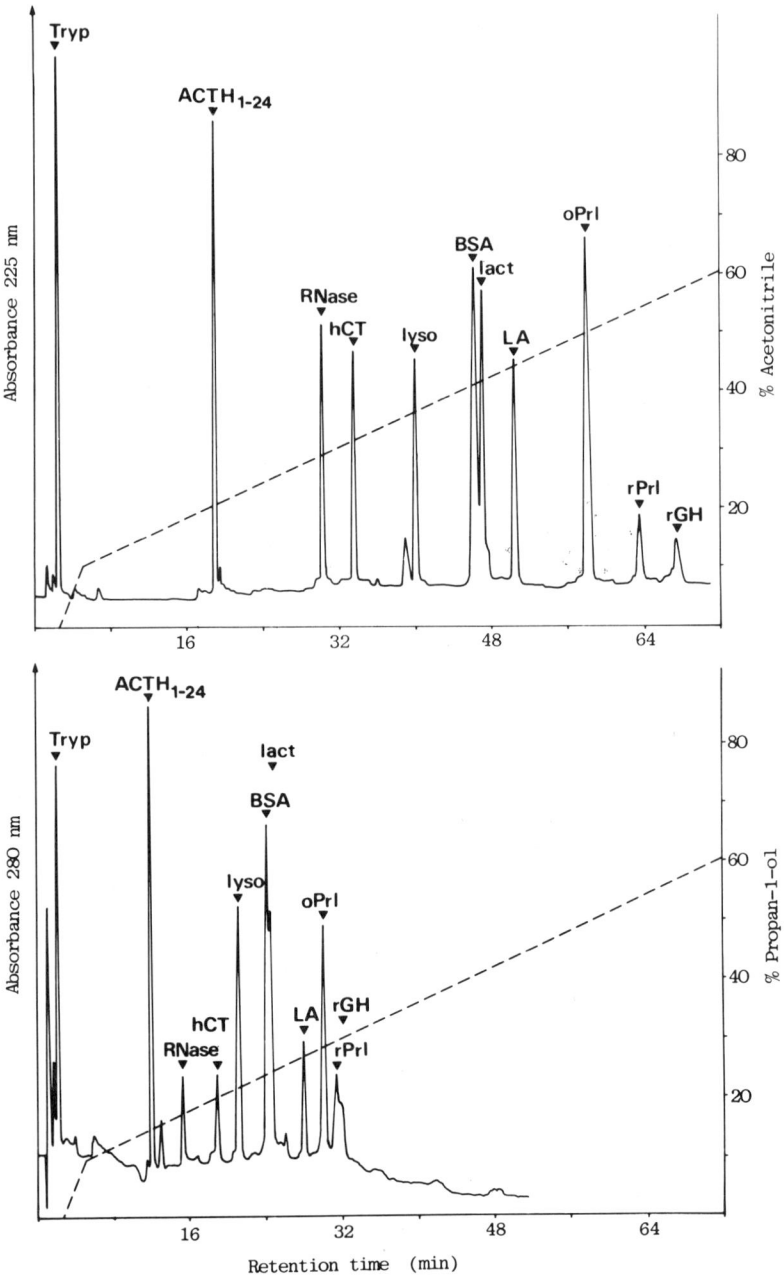

Fig. 3. Effect of organic modifier type on polypeptide/protein RP-HPLC with gradient elution. The eluent was 155 mM NaCl/10 mM HCl (pH 2.1) with acetonitrile (*upper trace*) or propan-2-ol (*lower trace*); % values are v/v.   *[continued opposite*

Table 1. Effect of mobile-phase composition on protein recoveries from short-chain (C-3) RP packings of large pore size (Beckman Ultrapore RPSC). Each tabulated primary component was 10 mM except for NaCl, which was 155 mM. Runs were at 30° and 1 ml/min flow-rate, with a continuous linear gradient changing by 1.0%/min with acetonitrile or 0.6%/min with propan-1-ol. Each run was with 10 µg of the protein; duplicates agreed within ±10%. *Data from ref. [10].*

Primary component	Secondary component	BSA, % rec.	Ovalbumin, % rec.
HCl/NaCl	Acetonitrile (no NaCl)	88	<1
HCl/NaCl	Propan-1-ol (no NaCl)	85	23
TFA	Acetonitrile + TFA	99	86
TFA	Propan-1-ol + TFA	98	96
HCl	Acetonitrile + HCl	100	82
HCl	Propan-1-ol + HCl	106	82
H_3PO_4	Acetonitrile + H_3PO_4	97	61
H_3PO_4	Propan-1-ol + H_3PO_4	92	86
TFA/NaCl	Acetonitrile + TFA	88	2
TFA/NaCl	Propan-1-ol + TFA	81	19

Mobile-phase effects: primary solvent

Our original studies [4, 8] explored the effect of different aqueous mobile phases, in particular those of different molarity and pH. In essence they showed that a relatively high molarity (0.2 M) and low pH (2 to 3) were necessary if maximum chromatographic efficiencies were to be obtained with all polypeptides, although the nature of the salt-acid used did not appear crucial. We opted for acid-saline (0.155 M NaCl/0.01 M HCl) as it afforded compatibility with a variety of bioassays. There were, however, some exceptions to this general rule, and some proteins can be chromatographed at pH's close to neutrality or under mildly alkaline conditions [4]. Reducing the molarity of the primary component also impaired efficiency for some polypeptides. Table 1, relating to recoveries (as considered below), indicates types of acidic systems studied besides NaCl/HCl as chosen.

Fig. 3, *continued from opposite.-* Column: C-4 (Altex), 75×4.6 mm i.d. and similar to the RPSC type (see text) except that particle size was 10 µm; operated at 45°. Flow-rate 1 ml/min. Compounds tested, besides tryptophan, ACTH 1-24 (Synacthen) and ribonuclease, *with prefixes* h = human, o = ovine, r = rat: CT, calcitonin; lyso, lysozyme; BSA, bovine serum albumin; lact, bovine α-lactalbumin; LA, lactoglobulin A; Prl, prolactin; GH, growth hormone.

The use of much favoured primary eluting solutions such as 0.1% (v/v) TFA, with its advantages of UV-transparency and presumed volatility, does incur penalties in respect of efficiency, when compared with acid saline [10]. High salt concentrations minimize adsorptive interactions with residual silanol groups, and low pH ensures their total protonation. The utility of low molarity or high pH therefore depends to some extent on packing coverage, and its stability, as well as on the nature of the polypeptide itself. A penalty of high-molarity systems is reduced recoveries of more hydrophobic proteins, as shown in Table 1 (some values for ovalbumin being notably low). However, this can be overcome to some extent by the choice of an appropriate organic modifier (see below).

With low-molarity systems, the choice of an inappropriate (i.e. incompletely capped, or uncapped) column can substantially reduce the chromatographic efficiency for a protein such as lysozyme, while that for another protein such as EGF can be preserved [11]. Using maximum-coverage RPSC packings, mouse EGF (J.A. Smith, unpublished) and rat EGF [2] can be chromatographed at pH 6.8. Closely-eluting proteins contaminating the EGF show markedly reduced efficiency with very broad peaks, thus providing one means of enriching samples in a desired protein. Initial extraction and fractionation should, however, be carried out under acid conditions [1] and with proteolytic inhibitors present to minimize the artifactual N-terminal clipping of the protein which otherwise occurs [12].

The use of strongly alkaline conditions (pH >8.5) is not feasible with silica-based packings because of their tendency to dissolve rapidly; the newer polymer-based RP supports may yield useful separations at high pH.

Mobile-phase effects: organic modifier

Unlike RP-HPLC of small molecules, e.g. steroid hormones [13], there are few selective effects to be obtained in protein RP-HPLC by the use of different types of organic modifier [4], once gradient profiles have been adjusted to take into account differing solvent strengths (see Fig. 3). In certain cases the use of mixed organic modifiers has afforded a marginal improvement in resolution [12]. However, the magnitude of these effects does not provide any incentive to use the computer-aided methods of selecting multi-component mobile phases that have been developed for 'classical' RP-HPLC [14]. Yet different organic modifiers do have important consequences for protein chromatography insofar as both efficiency and recovery are concerned. As is evident from Table 1, stronger organic modifiers such as propan-1-ol give significantly higher recoveries of hydrophobic proteins such as ovalbumin, when used in conjunction with high-molarity primary solvents [10]. Furthermore, this modifier reduces the loss in efficiency seen when proteins are chromatographed on poorly covered stationary phases, as compared with acetonitrile [9]. Small amounts of n-butanol, t-butanol and t-pentanol have been used admixed with acetonitrile for the same purpose [15].

As is well known, many proteins are reversibly or irreversibly denatured by organic solvents, and this may influence the choice. Some form of configurational change may, however, be involved in the elution process itself, albeit not necessarily irreversible insofar as the native aqueous configuration is concerned. Acetonitrile has tended to be favoured on the whole, by virtue of its UV-transparency and low viscosity, and it certainly suffices for growth factors such as EGF [1] and FGF [16].

Mobile-phase effects: ion-pairing additives

The impression conveyed up to now of protein RP-HPLC has been of a very rigidly determined chromatographic process in which only efficiency and recovery are markedly influenced by changes in either stationary-phase or mobile-phase composition, and in which few specific selective effects are available to manipulate separations of closely running or incompletely resolved proteins. This holds to some extent when compared with small-molecule HPLC. There is, however, one approach which does afford some flexibility, namely the introduction of hydrophobic ion-pairing additives into both aqueous and organic modifier-containing mobile phases.

Strictly speaking, all ionic components of the mobile phase are potential ion-pairing reagents, capable of interacting with oppositely charged amino acids in the protein. Thus, hydrophilic ions such as Cl^- or PO_4^{3-} significantly alter the behaviour of the protein itself, rendering it more hydrophilic and thus elutable from the stationary phase. In their absence, e.g. with water alone as the aqueous phase, complete retention results for all except the smallest and the least hydrophobic peptides. These ions do not, however, individually confer marked selective effects, nor do they interact with the hydrophobic stationary phase, for which they have no affinity. If, however, the ion-pairing additive has significant hydrophobic characteristics, it can both alter the relative retention of a protein with which it associates and, moreover, can create a kind of dynamically coated ion-exchanger by 'dissolving' in the stationary phase itself. While the relative importance of these mechanisms is, like many theoretical aspects of HPLC, subject to dispute, their practical utility is not.

Depending on the number of protonated residues in the protein, useful selective effects may be obtained by the use of hydrophobic additives, as in Fig. 4, at low concentrations (e.g. [10]). The use of such additives as the sole supplement in the water-based mobile phase does, however, have significant disadvantages. Compared with, say, acid-saline, it leads to greatly extended retention times and, moreover – as shown by the 'elutability' values in Fig. 5 – substantial

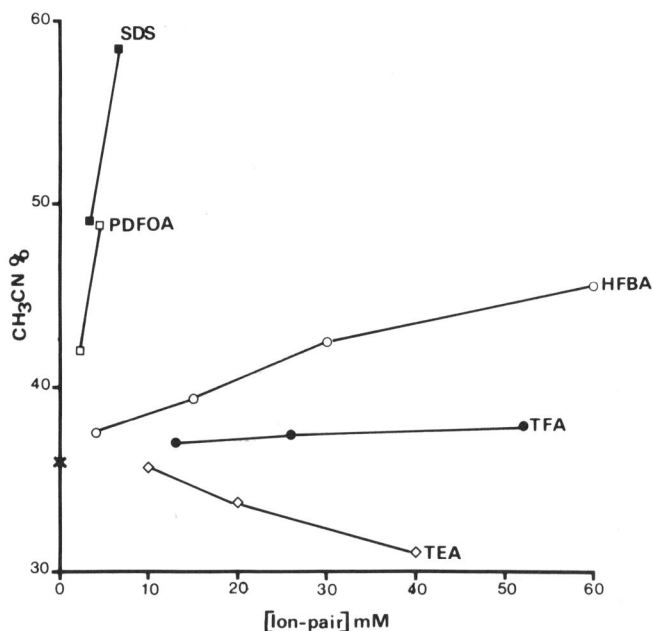

Fig. 4. Effect of different ion-pairing additives. The concentrations of acetonitrile (v/v) required to elute lysozyme from a 15 cm
× i.d. 4.6 mm Spherisorb ODS-2 column (45°; 1 ml/min flow-rate) are
shown for the different additives (abbreviations in footnote at
start of article). The point on the ordinate marked **x** indicates
the acetonitrile concentration required to elute the protein with
155 mM NaCl/10 mM HCl present (NaCl was likewise used for all test
points) but no ion-pairing additives.

concentrations (e.g. >30 mM HFBA) are required to compensate for
residual adsorptive effects of the packings and so enable reproducible
retention times and reasonable peak efficiencies to be obtained.

To counteract these effects we have explored the conjoint use
of such hydrophobic additives and various salt concentrations in
the primary eluent, in the hope of combining the advantages of both.
As reflected in Fig. 5 which shows 'elutability', if NaCl is present
at 0.05 M or higher, retention values for lysozyme are directly
correlated with HFBA concentrations in a reproducible and predictable
manner.   However, with NaCl at 0.005 M (Fig. 5) or lower, the protein
shows an augmented requirement (with an altered influence of HFBA
concentration) for acetonitrile to achieve elution; indeed, with the
lowest HFBA concentration (0.05% v/v) it was indefinitely retained.

By reference to Fig. 4 it can be seen that impeded elution is
especially marked with more strongly hydrophobic additives such

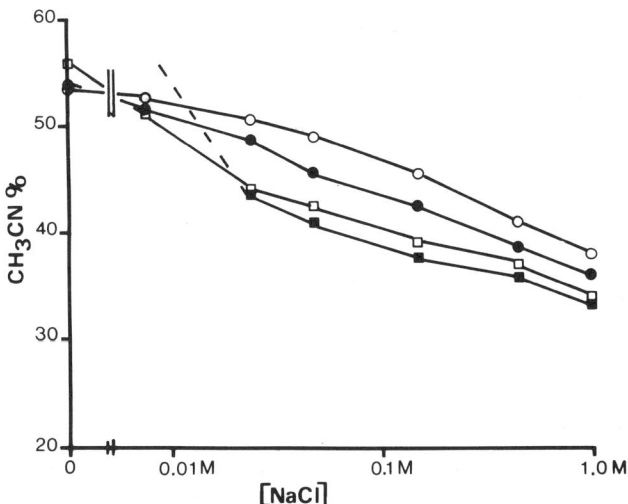

Fig. 5. Effect of HFBA at various concentrations as an ion-pairing additive in the presence of different NaCl concentrations on the tenacity with which lysozyme is held, judged by the acetonitrile concentration (v/v) needed to elute the protein. Separations were performed at 45° using a maximum-coverage Spherisorb ODS-2 column, 15 cm × 4.6 mm i.d. HFBA strength: o, 60 mM (0.8% v/v); ●, 30 mM (0.4%); □, 15 mM (0.2%); ■, 3.8 mM (0.05%). The NaCl concentrations refer to the solvent mixture. (HCl was absent.)

as PDFOA and SDS, whilst TFA - only weakly hydrophobic - impedes elution only slightly, as one would predict. When, however, hydrophobic cations such as TEA are used, retention is reduced (Fig. 4). This cannot be due to an ion-pairing mechanism, as TEA is at least as hydrophobic as TFA and in any event should not pair with negatively charged residues in the protein as these will be protonated at the pH employed (pH 2-3). The primary mode of action of these cations is probably the modification of the stationary phase to form a dynamic ion-exchange system, which being positively charged repels the protonated protein residues at an acid pH. Their action is, therefore, counter to the retention-enhancing effects of the hydrophobic anions; thus, as for NaCl addition, overall retention is decreased so that elution is obtained at lower overall organic-modifier concentrations, with the likelihood of improved recoveries and reduced risk of denaturation. Selectivities conferred by differential association of the hydrophobic anion with protonated protein residues are nevertheless preserved when hydrophobic anions and cations are used conjointly.

The practical exploitation of these effects is exemplified in Fig. 6, which shows the chromatography of a complex mixture of mouse EGF and its congeners in the presence of PDFOA plus TEA, compared

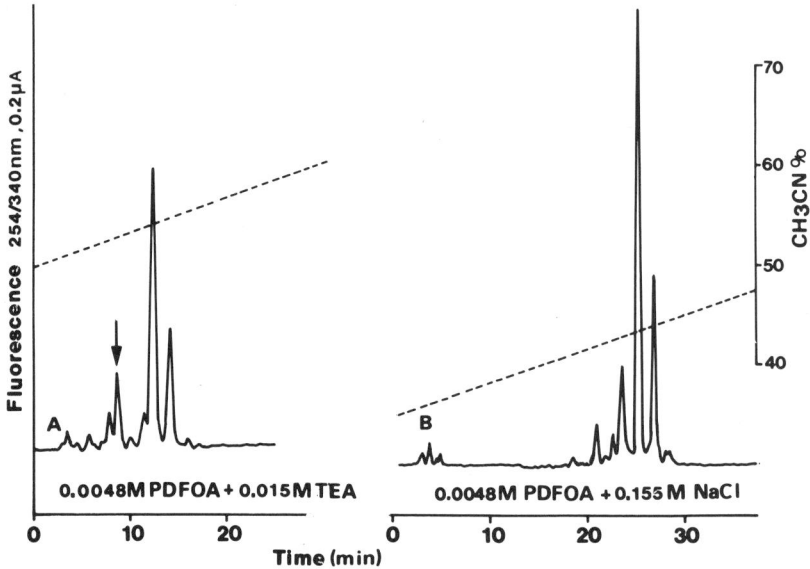

Fig. 6. Effect of ion-pairing additives on the separation of components in a mixture of mouse EGF$_{1-53}$ and congeners including mouse EGF$_{2-53}$ as well as oxidized (and probably deamidated) forms, present in a crude commercial product prepared by conventional (non-HPLC) methods. *Left*, **A**: Spherisorb ODS-2 column (15 cm × 4.6 mm i.d.); mobile phase 0.2% (w/v) PDFOA with 0.2% TEA. *Right*, **B**, as on left but with 0.155 M NaCl as well as TEA. *Interrupted lines* denote acetonitrile gradient (note the different v/v concentrations used). Although overall peak patterns are similar, evidently there are differences in the relative separation of some components, e.g. that marked in **A** with an *arrow*, evident in **B** at 23 min.

with PDFOA with 0.155 M NaCl and TEA.   Interestingly, although the overall patterns are similar for the two elution mixtures, with good resolution and high efficiencies, they are not identical. Some differences in selectivity are conferred by the use of the anionic and cationic additives conjointly. In contrast, with PDFOA alone (no TEA or HCl), EGF is still retained even with 60% acetonitrile, and with acid-saline alone none of the major peaks is resolved [11]. The similarity in RP elution profiles of EGF-related materials using quite different ion-pairing agents (PDFOA and SDS) [17] suggests that for an ion-pairing agent of a particular charge there is only one net effect, although its extent may differ.

Mobile-phase effects: flow rates and gradient profiles

Flow rates have important effects on protein RP-HPLC. The slow rates of diffusion associated with large molecules would theoretically indicate that low flow rates should enhance efficiency. This is indeed the case (e.g. for RNase run with acetonitrile/TFA on an RPSC column: HETP increased 2.5-fold with increase in flow-rate from 0.2 to 2 ml/min [Archer & Cooke, cited in Beckman literature]). However, low flow rates can also result in reduced recoveries as solubility limits are exceeded in small eluent volumes. The influence of flow rate on separation also reflects the gradient profile, i.e. the rate of change in the organic modifier concentration [9] which, if rapid, can also reduce recoveries. Complex trade-offs are therefore involved in optimizing resolution and recovery, and no general rules can be laid down. However, flow rate and gradient profile (commonly 1 ml/min and 0.5-1%/min respectively) can be varied quite widely in seeking to optimize a given separation, possibly with a resolution *vs.* separation-speed compromise.

Detectability can be enhanced by a low flow rate in particular. Microbore columns (1 mm i.d.) are used with flow rates of 10-20 μl/min, giving an equivalent linear solvent velocity to conventional analytical columns (4-5 mm i.d.) operated at 1 ml/min, but require specialized equipment. Thereby sensitivity is enhanced (by over an order of magnitude for small-molecular analytes), the analyte being at high concentration in the eluate, whilst efficiency remains optimal. Similar effects can be obtained with proteins, giving sensitivities of 5-10 ng/peak; thus, the mass and thence the specific radioactivity of ^{125}I-labelled EGF can be directly determined [18]. Almost as great an enhancement in detection can, however, be obtained using columns of 4-5 mm i.d. merely by reducing flow rates to the 25-50 μl/min range, provided that the pumps remain accurate and the detector has a low noise/signal ratio. The efficiency losses then associated with the resulting non-optimal (reduced) linear velocity of the mobile phase seldom jeopardize separations because of the very limited period of true chromatography occurring under gradient-elution conditions with proteins, as explained above.

Mobile-phase effects: temperature and dwell time

The effects of temperature on HPLC are complex. Increased temperatures will increase rates of mass transfer and thus tend to improve efficiencies, but at the same time rates of axial diffusion will be enhanced and counteract such improvements. For most analytes there is an optimum temperature for highest efficiency. Increased temperatures tend to decrease retentions of smaller, early-eluting polypeptides, but increase those of later-eluting compounds such as BSA and prolactin [10]. This effect tends to decrease recoveries of the more hydrophobic materials. Some limited selective effects can be obtained by adjusting temperature [10], even possibly by temperature programming. However, the temperature differential required is large (up to 60°) and thermal denaturation becomes a distinct hazard.

Karger and his colleagues [19] have shown for papain, a globular enzyme of M_r 30,000, that two peaks appear, one early-eluting and biologically active, the second later-eluting and irreversibly denatured. The amount of the second, inactive peak increases with increased column temperature. The duration of exposure of the protein to the stationary phase itself (dwell time) can also influence the extent of *in situ* denaturation, even in the absence of an organic modifier, as was also found in Karger's group [19]. β-HCG likewise chromatographs as two peaks in acid conditions [20], identical in amino acid composition [21]; peak doubling here may be due to differences in carbohydrate content.

For smaller proteins such as EGF and lysozyme in which structure is determined largely by internal disulphide bonds, such effects are not as likely to be important, and full bioactivity is retained even at column temperatures of up to 45° [1, 5]. Each case must, however, be examined separately with respect to temperature, dwell time and mobile-phase conditions, including organic-modifier type, bearing in mind that some conformational changes take place over quite extended time scales and that not all such changes need be irreversible.

HYDROPHOBIC INTERACTION HPLC (HIC)

The major drawback of all RP-HPLC systems is the requirement for an organic modifier to elute the protein, with the consequent risk of *in situ* denaturation. This risk is enhanced with larger proteins whose tertiary structures and hence bioactivity depend on internal hydrophobic interactions that are likely to be disrupted by the dense alkyl-bonded stationary phase. In an attempt to overcome these problems, packings have been developed in which a much lower density of hydrophobic moieties is created by interspersing them through a stable hydrophilic bonded phase similar to that used for size-exclusion or ion-exchange packings.

Two company-produced examples of such packings are the Synchropak Propyl matrix which is silica-based and the TSK Phenyl, based on a macroporous styrene-divinylbenzene copolymer. We have not yet used the former, but from published chromatograms it appears that while large proteins can be eluted using reverse salt gradients with no organic modifier, several proteins tested seemed to elute together. HIC packings of this nature can, however, resolve smaller compounds [22] and, unlike RP-HPLC, protein retentions are strongly influenced by alkyl chain-length which allows some flexibility. It is assumed that the matrix-protein interactions take place with externally located hydrophobic domains only (Fig. 7); certainly retention orders greatly differ from those obtained by RP-HPLC [4, 22]. Acyl ligand densities on these HIC packings are 1-1.5 μmol/m^2; as, however, they are based on a polyamine-bonded silica matrix they also possess weak anion-exchange properties which may contribute to separations. Irrespective of the mechanisms that operate, the main advantages of these HIC-type HPLC packings lie in their different selectivities compared with RP-systems and the fact that no organic modifiers are required.

Fig. 7. Schematic representation
of the interaction of a protein
with the packing in RP chromatography and in hydrophobic interaction chromatography (HIC),
where ●●● represent hydrophobic
residues or domains.

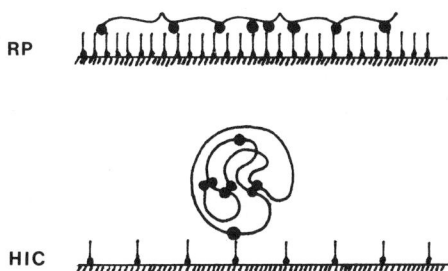

The other above-mentioned type of HIC packing, TSK Phenyl [23],
is able to resolve a variety of proteins under conditions - such
as those of Regnier's group [22] - that are compatible with full
bioactivity. For EGF these columns offer no particular advantage, as
full activity of this relatively small protein is retained after
RP-HPLC [1]. For FGF, however, despite its relatively small size we
have observed substantial loss of activity after RP-HPLC. It can,
however, be eluted with full activity from TSK Phenyl 5PW columns.
HIC gave enhanced selectivity for a natural growth hormone and a
genetically engineered analogue (identical with the former except
that it possesses one extra N-terminal residue, the weakly hydrophobic
methionine). With conventional RP-HPLC we were unable to separate
these two forms (Fig. 8) even when using the high-resolution PDFOA-
saline system with a very shallow acetonitrile gradient. With the TSK
Phenyl column, however, baseline separation was obtained, the synthetic
analogue eluting later (Fig. 8). These results lend some credence to
the supposition that hydrophobic interactions are confined to external
protein residues in this system.

ION-EXCHANGE HPLC (IEC)

Although IEC (originally not HPLC) is one of the traditional means
of separating proteins, until recently the available IE-HPLC packings
have been suitable only for small peptides [15]. The recent advent of
packings suitable for large proteins (CM- and DEAE-bonded, TSK;
Mono Q & S, Pharmacia; IE packings, Synchropak) has enabled conventional
IEC conditions to be transposed to HPLC, to achieve enhanced resolution. IEC principles are well established. The major variables are
the steepness of the displacing-salt gradient and the elution pH;
one option is to make use of a pH gradient to displace the protein
[24].

However, just as RP-HPLC seldom involves hydrophobic interactions
alone, IEC does not operate solely through charge interactions. Mixed
hydrophobic/IE interactions were studied by Hofstee [25] using alkyl-
amine-substituted agaroses, and by Kopaciewicz et al. [26] with HPLC
IE packings varying in hydrophobicity. Mixed-mode chromatography was

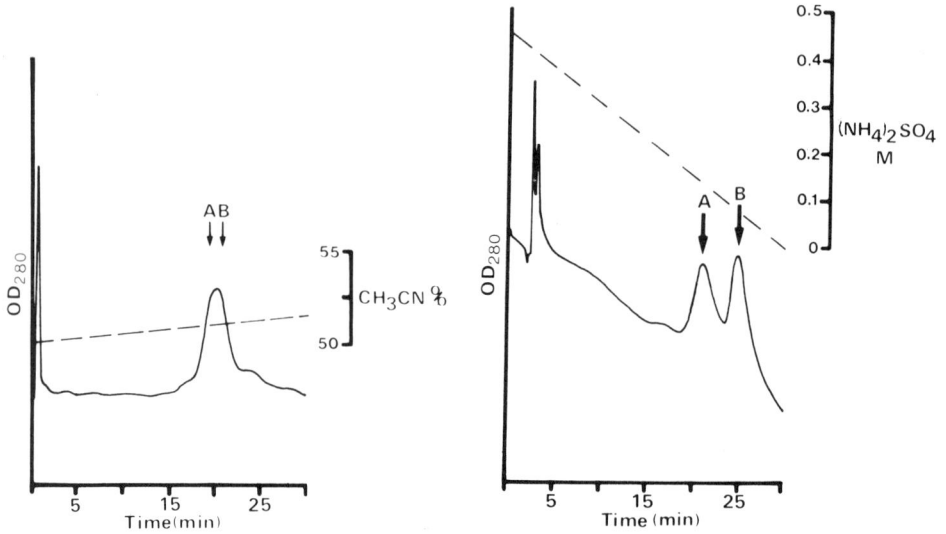

Fig. 8. Patterns for a mixture of natural (**A**) and synthetic (**B**) human Met-growth hormone. *Left:* Conventional RP-HPLC on a RPSC column (Altex Beckman; 7.5 cm × 4.6 mm i.d.) at 45° with 0.155 M NaCl/0.2% w/v PDFOA (pH 3.0) initially and an increasing admixture (% v/v) of acetonitrile. The two species do not separate although the gradient (— — —) is very shallow. *Right:* HIC on a TSK Phenyl column (15 cm × 8 mm i.d.) at ambient temperature with a gradient of ammonium sulphate in 0.1 M phosphate buffer, pH 8. Evidently there is complete separation.

shown to operate when mouse EGF was chromatographed on a silica-based stationary phase with bonded DEAE [17]. If the hydrophobic interaction is minimized by chromatographing with acetonitrile present, the elution profile may be deliberately altered by the presence of hydrophobic ion-pairing agents, with improved resolution (Fig. 9).

The full range of possibilities for IEC and HIC of proteins has not yet been explored. However, the much milder conditions used, compared with those generally used for RP-HPLC, and the consequent improved likelihood of retaining bioactivity, make these HPLC modes a method of choice for larger proteins which possess tertiary structure.

SIZE-EXCLUSION HPLC (SEC)

Conventional SEC has been used for many years to separate proteins. HPLC in the SEC mode under similar conditions is now feasible since a number of suitable packings are on the market.   Its main advantage is speed of separation. In principle there should be no interaction

Fig. 9. Effect of ion-pairing
additive on IEC of mouse EGF
(a crude preparation containing
multiple molecular forms as
well as deamidated material).
Column: TSK-IEX 545K, 15 cm ×
7.5 mm i.d. Mobile phase
initially 50 mM Tris-HCl,
pH 8.0, with NaCl (linear gradient)
to attain 0.25 M NaCl (+ Tris-HCl) at
60 min; both solutions contained
20% (v/v) acetonitrile to minimize adsorptive interactions.
With 25 mM octylamine present
(A) there was better separation
than in its absence **(B)**.

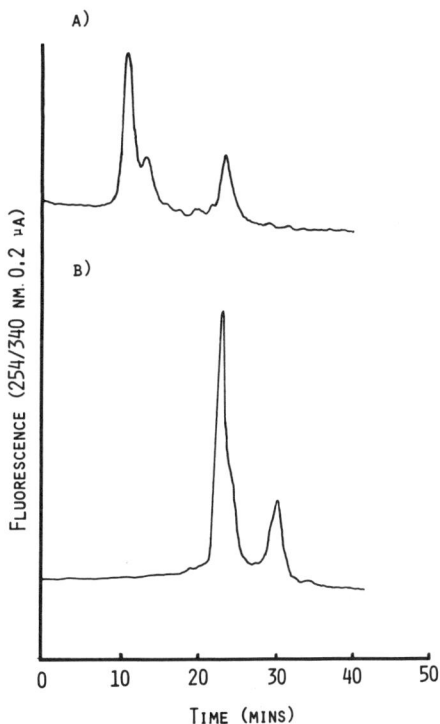

between protein and the matrix.   In practice, however, both ionic
and hydrophobic interactions have been found with typical hydrophilic
bonded phases used for SEC [27].   The TSK silica-based SEC packings
have been found to exhibit both types of interaction in this laboratory, the ionic interactions increasing rapidly as the column ages
(J.A. Smith, unpublished).   The new zirconia-stabilized GF250 column
from Du Pont carries a weak negative charge.   Hydrophobic and ionic
interactions may be suppressed using an organic modifier (e.g. 20%
v/v acetonitrile) or a salt (at 0.3 M) respectively.

The resolution achievable on most   SE-HPLC   packings is less
than that using conventional narrow-range gel-permeation matrices,
probably because of the heterogeneity of pore size which with typical
columns spans a separation range of 1.5-2 mol. wt. decades [28].
In contrast to IE- and RP-HPLC modes with which trace enrichment
is feasible, the capacity of typical SEC columns is generally too low
to be of use for the direct HPLC analysis of growth factors.   A
separation, of academic interest at least, of rat and mouse EGF has
been carried out in this laboratory using TSK G3000SW in the presence
of 0.3 M NaCl but without organic modifier.   The mouse EGF, which
possesses two tryptophan residues near its C-terminus, showed anomalous
retention owing to its hydrophobic interactions with the stationary
phase, whereas the rat EGF (or the mouse-EGF major tryptic fragment)

which lacks tryptophan did not.   This effect is virtually absent in
the presence of 20% (v/v) acetonitrile [1].

APPLICABILITY OF THE HPLC APPROACHES

The polypeptide and protein growth factors are generally present
in biological samples only in minute quantities; hence chromatography
cannot be used alone as a means of analysis with simultaneous quantitation and identification.   HPLC is, however, routinely used in
the purification of growth factors, e.g. EGF [1, 2], FGF [16, 29],
PDGF (platelet-derived growth factor) [30] and G-CSF (granulocyte
colony-stimulating factor) [31].   HPLC is a necessary adjunct to
immunoassay and receptor-binding assays in the analysis of closely
related growth factors such as EGF and α-TGF (a transforming growth
factor) [32, 33], and serves as a means of distinguishing new factors
related to them, e.g. VGF (vaccinia virus-induced growth factor) [34].

HPLC has also shown that the supposed growth-promoting properties of a number of substances actually reside in other proteins co-
purified with them.   For example, FGF is responsible for the apparent
effects of a number of pituitary hormones on fibroblasts [16], and
PDGF for some of the mitogenic activity of fetuin on aortic smooth
muscle cells [35].   Thus, within a relatively short space of time,
HPLC has become a standard tool in the isolation, identification
and analysis of protein growth factors.

Acknowledgements

We are grateful to various colleagues who have participated in some
of the work described here, notably E.C. Nice and M.W. Capp, both
previously on the staff of our Institute's London Branch, and B. Archer
and N. Cooke of Beckman Instruments Inc. (Berkeley, CA).   We are
particularly grateful to Drs. Archer and Cooke for permission to
use data from their laboratory, especially in Fig. 2, and to Dr.
D. Schulster (National Institute for Biological Standards and Control)
for the gift of human growth hormones.

References

1.   Smith, J.A., Ham, J., Winslow, D.P., O'Hare, M.J. & Rudland, P.S.
     (1984) *J. Chromatog. 305*, 295-308.
2.   Simpson, A.J., Smith, J.A., Moritz, R.L., O'Hare, M.J.,
     Rudland, P.S., Morrison, J.R., Lloyd, C.J., Grego, B.,
     Burgess, A.W. & Nice, E.C. (1985) *Eur. J. Biochem. 153*, 629-637.
3.   Unger, K.K. (1979) *Porous Silica: its Properties and Use as a
     Support in Column Liquid Chromatography*, Elsevier, Amsterdam.
4.   O'Hare, M.J. & Nice, E.C. (1979) *J. Chromatog. 171*, 209-226.
5.   Nice, E.C., Capp, M., Cooke, N. & O'Hare, M.J. (1981) *J.
     Chromatog. 218*, 569-580.
6.   Meek, J.L. (1980) *Proc. Nat. Acad. Sci. 77*, 1632-1636.

7. Browne, C.A., Bennett, H.P.J. & Solomon, S. (1982) *Anal. Biochem. 124*, 201-208.
8. Nice, E.C., Capp, M. & O'Hare, M.J. (1979) *J. Chromatog. 185*, 413-427.
9. Cooke, N., Archer, B.G., O'Hare, M.J., Nice, E.C. & Capp, M. (1983) *J. Chromatog. 225*, 115-123.
10. O'Hare, M.J., Capp, M., Nice, E.C., Cooke, N. & Archer, B.G. (1982) *Anal. Biochem. 126*, 17-28.
11. O'Hare, M.J., Smith, J.A., Archer, B.G., Cooke, N. & Nice, E.C. (1983) in *Protides of Biological Fluids Colloquium 30* (Peeters, H., ed.), Pergamon, Oxford, pp.723-726.
12. Smith, J.A. & O'Hare, M.J. (1984) *J. Chromatog. 299*, 13-28.
13. D'Agostino, G., Mitchell, F., Castagnetta, L. & O'Hare, M.J. (1984) *J. Chromatog. 305*, 13-26.
14. D'Agostino, G., Castagnetta, L., Mitchell, F. & O'Hare, M.J. (1985) *J. Chromatog. 338*, 1-23.
15. Hearn, M.T.W. (1983) in *High Performance Liquid Chromatography - Advances and Perspectives*, Vol. 3 (Horvath, C.S., ed.), Academic Press, New York, pp. 87-155.
16. Smith, J.A., Winslow, D.P., O'Hare, M.J. & Rudland, P.S. (1984) *Biochem. Biophys. Res. Comm. 119*, 311-318.
17. Smith, J.A. & O'Hare, M.J. (1985) *J. Chromatog. 345*, 168-172.
18. Nice, E.C., Lloyd, C. & Burgess, A.W. (1984) *J. Chromatog. 296*, 153-170.
19. Cohen, S.A., Benedek, K.P., Dong, S., Tapuhi, Y. & Karger, B.L. (1984) *Anal. Chem. 56*, 217-221.
20. Cowley, G., Smith, J.A., Ellison, M. & Gusterson, B. (1985) *Internat. J. Cancer 35*, 575-579.
21. Grego, B. & Hearn, M.T.W. (1984) *J. Chromatog. 336*, 25-40.
22. Fausnaugh, J.L., Pfannkoch, E., Gupta, S. & Regnier, F.G. (1984) *Anal. Biochem 137*, 464-472.
23. Kato, Y., Kitamura, T. & Hashimoto, T. (1984) *J. Chromatog. 292*, 418-426.
24. Regnier, F.G. (1984) *Meths. Enzymol. 104*, 170-189.
25. Hofstee, B.H.J. (1973) *Biochem. Biophys. Res. Comm. 50*, 751-757.
26. Kopaciewicz, W., Rounds, M.A. & Regnier, F.G. (1985) *J. Chromatog. 318*, 157-172.
27. Schmidt, D.E., Giese, R.W., Conron, D. & Karger, B.L. (1980) *Anal. Chem. 52*, 177-182.
28. Unger, K. (1984) *Meths. Enzymol. 104*, 154-169.
29. Bohlen, P., Baird, A., Esch, F., Ling, N. & Gospodarowicz, D. (1984) *Proc. Nat. Acad. Sci. 81*, 5364-5368.
30. Stroobant, P. & Waterfield, M.D. (1984) *EMBO J. 3*, 2963-2967.
31. Nicola, N.A., Metcalf, D., Matsumoto, M. & Johnson, G.R. (1983) *J. Biol. Chem. 258*, 9017-9023.
32. Kimball, E.S., Bohn, W.H., Cockley, K.D., Warren, T.C. & Sherwin, S.A. (1984) *Cancer Res. 44*, 3613-3619.
33. Twardzik, D.R., Kimball, E.S., Sherwin, S.A., Ranchalis, J.E. & Todaro, G. (1985) *Cancer Res. 45*, 1934-1939.

34. Twardzik,D.R., Brown, J.P., Ranchalis, J.E., Todaro, G.J. &
    Mors, B. (1985) *Proc. Nat. Acad. Sci. 82*, 5300-5304.
35. Libby, P., Raines, E.W., Cullinane, P.M. & Ross, R. (1985)
    J. Cell Physiol. 125, 357-366.

#A-4

HPLC-EC MEASUREMENT OF NEUROPEPTIDES IN BIOLOGICAL SAMPLES

G.W. Bennett, J.V. Johnson and C.A. Marsden

Department of Physiology and Pharmacology
Medical School, Queen's Medical Centre
Clifton Boulevard, Nottingham NG7 2UH, U.K.

Neuropeptides which contain one or more of the amino acids tyrosine, tryptophan and cysteine are electroactive and can be analyzed in biological samples using an electrochemical (EC) detector coupled with a suitable HPLC system. Peptides are generally measured by immunological procedures (e.g. RIA) which achieve high sensitivities, but can also produce false-positive measurements due to antibody (Ab) cross-reactivity with structurally related peptides present in the samples. The HPLC-EC technique avoids such specificity problems and enables the rapid assay of several peptides in appropriate samples. Recent developments to improve the sensitivity of the HPLC-EC procedure are described, and a comparison presented of the brain and pituitary tissue levels of the neuropeptide, vasopressin (AVP) measured by HPLC-EC and HPLC-RIA.

Most amino acids lack intrinsic electrochemical activity. Accordingly, HPLC-EC analytical methods for these and for peptides made up of these require pre-column derivatization to electroactive forms, using o-phthalaldehyde/mercaptoethanol [1] or o-phthalaldehyde/t-butyl thiol [2]. However, tyrosine, tryptophan and cysteine are electroactive without derivatization [3], and one or more of these residues are present in a number of important neuropeptides – including vasopresssin (AVP), oxytocin, neurotensin, somatostatin, cholecystokinin (CCK-8) and various opioid peptides – which can therefore be directly monitored using HPLC-EC [4-8], as is discussed in this article. HPLC has been widely used to separate neuropeptides prior to measurement of peptide content using sensitive RIA techniques [8, 9].

Neuropeptides are most commonly quantified by RIA's that achieve sensitivities lying in the pM to fM range, but all neuropeptide Ab's used in RIA's show significant cross-reactivity with closely related

peptides, resulting in false-positive values. Such specificity
problems are particularly pertinent where there is a need to separate
the peptide from metabolites which may have biological activity [10],
and also where structurally related but distinct forms of endogenous
neuropeptides undergo intracellular processing in the tissues concerned
[11]. Whilst high-resolution HPLC will help obviate immunoassay specificity problems, the use of an on-line detection system offers various
practical advantages. Generally, UV and fluorimetric on-line detection
methods are insufficiently sensitive to measure the low amounts
of neuropeptide in small biological samples; but recent EC detectors can
furnish sensitivities approaching those of RIA's.

In our own recent studies, the HPLC-EC method for peptides
has been significantly improved in comparison with earlier methods
[4, 5] with respect to both sensitivity and specificity by using a
radial compression HPLC system (Waters Z module) in place of a column,
and a dual-channel EC detector (ESA Coulochem 5100A) in place of a
small-surface single-detector system [8].

The HPLC-EC method has been applied to measure levels of AVP and
other neuropeptides, as shown, in brain and endocrine-tissue extracts.

Vasopressin (AVP)	H_2N-Cys-$\underline{Tyr}$-Phe-Gln-Asn-Cys-Pro-Arg-Gly-NH_2
Oxytocin	H_2N-Cys-$\underline{Tyr}$-Ile-Gln-Asn-Cys-Pro-Leu-Gly-NH_2
Met-enkephalin	H_2N-$\underline{Tyr}$-Gly-Gly-Phe-Met-OH
Leu-enkephalin	H_2N-$\underline{Tyr}$-Gly-Gly-Phe-Leu-OH
Angiotensin II	H_2N-Asp-Arg-Val-$\underline{Tyr}$-Ile-His-Pro-Phe-OH
Neurotensin	pGlu-Leu-$\underline{Tyr}$-Glu-Asn-Lys-Pro-Arg-Arg-Pro-$\underline{Tyr}$-Ile-Leu-OH

In particular, the improved HPLC-EC technique has been used to measure
immediate and chronic changes after adrenalectomy in AVP levels in
discrete brain and pituitary regions [6, 12]. The HPLC-EC values have
been compared with HPLC-RIA values, and observed differences have indicated the superior specificity and accuracy of the HPLC-EC method
in comparison with immunological techniques applied to HPLC fractions.

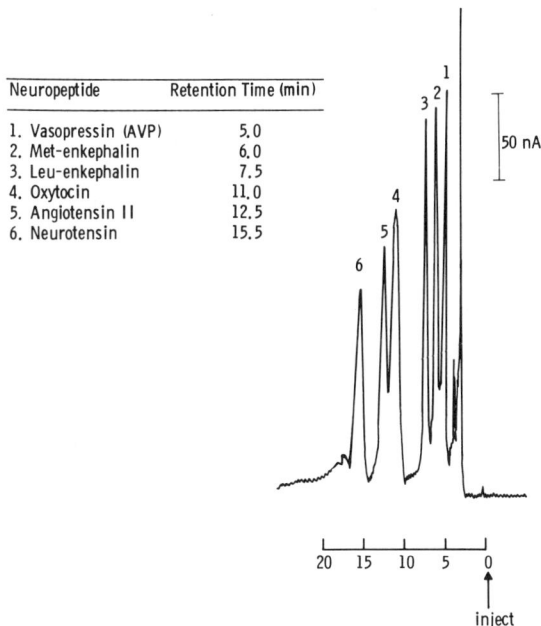

Neuropeptide	Retention Time (min)
1. Vasopressin (AVP)	5.0
2. Met-enkephalin	6.0
3. Leu-enkephalin	7.5
4. Oxytocin	11.0
5. Angiotensin II	12.5
6. Neurotensin	15.5

Fig. 1. RP-HPLC separation of neuropeptide standards (20 pmol injected). For conditions, see text.

HPLC–EC SYSTEM

Various neuropeptides were separated (Fig. 1) by isocratic RP-HPLC using the Waters Z module radial compression system containing a Radial-pak C-18, 10 μm cartridge. The ESA Coulochem 5100A dual channel detector with two porous-graphite in-line working electrodes was used in the screening mode with the second detector electrode set at a working potential of 0.85 V and the screening potential of the first set at 0.40 V. These settings were based on a current/voltage curve for AVP (20 pmol injected) in which the peak height at the second electrode plateaued at 800 nA between 0.80 V and 0.90 V, and rose from a base level of 100 nA at an applied potential of 0.40 V.

Similar electrode conditions were found to be optimal for the other neuropeptides investigated. The system also incorporated a guard cell detector prior to the injector, set at 0.90 V to act as a scrubber for the mobile phase. Using these conditions, and a mobile phase of 0.15 M NaH_2PO_4/methanol (60:40 by vol.), pH 5.8, delivered at a constant flow rate of 1.5 ml/min by a Waters 510 pump, the retention times of the peptide standards were as shown in Fig. 1. For each a calibration curve was constructed, from 0.2 to 200 pmol injected, by measuring peak area in nA/min, and the detection limit was <200 fmol at a 3:1 signal-to-noise ratio (Fig. 2).

Fig. 2. Dose-response
curves for vasopressin
(AVP; Δ) and oxytocin (▲).
Similar curves were
obtained for the other
neuropeptides studied.
The detection limit is
<0.2 pmol (signal-to-
noise 3:1).

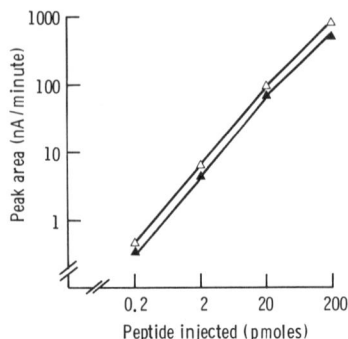

SAMPLE PREPARATION

Brain or pituitary tissues were dissected and homogenized by
sonication (Ultrasonics Rapides Ltd., 100 W for 1 min) in 1 M acetic
acid. The supernatants obtained by centrifugation (4000 **g**, 20 min)
were dried down in a vortex evaporator (Buchler) and stored at -20°.
The centrifugal pellet was similarly stored pending protein determination [13]. Samples were taken up in the HPLC mobile phase and filt-
ered prior to injection.

PEAK IDENTIFICATION, AND BEHAVIOUR OF 'COLUMN' AND DETECTOR

Tentative identification of peaks observed in brain extracts
was made by R_T comparisons with synthetic standards, and confirmed by
spiking standards into the original extract. To check each peak
for peptide heterogeneity, two oxidation peaks were generated for each
peptide and the ratio of the two peak heights ascertained. For
example, when pure AVP was applied, some was oxidized at the first
detector, set at 0.60 V, and the remainder at the second, set at 0.90 V;
the ratio of the two peak heights was 1.255 ±0.005 (SEM; n = 10). On
repeating the procedure with AVP-containing extracts of neurointermedi-
ate lobe the ratio was 1.300 ±0.020 (n = 10). There was no significant
difference between these two values (p <0.05), suggesting that the
AVP peak measured in the tissue extracts did not include other peptides
with similar R_T. For other brain extracts and other peptides, similar
verification of identity was made.

The use of the Z module offered a number of advantages compared
with a conventional column. Firstly, the uniformly compressed cartridge
improved peak separation and reduced the normal peak 'tailing' that
results from surface properties. Secondly, the lessened flow resistance
of a cartridge compared with a column (with equivalent packing material)

enabled more rapid analysis at lower back-pressures. Finally, use of the Z module cartridge contributed towards improvements in the signal-to-noise ratio and hence to the overall gain in sensitivity.

The use of the dual-electrode coulometric detector also improved the signal-to-noise ratio. 'Screen mode' operation enabled peptide oxidations to be monitored within the range 0.40-0.85 V, thereby excluding other analytes in the samples which are oxidized outside this range. This screening was feasible since with their large surface area the porous-graphite detectors oxidized most of the analyte, in contrast with detectors having a more conventional single surface. Reproducibility was also improved since peptide adsorption to the larger surface area was less prone to reduce electrode sensitivity.

COMPARISON OF EC AND RIA ANALYTICAL APPROACHES

Rats were adrenalectomized and AVP measured in brain and pituitary regions by HPLC-EC [12]. Aliquots of identical samples were stored at -80° for parallel measurement of HPLC effluents by RIA using the method and antiserum of Jenkins et al. [14]. AVP standards were spiked in and similarly treated; AVP levels were thereby shown not to alter significantly during storage (up to 7 months) when measured by either HPLC-EC or RIA without HPLC.

Adrenalectomy caused regional specific changes in AVP content as measured by HPLC-EC [12]. Parallel measurement by RIA showed qualitatively similar changes in AVP content; but the values by RIA were ~2-3 times the HPLC-EC values [8]. This was particularly evident in pituitary and brain regions where AVP is stored in nerve terminals prior to release. The most likely explanation for the higher levels with RIA compared with HPLC-EC is over-estimation because of non-specific binding of the antibody to 'AVP-like' peptides present in the tissue extracts of regions where AVP is processed and stored.

RIA following HPLC.- Selected groups of tissue extracts from these regions (e.g. median eminence) were run through the HPLC procedure prior to RIA, with HPLC conditions identical to those for HPLC-EC. Fractions were collected during successive 1-min periods (with the EC detector switched off), and their AVP content was measured by RIA. This HPLC-RIA approach enabled (a) a direct comparison to be made with HPLC-EC measurements on similar aliquots, and (b) an assessment of the recovery of AVP-like immunoreactivity from the HPLC run. The AVP measured by HPLC-EC in median-eminence extracts occurred as a sharp peak at 5 min (917 ±69 pg, SEM; n =6), shown in Fig. 3. In contrast, significant AVP immunoreactivity was manifest in three HPLC fractions (4-7 min) as a large, broad peak; but the value by immunoreactivity in the peak fraction at 5-6 min (953 ±158 pg; n = 6) was not significantly different from the EC value (Fig. 3). Moreover, the total AVP immunoreactivity eluted in the 10-min HPLC collection

Fig. 3. Vasopressin (AVP) levels in median eminence (ME) extracts: HPLC-RIA value (**b**) compared with HPLC-EC value (**a**) for the fraction containing the peak revealed by the on-line EC trace. The EC value was negligible on either side of the peak fraction.

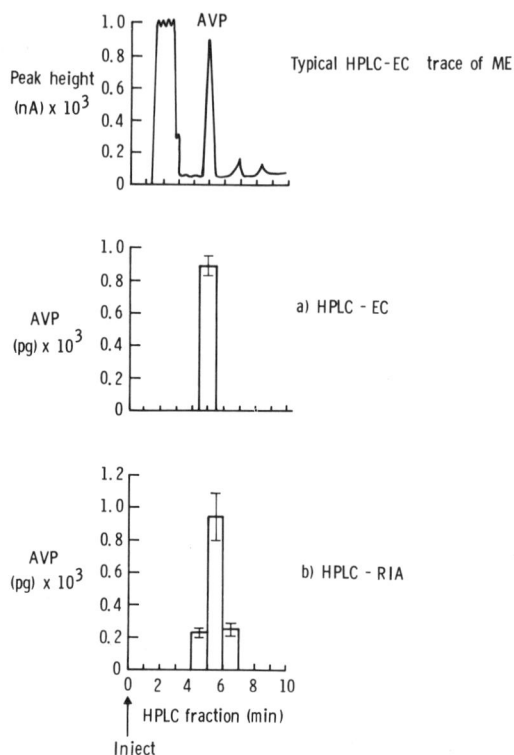

period was 1704 ±208 pg (n = 6), which represented only 75% of the AVP immunoreactivity present in the sample before HPLC (2234 ±126 pg; n = 6). These results suggest that the non-specific 'AVP-like' immunoreactivity in acetic acid extracts of rat median eminence is due to natural or generated molecules chemically similar to AVP, which co-elute with 'true AVP', and also to other 'AVP-like' material, possibly larger precursor molecular forms, which does not elute with our HPLC conditions during the 10-min fraction-collection period.

CONCLUDING COMMENTS

With a dual rather than a single channel detector one can be more confident that a peptide peak measured by HPLC-EC represents a single molecular component; thus HPLC-EC may provide a more specific method of measuring neuropeptide levels than HPLC-RIA. Therefore, with the recent improvements in sensitivity here described for HPLC-EC, this technique may offer an attractive method for measuring various peptides in common biological samples. Blood plasma samples require prior extraction with Fluorisil to eliminate interferences.

Further improvements may involve the application of gradient elution HPLC-EC. In recent studies in our laboratory of the neuro-peptides present in the hypothalamus of the Brattleboro-strain rat (which lacks central synthesis and release of AVP), a non-AVP peak has been observed close to the position of AVP. It is hoped that by using simple gradient elution HPLC with EC detection,   such AVP-like and other peptides may be isolated and identified.

References

1. Joseph, M.M. & Davies, P. (1983) *J. Chromatog. 277*, 125-136.
2. Allison, L.A., Meyer, G.S. & Shoup, R.E. (1984) *Anal. Chem. 56*, 1089-1096.
3. Bennett, G.W., Brazell, M.P. & Marsden, C.A. (1981) *Life Sci. 29*, 1001-1007.
4. Meek, J.L., Yang, H.Y.T.& Costa, E. (1977) *Neuropharmacol. 16*, 151-154.
5. Sauter, A. & Frick, W. (1983) *Anal. Biochem. 133*, 307-313.
6. Johnson, J.V., Bennett, G.W., Marsden, C.A., Gardiner, S.M. & Bennett, T. (1984) *Regul. Peptides 9*, 335.
7. Marsden, C.A. (1984) in *Drug Determination in Therapeutic and Forensic Contexts* [Vol. 14, this series] (Reid, E. & Wilson, I.D., eds.), Plenum, New York, pp. 319-330.
8. Bennett, G.W., Johnson, J.V. & Marsden, C.A. (1986) in *Monitoring Neurotransmitter Release during Behaviour* (Joseph, M.H., Fillenz, M., Macdonald, I.A. & Marsden, C.A., eds.), Horwood, Chichester⊗.
9. Morris, H.R., Etienne, A.T., Dell, A., Albuquesque, R. (1980) *J. Neurochem. 34*,   574-582.
10. Griffiths, E.C. & McDermott, J.R. (1984) *Neuroendocrinol. 39*, 573-587.
11. Hammar, A.J. (1984) *Trends Neurochem. Sci. 7*, 57-60.
12. Johnson, J.V., Bennett, G.W., Marsden, C.A., Gardiner, S.M. & Bennett, T. (1984) *Hypertension A6*, 1993-1998.
13. Lowry, O.H., Rosebrough, N.J.,   Farr, A.L. & Randall, R.J. (1951) *J. Biol. Chem. 193*, 265-275.
14. Jenkins, J.S., Ang, V.T.Y., Hawthorn, J., Rossor, M.N. & Iversen, L.L. (1983) *Prog. Brain Res. 60*, 123-128.

⊗ in press

#A-5

DETERMINATION OF SUBSTANCE P AND NEUROKININS BY A COMBINED HPLC/RIA PROCEDURE

J.M. Conlon and C.F. Deacon

Clinical Research Group for Gastrointestinal
   Endocrinology of the Max-Planck-Gesellschaft
University of Göttingen, Gosslerstrasse 10d
D-3400 Göttingen, W. Germany (FRG)

Problems in the measurement by radioimmunoassay (RIA) of the mammalian tachykinins (substance P, neurokinin A, neurokinin B) arise from (1) lack of immunogenicity, particularly for neurokinin B, (2) non-specificity of antisera raised against an individual tachykinin, and (3) molecular heterogeneity derived from the presence of biosynthetic precursors, catabolites and components with oxidized methionine residues. These problems have been overcome by separating the immunoreactive components by reverse-phase (RP) HPLC followed by quantitation using antisera of defined regional specificity.

RIA's have been devised for substance P using antisera directed against the COOH-terminal and NH_2-terminal regions with <0.4% cross-reactivity towards the neurokinins. For the neurokinins an antiserum raised against A that shows 22% cross-reactivity with B but only 0.6% towards substance P has been used. With a C-18 column and gradient elution, various peptides - cf. (3) above - were resolved. Post-mortem formation of oxidized forms is unavoidable, but mercaptoethanol or dithiothreitol addition to extracting solvents is helpful.

Substance P-like and neurokinin A-like immunoreactivities were high in extracts of metastases from human mid-gut tumours. HPLC has disclosed components corresponding chromatographically and immunochemically to substance P and neurokinin A and their oxidized forms, to a metabolite that may be [pGlu^5] substance P (5-11), and to an NKA-LI component more hydrophobic than neurokinin A but distinct from neurokinin B. Neurokinin A and substance P immunoreactivities are below the RIA detection limits in normal peripheral plasma, but were high in patients with carcinoid tumours.

The tachykinins are a family of polypeptides that share a common C-terminal sequence, represented by Phe.X.Gly.Leu.Met.NH_2, and display a similar spectrum of biological activities, e.g. contraction of smooth muscle and vasodilation (as reviewed [1, 2]). Until quite recently, substance P was regarded as the only tachykinin present in mammalian tissues where it is distributed throughout the central and autonomic nervous systems. The other tachykinins were isolated from amphibian skin and from a mollusc. The isolation from porcine spinal cord of the kassinin-related peptides, neurokinin A [3] and neurokinin B [4], has greatly stimulated interest in the field of tachykinin research. Table 1 shows the structures of these tachykinins.

Sequence analysis of a cloned cDNA for a substance P precursor from bovine brain [5] has shown that synthesis of neurokinin A and substance P is directed by the same mRNA. This article presents approaches to the solution of methodological problems associated with the simultaneous measurement of substance P and neurokinins in biological samples. HPLC combined with RIA's, using antisera of defined regional specificity, has been used to quantify and partially characterize the immunoreactive components of substance P and neurokinin A in extracts of carcinoid tumours.

NOMENCLATURE

Neurokinin A, the term recommended by the Nomenclature Committee of the IUPHAR (August 1984), has also been referred to as substance K, neurokinin α and neuromedin L. Similarly, neurokinin B has been referred to as neurokinin β and neuromedin K. In this article, substance P-like immunoreactivity measured by RIA using an antibody directed against the C-terminal region of the molecule is termed C-SPLI. Similarly, N-SPLI refers to measurements with an N-terminally directed antibody.

METHODOLOGICAL PROBLEMS

(a) **Lack of immunogenicity.**– The tachykinins, coupled to a suitable protein such as haemocyanin or thyroglobulin, vary in their ability to produce high affinity antisera suitable for use in RIA. Substance P and neurokinin A are fortunately highly immunogenic, but attempts in the authors' laboratories to raise antisera against neurokinin B or against Lys.Phe.Ile.Gly.Leu.Met.NH_2, a synthetic hexapeptide, were unsuccessful.

(b) **Lack of specificity of antisera.**– The tachykinins contain an amidated C-terminal residue (Table 1), such that coupling to a carrier protein must proceed by way of the free α-amino group or through the ε-amino group of lysine. Hence most antisera raised against tachykinin-protein conjugates are directed towards a site in the exposed homologous C-terminal region of the peptides. Antisera raised against a particular tachykinin generally display appreciable cross-reactivity towards other tachykinins.

Table 1. Amino acid sequences of some tachykinins (C-terminal amide; pGlu denotes pyroglutamic acid).

Substance P	Arg-Pro-Lys-Pro-Gln-Gln-Phe-Phe-Gly-Leu-Met.NH$_2$
Kassinin	Asp-Val-Pro-Lys-Ser-Asp-Gln-Phe-Val-Gly-Leu-Met.NH$_2$
Eledoisin	pGlu-Pro-Ser-Lys-Asp-Ala-Phe-Ile-Gly-Leu-Met.NH$_2$
Physalaemin	pGlu-Ala-Asp-Pro-Asn-Lys-Phe-Tyr-Gly-Leu-Met.NH$_2$
Neurokinin A	His-Lys-Thr-Asp-Ser-Phe-Val-Gly-Leu-Met.NH$_2$
Neurokinin B	Asp-Met-His-Asp-Phe-Phe-Val-Gly-Leu-Met.NH$_2$

(c) **Non-specific interference effects in RIA.**- Problems arise during the measurement of tachykinin-like immunoreactivity in biological samples, e.g. plasma, CSF and tissue extracts, from the presence of high mol. wt. substances that non-specifically inhibit the binding of tracer to antibody [6] and from the presence of tracer-degrading peptidases. Extraction of immunoreactive peptides before quantitation by RIA is thus mandatory.

(d) **Heterogeneity of the immunoreactive components.**- In common with most endocrine- and neuro-peptides, the tachykinins exist in multiple molecular forms which reflect different pathways of post-translational processing of a biosynthetic precursor. For example, the sequence of neurokinin A is found at the C-terminus of a 36-amino acid residue peptide, neuropeptide K isolated from porcine brain [7]; moreover, higher mol. wt. forms of immunoreactive substance P have been detected in human brain tissue [8].

Further heterogeneity arises from the presence in tissues or in the circulation of proteolytic fragments that retain the ability to bind to antibody, and from the presence of oxidized forms of the peptides. Substance P and neurokinin A contain one methionine residue and neurokinin B two methionine residues that are susceptible to oxidation, particularly in dilute solution at near-neutral pH. The resulting sulphoxide (or sulphone) derivatives show reduced reactivity towards C-terminally directed antisera [9] and elute from RP (C-18 silica) columns before the reduced form.

DEVELOPMENT OF SEQUENCE-SPECIFIC RADIOIMMUNOASSAYS

(1) Measurement of NKA-LI

Antibodies were raised in rabbits (n = 5) against a conjugate of neurokinin A coupled to keyhole limpet haemocyanin using a water-soluble carbodiimide. Within 3 months, all animals produced antisera that were of sufficiently high titre (>10,000 final dilution) to be

Table 2. Cross-reactivities of antisera raised against neurokinin A with some tachykinins. Values represent % binding of label, with no tachykinin addition or with 10 ng/ml of the named tachykinin present.

Anti-serum	Final dilution	Alone	+ Neuro-kinin A	+ Neuro-kinin B	+ Subs-tance P	+ Kassinin
NKA 1	1:20,000	33.6	1.9	3.0	19.8	3.5
NKA 2	1:20,000	39.7	1.9	7.1	39.7	12.6
NKA 3	1:40,000	26.2	0.5	1.0	15.7	0.8
NKA 4	1:20,000	35.4	2.9	7.8	32.1	11.7
NKA 5	1:10,000	30.1	1.4	10.9	28.2	10.1

of potential use in RIA. The ability of neurokinin A, neurokinin B, kassinin and substance P to inhibit the binding of (2-[^{125}I]iodohistidyl)neurokinin A (~2000 Ci/mmol; Amersham International) to the antisera [cf. K.G. McFarthing et al. -#A-7, this vol.- *Ed.*] is shown in Table 2.

Antiserum NKA2 showed the lowest cross-reactivity with substance P and so was used in developing a RIA. With a 72 h incubation period and separation of Ab-bound radioactivity by addition of polyethylene glycol, a sensitive RIA with mid-range (IC_{50}) of 270 pg/ml and a detectability down to 10 pg/ml was achieved. Serial dilutions of eledoisin, neurokinin B and kassinin gave rise to dilution slopes parallel to that of neurokinin A. The ratios of the IC_{50} values relative to neurokinin A as 1.0 were: eledoisin, 1.9; neurokinin B, 4.5; kassinin, 10.7. Substance P and physalaemin at 10 ng/ml inhibited binding of ^{125}I-labelled neurokinin A by an amount equivalent to that produced by 62 pg/ml and 54 pg/ml respectively of neurokinin A, i.e. cross-reactivities of 0.6% and 0.5%. Bombesin at concentrations up to 100 ng/ml produced no inhibition of binding.

(2) **Measurement of C-SPLI**

As previously described [9, 10], RIA conditions were established using antiserum P4, directed against a site in the residues 6-11 region of substance P and ^{125}I-[Tyr^8]substance P (s.a. 2200 Ci/mol; New England Nuclear). Compared with substance P as 1.0, reactivities under RIA conditions were as follows: [Met(O)^{11}]substance P, 0.69; substance P COOMe, 2×10^{-4}; physalaemin, 0.35; eledoisin, 5×10^{-4}; kassinin, 3×10^{-4}; neurokinin A, 8×10^{-4}; neurokinin B, 4×10^{-3}.

Fig. 1. RP-HPLC (see text for conditions) of: **a**, neurokinins A and B (synthetic); b-d, neurokinin A (**b**) or B treated with H_2O_2 (0.01%, room temp.) for the time indicated. *Arrows* show positions of substance P and its oxidized form.

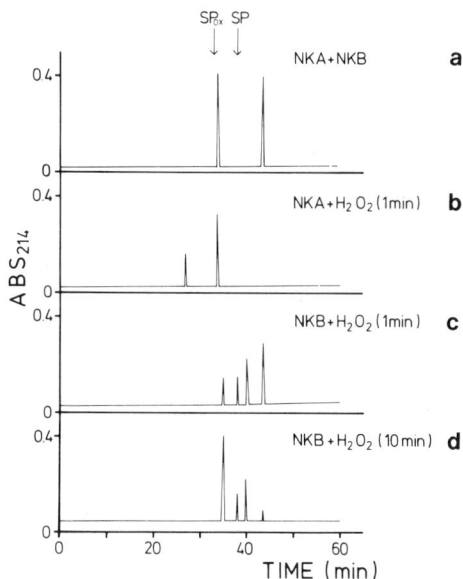

(3) Measurement of N-SPLI

RIA determination entailed use of antiserum R140 (supplied by Dr. P.C. Emson, MRC Neurochemical Pharmacology Unit, Cambridge, U.K.) directed against a site in the N-terminal region of substance P, and ^{125}I-$[Tyr^8]$substance P. This antiserum [11] shows no detectable cross-reactivity with other members of the tachykinin family.

HPLC SEPARATION OF SUBSTANCE P AND NEUROKININS A AND B

The oxidized forms of the tachykinins were prepared by H_2O_2 treatment by the method of Floor & Leeman [12]. As neurokinin B contains two methionine residues, H_2O_2 treatment generates the $[Met(O)^2]$, the $[Met(O)^{10}]$ and the $[Met(O)^2, Met(O)^{10}]$ derivatives. As shown in Fig. 1, a complete separation of the oxidized and reduced forms of neurokinins A and B and substance P was achieved using a C-18 silica column (Supelcosil LC-18-DB, 250x4.6 mm; run at 30°). The flow rate was 1.5 ml/min, with a linear gradient (67.5 ml total vol.) formed from 0.1% trifluoroacetic acid (TFA) and acetonitrile/water (38.5:61.5 by vol.) containing 0.1% TFA.

Prolonging the reaction time of neurokinin B with H_2O_2 to 10 min increased the magnitude of the earliest peak, suggesting that it represented $[Met(O)^2, Met(O)^{10}]$neurokinin B. Different commercially available C-18 columns were compared. With these chromatographic conditions, complete resolution of neurokinin A, substance P and neurokinin B was achieved with μ Bondapak C18 (10 μm; Waters Associates), Ultrasphere-ODS (5 μm; Beckman Insts.) and ODS-Hypersil (5 μm; Shandon

Labortechnik).   Only the ODS-Hypersil gave complete resolution of
substance P and (3-11) and (5-11) metabolites [13].

APPLICATION OF THE RIA PROCEDURES

(1) Measurement of SPLI and NKA-LI in human plasma

The reported concentrations of SPLI in the plasma of healthy
fasted subjects vary widely: e.g. 168±31 fmol/ml in supine subjects
and 401±51 fmol/ml when ambulant [14], 38±5 pg/ml [= 28±4 fmol/ml] in
pregnancy rising to 77±33 pg/ml immediately post-partum [15].

We found that human plasma strongly inhibited the binding of
radiolabelled substance P to both the C-terminally and the N-terminally
directed antisera.   The magnitude of the inhibition by a particular
sample was irreproducible and varied markedly with the RIA incubation
time.   After subjecting plasma to gel filtration (Biogel P-10 or
Sephadex G-50), it was found that only material that was eluted at
the void volume of the column was capable of inhibiting the binding of
tracer to antibody.   Fractions with the elution volume of synthetic
substance P did not display immunoreactivity.

Blood samples were taken from 9 healthy, fasted subjects and
at 15 min intervals following a 550 kCal breakfast; they were collected into EDTA (50 mM final concn.) and Trasylol (10,000 kIU) and
centrifuged immediately at 4°.   Plasma was extracted using Sep-Pak
C-18 cartridges (Waters Associates) as previously described [10,13]
using acetonitrile/water (70:30) containing 0.1% TFA for elution. The
recoveries of synthetic substance P and neurokinin A added to plasma
were >90%.   The Sep-Pak extracts of plasma, taken in the fasting
and post-prandial states, did not significantly inhibit binding of
tracer to either antibody against substance P or to the antibody
against neurokinin A.

It is concluded, therefore, that the concentrations of SPLI and
NKA-LI in the peripheral circulation of healthy subjects are below the
detection limits of the RIA's: SPLI, <10 fmol/ml; NKA-LI,<3 fmol/ml.
Attempts to measure SPLI and NKA-LI by RIA in unextracted plasma
samples are subject to non-specific interference effects, and the
resulting values will considerably over-estimate the true concentrations of the circulating peptides.

(2) Measurement of C-SPLI and NKA-LI in extracts of carcinoid tumours

The presence of substance P-like immunoreactivity (determined
by RIA and immunohistochemistry) in human carcinoid tumours has been
extensively documented (refs. in [9]).   In the authors' laboratories,
tissue from lymph node and liver metastases from patients with primary
tumours of the mid-gut have been investigated.   An examination of the
structures shown in Table 1 shows that substance P, with arginine and

lysine residues and no free carboxyl group, is a more strongly basic molecule (pI >10) than neurokinins A and B. Hence different conditions are needed for optimal extraction from tissues, depending on the component sought. In agreement with a previous report [16], maximum efficiency for extraction of substance P involves cutting tissue into small pieces while frozen and boiling for 10 min in 0.5 M acetic acid (~10 ml/g wet wt.). Boiling in water alone results in an appreciably lower efficiency of extraction. In contrast, it has been shown [17] for neurokinins that extraction with boiling water (10 min) followed by acidification (final concn. of acetic acid 0.5 M) and homogenization surpasses extraction by boiling acetic acid alone.

Fig. 2 shows the elution profile on a C-18 analytical (30×0.39 cm) column (μ Bondapak) of a boiling acetic acid extract of a biopsied liver metastasis, frozen in liquid nitrogen, from a carcinoid tumour; the levels of C-SPLI and N-SPLI were known to be 1176 and 1050 pmol/g respectively (~1 million times higher than in plasma). The immunoreactivity was resolved into two components with the retention times of substance P and [Met(O)[11]]substance P, measured with both C- and N-terminally directed antisera, and into a component not identified unambiguously: it may be [pGlu[5]]substance P (5-11) as judged by comparison of its retention time (with isocratic elution) with the times for several commercially available fragments of substance P.

Fig. 3 shows the profile with a C-18 semi-preparative (25× 1 cm; Ultrasphere-ODS) column for hepatic tumour tissue taken ~6 h postmortem; the extract contained 407 pmol/g of tissue. Evidently the the contribution of the oxidized form of substance P to total immunoreactivity is higher than for the biopsy specimen. Oxidation of substance P during the extraction procedure can be reduced, but not completely eliminated, by adding a reducing agent, e.g. 0.01 M dithiothreitol or 2-mercaptoethanol, to the solvents.

Extracts of mid-gut carcinoid tumour biopsies, prepared by the boiling water method [17], also contained neurokinin A-like immunoreactivity. Concentrations of NKA-LI in the range 210-2280 pmol/g wet wt. have been measured. Fig. 4 shows the elution profile on a Supelcosil LC-18-DB column (25×0.46 cm) for the NKA-LI in an extract of a hepatic metastasis from a primary mid-gut tumour. Components with the retention times of synthetic neurokinin A and its oxidized form were identified together with a more hydrophobic component that did not match neurokinin B in retention time. This component was eluted from a Sephadex G-50 column in the 3000-4000 mol. wt. zone, suggesting that it may represent an N-terminally extended form of neurokinin A analogous to neuropeptide K [7].

(3) Measurement of SPLI and NKA-LI in patients' plasma [cf. (2)]

In contrast with the situation in healthy subects, C-SPLI, N-SPLI and NKA-LI have been detected in Sep-Pak extracts of peripheral plasma

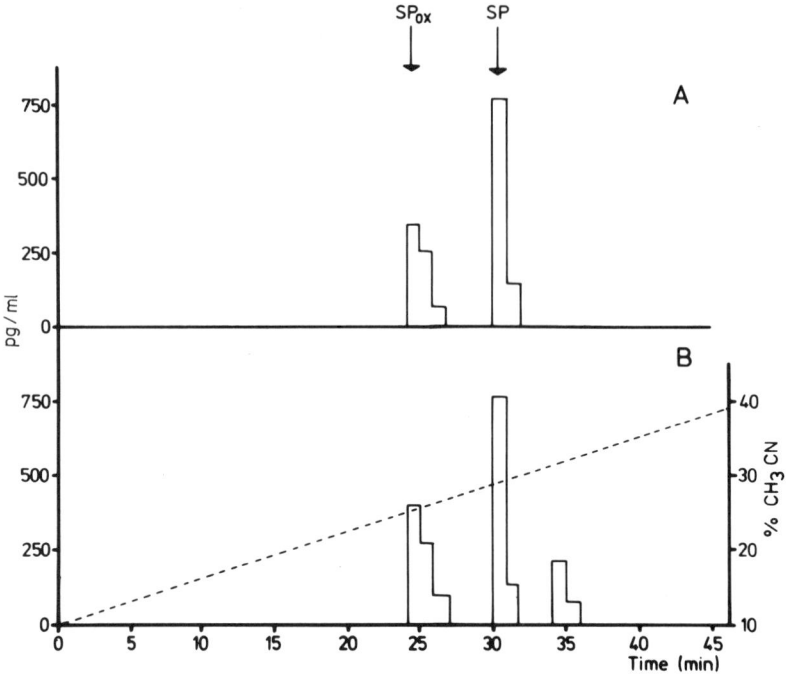

Fig. 2. RP-HPLC (with an acetonitrile gradient, ----) of an extract of a biopsy of a tumour metastasis from a patient with a carcinoid tumour of the mid-gut: substance P-like immunoreactivity measured with:- **A**, an N-terminally directed antiserum; **B**, a C-terminally directed antiserum.

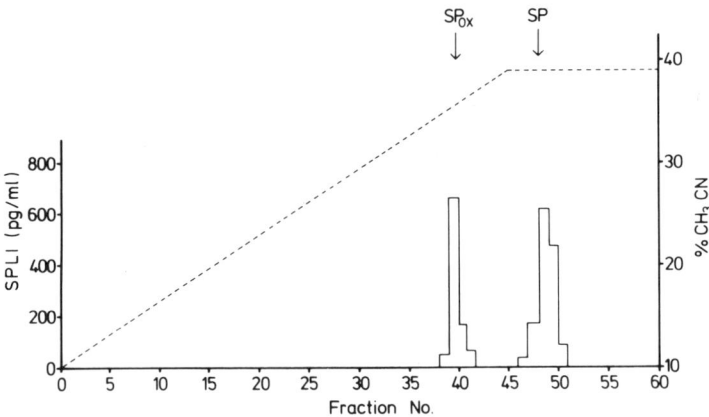

Fig. 3. As for **B** in Fig. 2 (same patient), but extract made from a metastasis taken post-mortem.

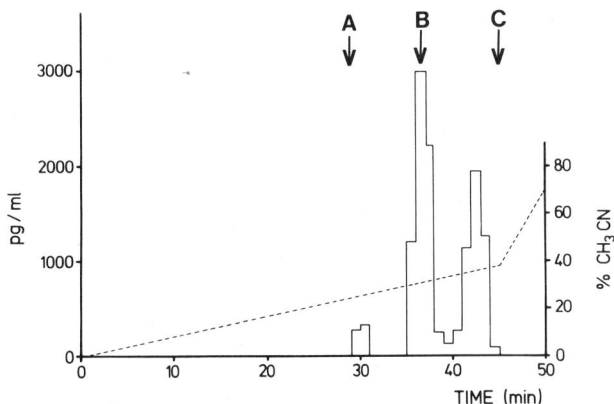

Fig. 4. RP-HPLC as for Fig. 2 (tumour biopsy), with RIA measurement of neurokinin A-like immunoreactivity. *Arrows* show retention
times: **A**, [Met(O)^{10}]neurokinin A; **B**, neurokinin A; **C**, neurokinin B.

from some patients – 5 out of 10 – with carcinoid tumours (histolo-
gically verified; mid-gut, with hepatic metastases).   C-SPLI and
NKA-LI concentrations up to 345 and 1034 fmol/ml respectively have
been observed by us in the fasted state, with significant rises in
response to food [18].   This result is consistent with and extends
the observations of Emson et al. [19].

Acknowledgements

This work was supported by the Stiftung Volkswagenwerk.   The
authors thank Prof. W. Creutzfeldt, Dept. of Medicine, University
of Göttingen, for his cooperation in studying patients under his care.

References

1. Erspamer, V. & Melchiorri, P. (1980) *Trends Pharmacol. Sci. 1*,
    391-395.
2. Iversen, L.L. (1982) *Br. Med. Bull. 38*, 277-282.
3. Minamino, N., Kangawa, K., Fukuda, A. & Matsuo, H. (1984)
    Neuropeptides 4, 157-166.
4. Kangawa, K., Minamino, N., Fukuda, A. & Matsuo, H. (1984)
    Biochem. Biophys. Res. Comm. 114, 533-540.
5. Nawa, H., Hirose, T., Takashima, H., Inayama, S. & Nakanishi, S.
    (1983) *Nature 306*, 32-36.
6. Conlon, J.M., Bridgeman, M. & Alberti, K.G.M.M. (1982) *Anal.
    Biochem. 125*, 243-252.
7. Tatemoto, K., Lundberg, J.M., Jörnvall, H. & Mutt, V. (1985)
    Biochem. Biophys. Res. Comm. 128, 947-953.
8. Nyberg, F., Le Grevés, P. & Terenius, L. (1985) *Proc. Nat.
    Acad. Sci. 82*, 3921-3924.

9. Conlon, J.M., Schäfer, G., Schmidt, W.E., Lazarus, L.H., Becker, H.D. & Creutzfeldt, W. (1985) *Regul. Peptides 11*, 117-132.

10. Conlon, J.M., Lahuerta, J., Miles, J. & Lipton, S. (1984) *Neuropeptides 4*, 227-236.

11. Lee, C.M., Emson, P.C. & Iversen, L.L. (1980) *Life Sci. 27*, 535-543.

12. Floor, E. & Leeman, S.E. (1980) *Anal. Biochem. 101*, 498-503.

13. Conlon, J.M. & Sheehan, L. (1983) *Regul. Peptides 7*, 335-345.

14. Kramer, H.J., Düsing, R., Stelkens, H., Heinrich, R., Kipmowski, J. & Glänzer, K. (1980) *Clin. Sci. 59*, 75-77.

15. Skrabanek, P., Balfe, A., McDonald, D., McKaigney, J. & Powell, D. (1980) *Eur. J. Obstet. Gynec. Reprod. Biol. 11*, 157-161.

16. McGregor, G.P. & Bloom, S.R. (1983) *Life Sci. 32*, 655-662.

17. Norheim, I., Theodorsson-Norheim, E., Brodin, E., Öberg, K., Lundqvist, G. & Rosell, S. (1984) *Regul. Peptides 9*, 245-257.

18. Conlon, J.M., Deacon, C.F., Richter, G., Schmidt, W.E., Stöckman, F. & Creutzfeldt, W. (1986) *Regul. Peptides 13*, 183-196.

19. Emson, P.C., Gilbert, R.F.T., Martensson, H. & Nobin, A. (1984) *Cancer 54*, 715-718.

#A-6

METHODS AND PROBLEMS IN THE ASSAY OF CSF
FOR β-ENDORPHIN AND OTHER ENDOGENOUS PEPTIDES

Richard F. Venn, Stephen J. Capper,
John S. Morley and John B. Miles

Pain Relief Foundation
Rice Lane, Liverpool L9 1AE, U.K.

RIA is a very sensitive technique for peptide assay but can suffer from the drawback of significant cross-reactivity between related peptides. We have developed techniques that allow specific analysis of many of the peptides found in cerebrospinal fluid (CSF) by combining HPLC with RIA. New methodology for raising antisera of high specificity has been developed, and used to determine the levels of peptides in CSF obtained from patients suffering pain.

One interest of the Neurochemistry Section of our Foundation is measurement in CSF of the endogenous peptides involved in the mechanism of pain transmission and perception. In particular we are interested in the analysis of the endogenous opioid peptides such as those in the enkephalin, endorphin and dynorphin families. This article concentrates on the problems encountered, and their solutions, in the development of specific assays for these peptides. The problems are of several types, as follows.

Low concentrations.- As the peptide levels are 0-500 fmol/ml, very high sensitivity is needed, obtainable with RIA provided that suitable antibodies (Ab's) are available.

Structural similarities.- As many of the peptides are structurally related, RIA is not as specific as would be desired. For example, the sequence Tyr-Gly-Gly-Phe is shared by methionine enkephalin (ME), leucine enkephalin (LE) and dynorphin (Fig. 1). Thus it is difficult to raise specific Ab's for RIA. Similarly, pro-opiomelanocortin (POMC) is the precursor of, and contains the sequences of ACTH, β-lipotrophin (LPH), β-endorphin (BE), ME, and the MSH family (Fig. 2). Any Ab that recognizes the C-terminal end of BE will also recognize LPH, while an N-terminally directed Ab would also recognize ME.

Tyr-Gly-Gly-Phe-Met   Met-enkephalin (ME)

Tyr-Gly-Gly-Phe-Leu   Leu-enkephalin (LE)

Tyr-Gly-Gly-Phe-Leu-Arg-*Arg-*Ile-Arg-*Pro-Lys-Leu-Lys-Trp-Asp-Asn-Gln

Dynorphin

Fig. 1. The amino acid sequences of enkephalins and dynorphin, with positions marked (*) where proteolytic action gives rise to smaller related peptides.

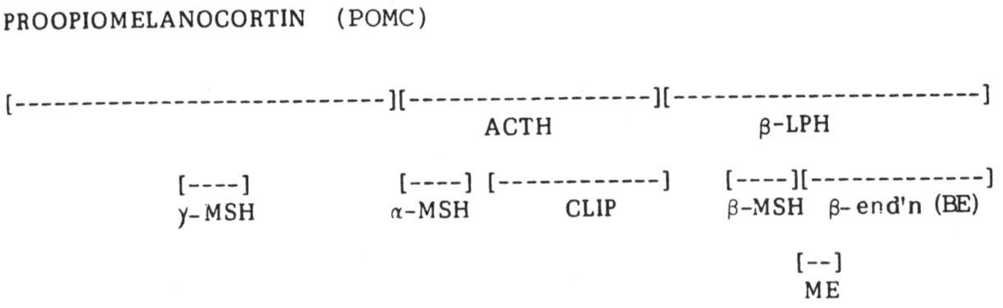

PROOPIOMELANOCORTIN (POMC)

[--------------------------][-----------------][---------------------]
                                  ACTH   β-LPH

        [----]   [----] [------------]   [----][------------]
        γ-MSH   α-MSH   CLIP   β-MSH β-end'n (BE)

                                                        [--]
                                                         ME

                          α-MSH
                          Ac-Ser—Tyr-Ser-Met-Glu-His-Phe-Arg-Trp-Gly-Lys-Pro-Val
   β-MSH
   Ala-Glu-Lys-Lys-Asp-Glu-Gly-Pro-Tyr-Arg-Met-Glu-His-Phe-Arg-Trp-Gly-Ser-Pro-Pro-Lys-Asp
                          γ-MSH
                          Tyr-Val-Met-Gly-His-Phe-Arg-Trp-Asp-Arg-Phe-NH$_2$

Fig. 2. Schematic representation of the structure of pro-opio-melanocortin, the precursor of ACTH, LPH, the MSH family (structures shown), β-endorphin (BE) and methionine encephalin (ME).

'β-Endorphin-like immunoreactivity' has been measured previously in CSF and plasma [1, 2]; however, these and other papers have not distinguished between BE and LPH or any other species that might cross-react with the antisera used.

Sample preparation.- Care must be taken to ensure that no losses are experienced in sample handling. Some of these peptides are labile and easily destroyed. There is also the problem of adhesion to glass. Some HPLC columns are now glass-lined and, if this glass is not silanized, large losses of peptides can occur.

Availability of standards.- This is not a trivial problem, as some of these low-concentration compounds are either unobtainable or extremely expensive. Authentic, good-quality peptides are necessary for assay and HPLC development.

Availability of sample.- Many of our samples are available only in small quantities and are irreplacable, coming as they do from patients undergoing some form of surgical treatment for pain. It is not always possible to complete a series of assays because of sample constraints. Thus more sensitive assays are required.

SAMPLE HANDLING, HPLC, AND REAGENTS

CSF samples were obtained from patients being treated for pain by surgery, e.g. cordotomy or pituitary ablation. CSF was collected into formic acid (90% w/w, 20 μl/ml CSF) in cooled tubes and frozen immediately. For analysis, the thawed samples were extracted using Sep-Pak C-18 cartridges, pre-wetted with methanol/0.1% w/v trichloro-acetic acid (TFA; 80:20 by vol.) and pre-washed with 3 ml 0.1% TFA. After the samples, further acidified by addition of 10 μl formic acid, had been applied to the cartridge, it was washed with 4 ml water and 2 ml 0.1% TFA. Peptides were eluted with 1.6 ml of methanol/0.1% TFA (80:20) into a polypropylene tube containing 30 μl of mercapto-ethanol to prevent ME oxidation.

HPLC was carried out using a Beckman two-pump system, consisting of a 420 controller, the pumps (112) and a Rheodyne 7125 injector. The detector was an LKB Ultrospec with flow cell of path 2.5 mm. The 'TEAP' solvent system comprised solvent A, a 10-fold dilution in water of 0.2 M orthophosphoric acid adjusted to pH 3.0 with triethylamine, and solvent B consisting of the foregoing stock solution diluted 10-fold in acetonitrile. The 'TFA' system comprised solvents A and B consisting respectively of 0.15% v/v TFA in   % v/v   acetonitrile and 0.15% TFA in 70% acetonitrile. Solvents were degassed by vacuum filtration (0.22 μm nylon filter) prior to use.

Acetonitrile (HPLC Grade 'S') and water were purchased from Rathburn Chemicals Ltd. (Walkerburn, Scotland). Other chemical reagents were the best available (Analar or Aristar) from BDH Chemicals Ltd. The HPLC columns were μ-Bondapak C-18 silica (300 × i.d. 4.0 mm; HPLC Technology Ltd.) and Partisil-5 C-8 silica (100 mm, i.d. 9.8 or 4.0 mm; Whatman). Biochemical reagents such as thimerosal and bovine serum albumin (BSA) were from Sigma Chemical Co. Anti-BE antiserum, ^{125}I-BE and Na^{125}I were from Amersham International, and BE from Cambridge Research Biochemicals. LPH was generously given by both Dr. D.G. Smyth and Dr. B.M. Austen.

RESULTS

Our primary concern in seeking to solve the problems listed above has been to increase the assay sensitivity. This has been achieved by development of superior Ab's (see below) and by improving the assay techniques. This has been done by (i) using purified Ab's obtained by affinity purification techniques; (ii) ensuring that

Table 1. Cross-reactivities of two Ab preparations [4] with various peptides and opiates.*   Any   unnamed   residue is as in first entry.

Peptide	%, Ab 614	%, Ab 629
H-**Tyr—Gly—Gly—Phe—Leu**	(100.0)	(100.0)
————————————————Met	30.0	35.0
Lys———————————————	0.046	
D–Asp———————————————	<0.001	0.0013
Arg————————————Met	0.74	
Boc———————————————	<0.001	
H–Tyr(SO₃H)—————————————	100.0	
——D–Ala ——— ———	49.6	
————— β–Ala————Nle	0.001	0.05
————————D–Ala————Nle	<0.001	
———————————————Nle	100.0	100.0
————————————Leu–NH₂	7.7	21.0
——————————————————Arg	0.64	1.0
H–Gly—Gly—Phe— Leu	0.0003	0.0
H–Tyr—Gly—Gly—Phe–OH	0.026	
α–endorphin	0.0	
BE	0.001	0.21
γ–endorphin	0.0	
morphine	0.0	

* Boc (on left) = t–butyl–oxycarbonyl protecting group; H = hydrogen.

care was taken over the glassware and plasticware used in the assays (e.g. polystyrene tubes should not be used for collecting HPLC fractions containing acetonitrile, hence we used polypropylene tubes; any glass tubes should be silanized);   (iii) employing a centrifugal Sephadex G-50 assay for BE, providing better quality assays [3].

We have also increased the specificity of the assays by improving our Ab's, developing the use of monoclonal Ab's (MAb's), and using HPLC to separate peptides in the first instance.

Antibody development

In order to improve our enkephalin assays, we developed new methodology for preparing peptide-hapten conjugates [4].   Fig. 3 shows the method used to synthetize an enkephalin-BSA antigen that would theoretically give better specificity and allow us to perform enkephalin assay in the presence of extended peptides.   That this was achieved can be seen from Table 1, where cross-reactivities of the two Ab's produced are listed.   Note that LE and the sulphated LE cross-react 100%, indicating that iodination of the peptide to serve as a tracer for the RIA procedure will not affect the assay adversely. Note also that ME cross-reacts by 50% in the assay, while C-terminally extended peptides cross-react to only a slight extent.   Fig. 4 shows

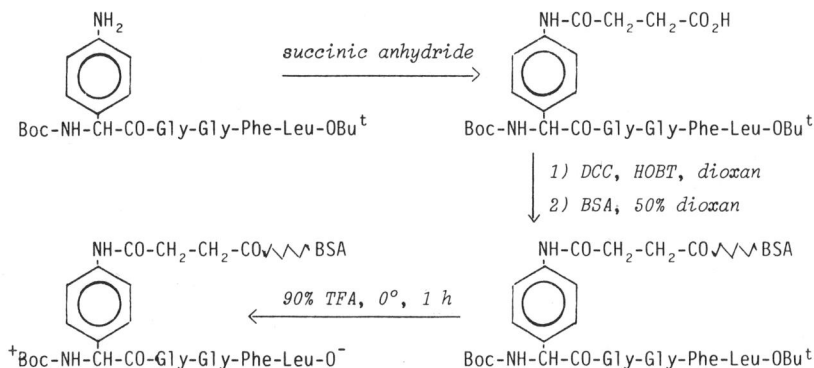

Fig. 3. Reaction scheme for the preparation of hapten-conjugated enkephalin to use in producing specific anti-enkephalin Ab's. The protected tyrosyl-amine derivative of [Leu]-enkephalin was succinylated, and the product coupled to BSA using the carbodiimide (DCC) method. The product was then de-protected with TFA and used as an immunogen in rabbits.

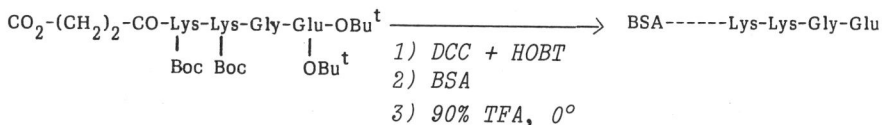

Fig. 4. Reaction scheme for the preparation of hapten-conjugated MPF [defined in text] to use in producing Ab's. Succinylated, fully protected MPF is coupled to BSA using carbodiimide. The reaction product is de-protected with TFA and used in rabbits as an immunogen.

a similar methodology used for the generation of Ab's against MPF, viz. Lys-Lys-Gly-Glu, the C-terminal tetrapeptide of BE and LPH, which we expect to cross-react with MPF, LPH and BE. The resulting Ab will not, of course, provide us with the specificity necessary to determine BE in the presence of LPH.

HPLC procedure development

In order to achieve specificity in the BE/LPH assay we used HPLC. This was also intended to overcome the problem that even if the cross-reactivity of a contaminating peptide is very low with a given Ab, there is an element of uncertainty in the final assay, since there may be a very high concentration of that peptide present. Our aim was to develop a single system that would separate every peptide of interest to us, allowing fractions to be assayed with

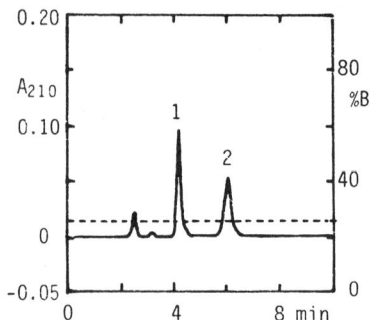

Fig. 5 *(left).* HPLC profile of ME (peak 1) and LE (peak 2) under isocratic conditions using system TEAP (---, % of solvent B pumped). Partisil column i.d. 4 mm; 0.5 ml/min flow-rate; 0.5 μg each of ME and LE loaded.

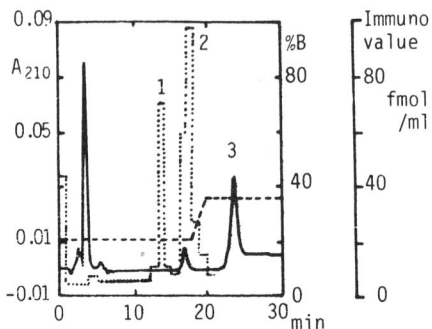

Fig. 6 *(right).* Typical HPLC profile for CSF with system TEAP (---, % of solvent B pumped), with Partisil column of 9.8 mm i.d. and C-18 pellicular guard column, 50 × 2 mm; 2 ml/min flow-rate. Loaded, in starting solvent: 1 ml (= 1 ml CSF; for added marker, see text) of material extracted by the Sep-Pak procedure. Peaks: no. 1, ME; 2, LE; 3, BE and LPH; ·····, enkephalin immunoreactivity.

the appropriate Ab. Such a system should ideally provide sharp peptide peaks, preferably in a volatile solvent system so that the solvent could be evaporated to dryness to permit RIA directly.

Several publications on methodology [5, 6] claim to separate BE from LPH but none provided an adequate separation in our hands. We adopted system TEAP to separate ME and LE in an isocratic elution (Fig. 5). Increasing the acetonitrile concentration late in the run (solvent B input raised to 35%; Fig. 6) allowed a fraction containing BE and LPH (peak 3) to be collected which was further separated using system TFA as considered below. Whereas Fig. 5 was a run with authentic compounds, a CSF sample was used for the run in Fig. 6, and enkephalin immunoreactivity was monitored. Fig. 7 shows the profile for a CSF extract spiked with BE and chromatographed as for the enkephalin separation with, till late in the run, 20% input of solvent B. Note in Fig. 6 that despite the extremely low cross-reactivity of the internal marker used in the RIA ([β-Ala^3-N-Leu^5]-enkephalin; cross-reactivity <0.001%), the assay still shows a very

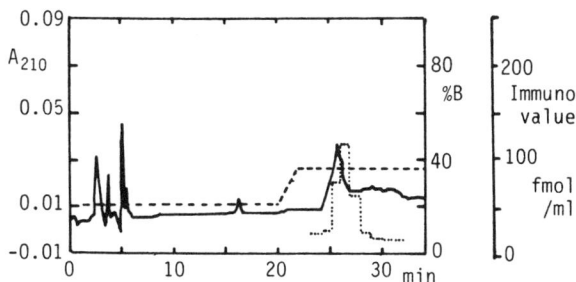

Fig. 7. HPLC profile of 'CSF', as in Fig. 6 (⋯⋯, BE immunoreactivity), but cartridge early eluate (no peptides) spiked with BE to give on-column load of 300 fmol.

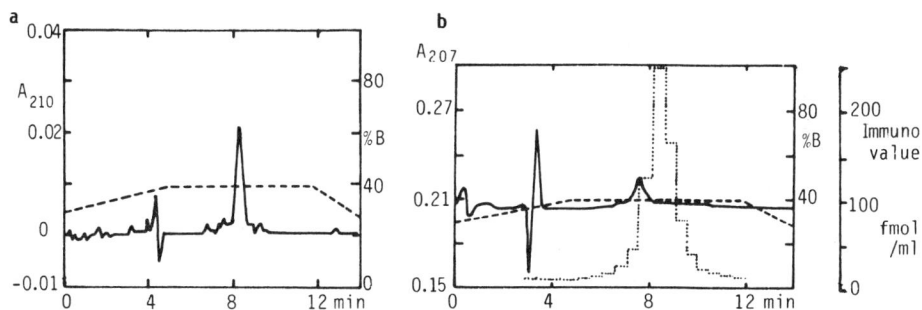

Fig. 8. HPLC of BE using system TFA: **a**, 2.5 μg BE in 5 μl water injected; **b**, as for **a** but with the RIA profile superimposed. Column: μ-Bondapak, with a C-18 pellicular guard column; 1 ml/min. (The dip-&-peak at ~4 min is 'solvent front'. For **a** *vs.* **b**, see text comment.)

large peak corresponding to the standard, since its concentration is so high. This is a good illustration of the problems that can be encountered with RIA.

System TFA was optimized by investigating the retention times of BE and LPH over the ranges 0.05–0.1% for TFA and 20–50% for acetonitrile. Fig. 8 shows elution results for BE and, in **b**, the RIA profile. The UV peak is broader than might be desired; but the column was overloaded due to the high amount of BE needed to allow UV detection. Elution of LPH is shown in Fig. 9: there is an effective separation of BE from LPH, which ran 3 min apart. Note that the LPH peak could be detected only by RIA, there being insufficient peptide to see on the 210 nm trace. (The runs shown in Figs. 8b and 9 were performed with the same column, different from that for Fig. 8a.)

Fig. 9. HPLC of LPH using
system TFA; 0.3 μg of LPH
in 100 μl solvent injected.
HPLC performed as in Fig. 8
legend; ······, LPH immunoreactivity.

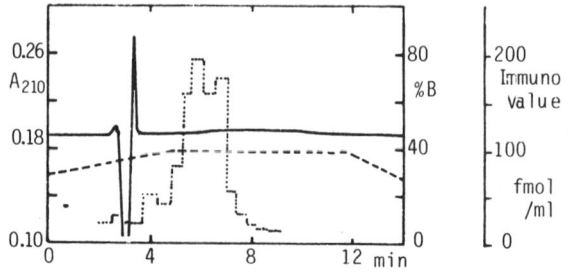

Fig. 10. Typical HPLC
profile with system TFA
of BE/LPH CSF fractions
previously separated with
system TEAP (legend to
Fig. 6; 1 ml CSF, Sep-Pak-
extracted). Peptide frac-
tions eluted 1 min after
the increase of solvent B
to 35% were dried, redissolved in 0.5 ml system TFA
solvent, and run as in Fig. 8
(······, BE immunoreactivity).

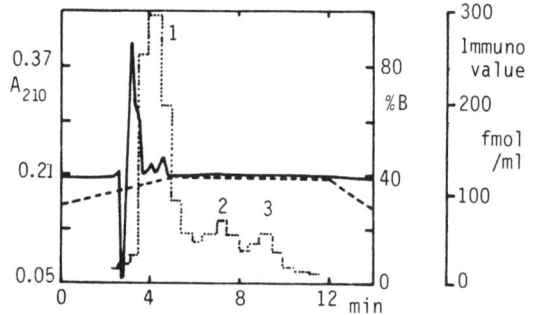

Applicability to patients

In combination, these two HPLC systems and the RIA methods using
Ab's developed as outlined above provide an effective assay system
for CSF peptides involved in the pain perception/modulation pathways.

Fig. 10 shows typical HPLC and RIA profiles, obtained with
system TFA after initial separation with system TEAP, for BE and LPH
in CSF from patients. The RIA profile shows 3 distinct peaks.
Peaks **2** and **3** correspond to LPH and BE. The large early peak
(**1**), which is at present unidentified, is not an artefact of the assay
system, since blank or standard runs do not show this peak. We have
tentatively identified it as POMC, the precursor of the BE/LPH
system, which would be expected to cross-react with the commercial
anti-BE Ab we have used.

Table 2 shows results obtained from 3 patients for LE, ME, BE
and LPH using these HPLC and RIA systems. Patients A and B underwent
treatment for severe cancer pain, which involved treatment of the
pituitary with alcohol. In patient C, with congenital analgesia (no
pain can be felt), there were no detectable enkephalins but a
high BE concentration. The alcohol injections had little or no
effect on enkephalin concentrations in the pain patients, while BE
and LPH concentrations both increased significantly. The 'POMC'

Table 2. Peptides in CSF from patients, as pmol/l. Conentrations were determined by a combination of two HPLC separations and RIA, to achieve sensitivity and specificity (see text). ud = undetectable.

Condition	Patient	ME	LE	BE	LPH
Before/after pituitary alcohol ablation	A	*0.5/22*	*61/64*	*ud/102*	*ud/104*
	B	*2/ud*	*59/64*	*10/188*	*34/428*
Congenital analgesia	C	ud	ud	200	20

concentrations (not shown) also increased, 60-fold in patient B. This may indicate that the operative procedure causes a release, or stimulation of synthesis, of POMC, causing in turn an elevation of LPH and BE concentrations. This flood of potent peptide into the CSF could explain the relief of pain experienced by these patients.

It should be noted that when sufficient CSF is available it is not necessary to combine the HPLC runs sequentially, and it may be preferable to use the two methods in parallel. This implies less sample handling with a lower risk of analyte loss.

Acknowledgements

R.F.V. was supported by the Medical Research Council (Grant no. G8311298N). We thank Turners of Liverpool, Merck Sharpe & Dohme, and Parke-Davies for their support, Drs. D.G. Smyth and B. Austen for their generous gifts of LPH, and Mr. D. Miles for technical assistance.

References

1. Tsubokawa, T., Yamamoto, T., Katayama, Y., Hirayama, T. & Sibuya, H. (1984) *Pain 18*, 115-126.
2. Cahill, C.A., Matthews, J.D. & Akil, H. (1983) *J. Clin. Endocrinol. Metab. 56*, 992-997.
3. Glasel, J.A., Bradbury, W.M. & Venn, R.F. (1983) *J. Immunol. Meths. 63*, 291-298.
4. Morley, J.S., Capper, S.J. & Miles, J.B. (1984) *Neuropeptides 4*, 477-482.
5. Seidah, N.G., Routhier, R., Benjannet, S., Larivière, N., Gossard, F. & Chrétien, M. (1980) *J. Chromatog. 193*, 291-299.
6. Bennett, H.J.P., Browne, C.A. & Solomon, S. (1981) *Biochemistry 20*, 4530-4538.

#A-7

THE IMPORTANCE OF DEFINED TRACERS IN RIA

K.G. McFarthing, M.R. Harris, A. Smith, R.J. Pither,
D. Silver, A.L. Hamilton, *D.G. Smyth and R.H. Jackson

Amersham International plc   *National Institute for
White Lion Road   Medical Research
Amersham, Bucks. HP7 9LL   The Ridgeway, Mill Hill
U.K.   London NW7 1AA, U.K.

*The radio-iodination of a peptide often leads to the production
of heterogeneous mixtures due to monoiodination at different residues,
iodination at more than one residue, di-iodination at single residues,
peptide damage (e.g. methionine oxidation), and the presence of underivatized peptide. Such mixtures often show chemical and radiochemical
variations between preparations, and sub-optimal sensitivity in RIA.
Regulatory peptides are often present in body tissues and fluids at
very low concentrations and in different forms, such that very sensitive
and specific assays are needed. These assays can be improved by the
use of defined tracers, the use of which is now described for a range
of iodinated peptides purified by RP-HPLC. These include human α-ANP®,
insulin, VIP, glucagon, β-endorphin, neurotensin, GRF, ACTH and
IGF-1. RP-HPLC can produce carrier-free labelled peptides which are
mono-iodinated at specific residues, leading to improved and consistent
performance in RIA's and RRA's.*

[125]-I is widely used in RIA and RRA. Many direct and indirect techniques are employed to attach it to peptides and proteins. Direct
methods usually depend on oxidation of I^- to I^+-type species by chloramine-T [1], lactoperoxidase and H_2O_2 or Iodogen† to produce electrophilic
attack at tyrosine and histidine residues. Indirect methods use conjugates such as the Bolton & Hunter reagent to attach radioactive
iodine-containing moieties to the amino groups of lysine or N-terminal
residues [2].

†® Pierce Chemical Co. ® α-ANP, α-atrial natriuretic peptide; GRF,
growth hormone-releasing factor; IGF, insulin-like growth factor;
VIP, vasoactive intestinal peptide; *see text for* CGRP, RCP; RRA,
radioreceptor (receptor-binding) assay; Ab, antibody; BSA, bovine
serum albumin; RP, reverse-phase; PMSF, phenylmethylsulphonyl fluoride.

Table 1. Purification of ^{125}I-peptides: efficiency of removal of unwanted substances by different techniques.

Technique (& time needed)	^{125}I-Iodide	Oxidized peptide	Unreacted peptide	Di- & multi-iodinated peptide	Aggregated peptide	Lacto-peroxidase	Mono-iodinated isomers
Gel filtration (1-24 h)	√	×	×	×	×	×	×
Ion exchange (1-24 h)	√	×	√	√	?	√	×
RP-HPLC (1-2 h)	√	√	√	√	√	√	√

Peptides often contain more than one amino acid that can be iodinated. This can lead to heterogeneity caused by iodination at different loci on the same residue or at loci in different residues. Even preparations of peptides iodinated at a single residue can be heterogeneous due to di-iodination and the presence of underivatized peptide. In addition chemical modification can occur, most often through the oxidation of methionine to methionine sulphoxide by chloramine-T. Fig. 1 shows a model peptide which contains two tyrosines and one methionine, as is the case with β-endorphin, VIP, glucagon and GRF. In this example there are potentially 17 products of the iodination. In practice, conditions can be adjusted to minimize the formation of multi-iodinated peptides, but in the case of β-endorphin, VIP, glucagon and GRF mono-iodination occurs in approximately equal proportions at each tyrosine residue (K.G. McFarthing et al., unpublished observations).

For both RIA's and RRA's a mono-iodinated peptide is the preferred tracer since it gives the minimum possible alterations to the peptide structure and since the avoidance of multi-iodinated peptides minimizes the formation during storage of labelled peptide fragments which can interfere in assays [3]. Several methods are commonly used to separate mono-iodinated peptide from other products of the iodination reaction. Table 1 summarizes three methods that are now considered.

Separation by molecular size using gel filtration removes products of small molecular size such as chloramine-T and [^{125}I]iodide, but mono-iodinated peptides co-chromatograph with unlabelled, di- and multi-iodinated peptides. Ion-exchange, which separates on the basis of charge, is potentially capable of removing unlabelled, di- and multi-iodinated peptides in addition to non-peptide reactants, but is unable to separate mono-iodinated species. However, RP-HPLC can

Fig. 1. Theoretical possibilities for pro- ducts from the iodination of a peptide containing two tyrosines and one methionine.

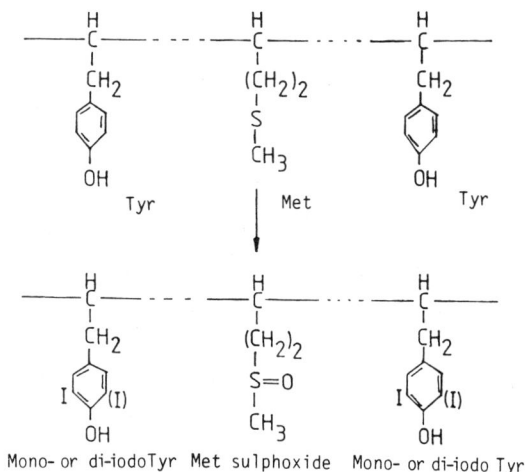

be used to separate peptides mono-iodinated at specific residues from all other products of the reaction, giving a carrier-free tracer of maximum specific activity (as below).

This article describes several examples of purified ^{125}I-labelled peptides, which are mono-iodinated at specific residues, and illus- trates the advantages that these tracers can give in both RIA's and RRA's.

HPLC

The iodination of a peptide with more than one possible position of labelling will normally give a mixture of products, one of which will be preferred as the tracer for an RIA or RRA. In order to select the optimum tracer we have used the resolving power of RP-HPLC. This technique has enabled the purification of mono-iodinated, speci- fically labelled peptides at specific radioactivities of ~74 TBq/mmol (~2000 Ci/mmol). Fig. 2 shows an example of the RP-HPLC purification of mono-iodinated isomers of human insulin. The mobile phase consisted of 0.2 M ammonium acetate, pH 5.5, containing 27% (v/v) acetonitrile, based on the method of Frank & co-workers [4]. Evidently this system was capable of separating unlabelled insulin, unreacted [125I]iodide and auto-iodinated lactoperoxidase in addition to the four mono- iodinated isomers of insulin labelled at tyrosine residues A14, A19, B16 and B26. Studies on insulin receptors using these peptides showed that the A14 and B26 isomers were particularly useful for assisting in the characterization of insulin receptors from different tissues [4]. These two isomers were further assessed for their suitability in RIA.

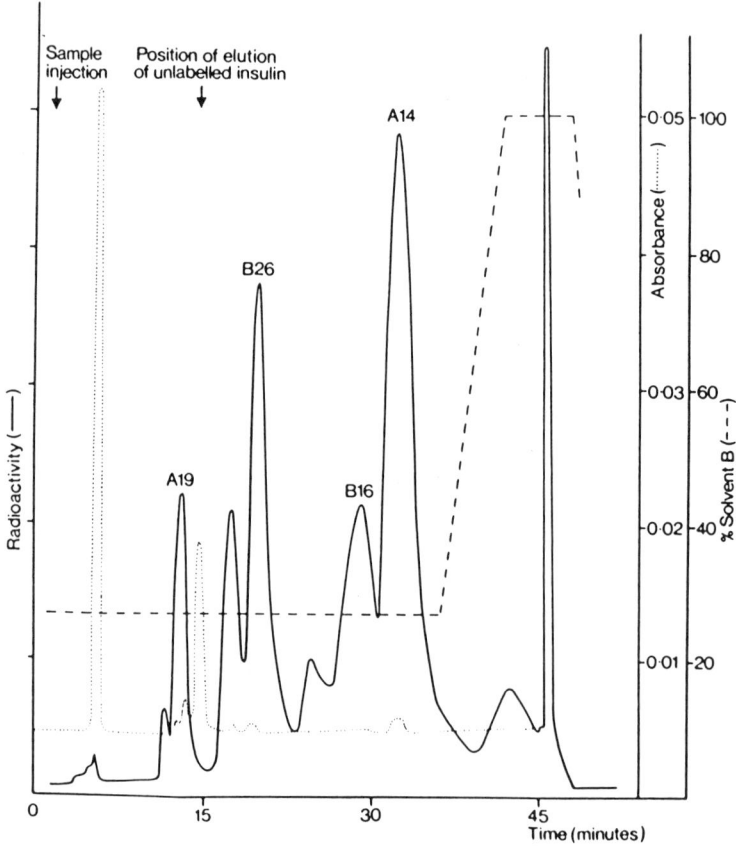

Fig. 2. RP-HPLC of the iodination reaction mixture of human insulin (details in text; lactoperoxidase used for iodination).

RIA

Fig. 3 shows the standard curves obtained using ^{125}I-(TyrA14) and ^{125}I-(TyrB26) human insulin in RIA with an antiserum raised in guinea pig to porcine insulin. Recombinant human insulin (Eli Lilly) was used as standard. The incubation buffer was 50 mM Na phosphate, pH 7.4, containing 10 mM EDTA and 0.25% (w/v) BSA. After incubation at 4° for 24 h, Ab-bound tracer was separated from free tracer using dextran-coated charcoal. The (TyrA14)-labelled insulin gave a higher zero standard binding than a similar mass of the (TyrB26) form (Fig. 3).

Fig. 4 shows the result of using three different ^{125}I-glucagon tracers in RIA with a C-terminally directed rabbit antiserum, porcine glucagon being used as standard. The two tracers purified by RP-HPLC gave standard curves which were virtually indistinguishable. However, the ^{125}I-glucagon purified by ion-exchange chromatography gave a

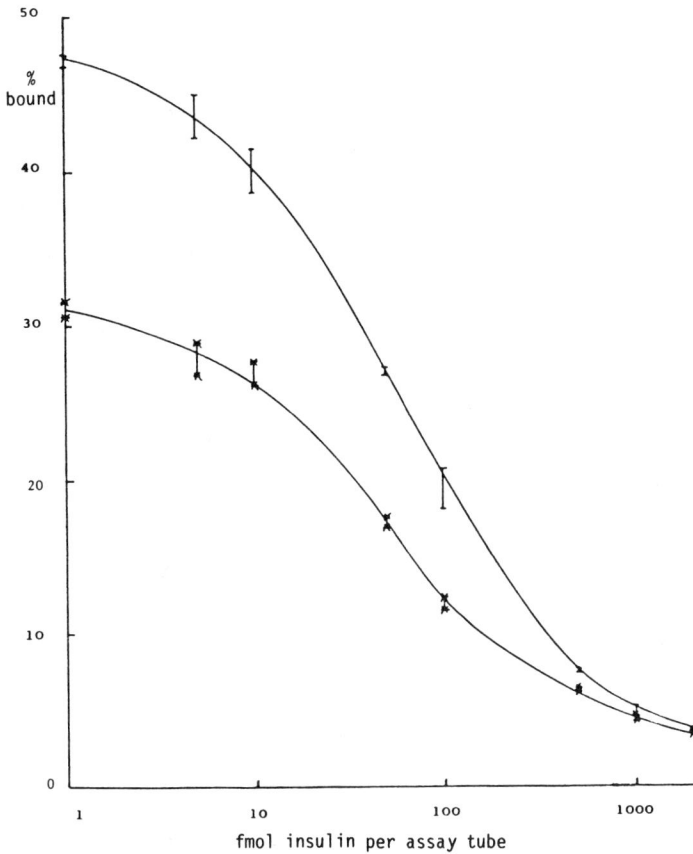

Fig. 3. RIA of ^{125}I-(TyrA14) insulin and ^{125}I-(TyrB26) insulin (details in text).

poor standard curve with much lower sensitivity. Glucagon contains a methionine residue near to the C-terminus, and this was present intact (not oxidized) in the HPLC-purified tracers.   However, the tracer purified by ion-exchange had an oxidized methionine-27. The results suggest that the antiserum had a higher affinity for glucagon containing a native as compared with an oxidized methionine residue.

RP-HPLC of human α-ANP gave four major peaks (1-4).   Each was examined for its suitability as the tracer in RIA using a rabbit antiserum raised against human α-ANP covalently conjugated to BSA, with procedures similar to those described above for insulin.   As shown in Fig. 5, peaks 1-3 gave good displacement of unlabelled human α-ANP, evidenced by satisfactory dose-response curves, whereas peak 4 gave no dose-response curve. Immunoreactivity was highest for peaks 1 and 3.   In the legend to Fig. 5 are shown the identities established for the peaks (M.R. Harris et al., unpublished observations).

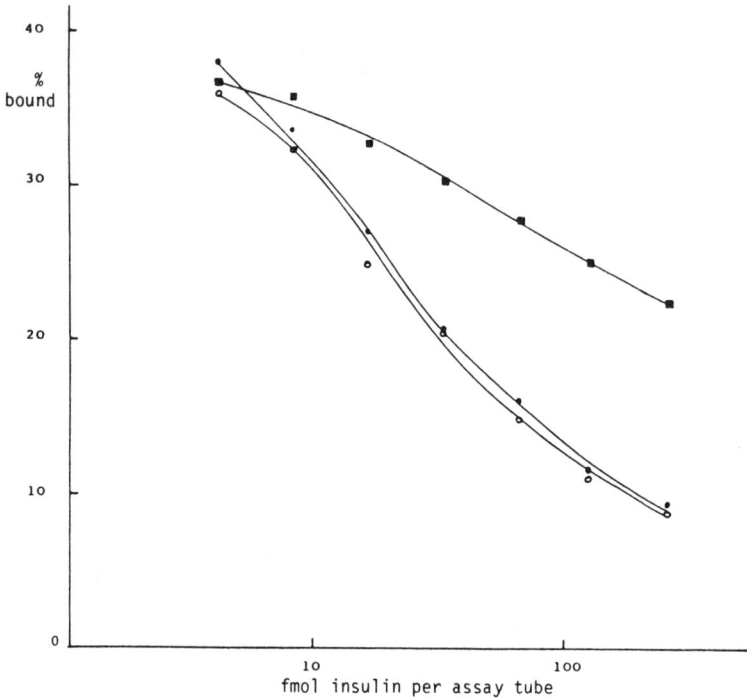

Fig. 4. RIA of glucagon using ^{125}I-glucagon purified by RP-HPLC
- giving ^{125}I-(Tyr13) glucagon, ● and ^{125}I-(Tyr10) glucagon, o-
or by ion-exchange chromatography, ■. [*Risk of typographical confusion; e.g.* Tyr13 = Tyr^{13}, *(in text)* Tyr1 = Tyr^1. - *Ed.*]

RRA

Iodine-125 offers several advantages over tritium in receptor-
binding assays, most notably higher specific activity and ease of
counting. However, as a large atom, iodine introduced into a peptide
sequence gives an unnatural biological structure. Thus ^{125}I-labelled
peptides to be used to study binding sites need to be highly defined,
and if possible the substitution of iodine-125 should be at a residue
not directly involved in the interaction with the receptor. We
have applied these criteria to several peptides that contain two
or more tyrosines - VIP [5], glucagon, β-endorphin, neurotensin,
insulin, IGF-I, GRF and ACTH. Taking β-endorphin as an example,
we illustrate the principle further.

Human β-endorphin contains two tyrosine residues, at positions
1 and 27. Tyrosine-1 is essential for binding to the opiate receptor.
The inhibition of binding of both ^{125}I-(Tyr1) β-endorphin and ^{125}I-
(Tyr27) β-endorphin by unlabelled β-endorphin to rat-brain cortex

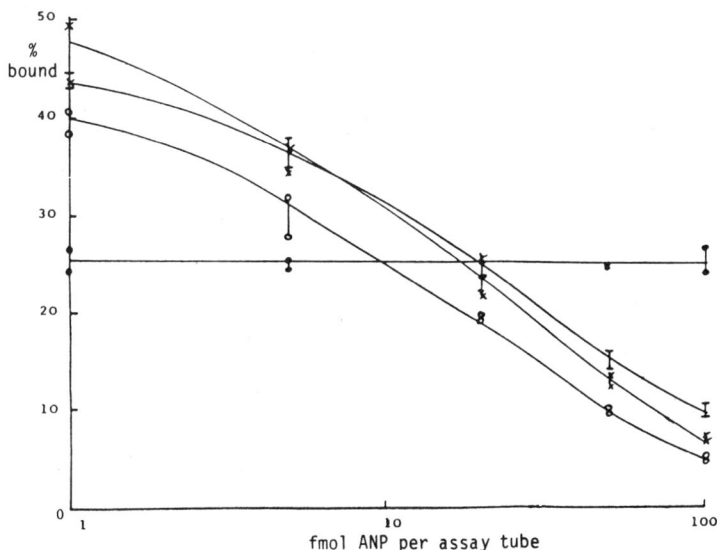

Fig. 5. RIA of 4 radioactive peaks from the RP-HPLC purification of ^{125}I-human α-ANP (details in text). Identifications: peak 1, *no symbol*: mono-iodinated oxidized ^{125}I-α-ANP; peak 2, o: di-iodinated oxidized ^{125}I-α-ANP; peak 3, x: mono-iodinated ^{125}-I-α-ANP; peak 4, •: iodinated lactoperoxidase. [Throughout, 'α-ANP' = hα-ANP, i.e. human.- *Ed.'s excision.*]

membranes was studied as follows. Membranes (1 mg protein) and labelled β-endorphin (10 fmol, 3×10^4 cpm; 4.4×10^4 dpm) were incubated at 30° for 90 min in 1.0 ml of 20 mM HEPES, pH 7.6, containing $MgSO_4$ (3 mM), PMSF (0.1% w/v), and (all 0.005%) aprotinin, bacitracin, chymostatin, pepstatin, leupeptin and antipain. The binding reaction was terminated by centrifugation for 5 min in a Beckman Microfuge and rinsing of the pellet in 50 mM Na phosphate pH 7.4 containing 0.1 M NaCl.

Under these conditions the apparent affinity of the specific binding site for ^{125}I-(Tyr1)[⊗] β-endorphin was ~10 times lower than that for ^{125}I-(Tyr27) β-endorphin ($Ka = 3\times10^9$ M^{-1}). The inhibition of binding was further studied using C-terminally shortened forms of β-endorphin (Fig. 6). This demonstrated the specificity of the binding site for β-endorphin 1-31. Further experiments showed that non-radioactive ^{127}I-(Tyr27) β-endorphin had a similar IC_{50} displacement to β-endorphin itself, suggesting that the binding site did not distinguish between the two [6].

⊗ 'Tyr1' could advantageously have been rendered as 'Tyr$^{1'}$'.- *Ed.*

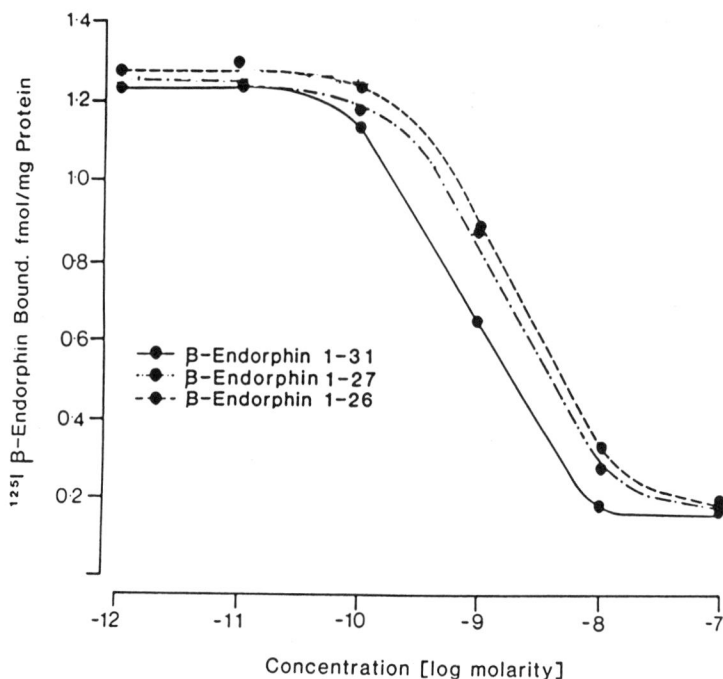

Fig. 6. The binding of ^{125}I-(Tyr27) β-endorphin to specific sites in rat brain cortex membranes, and inhibition of binding by C-terminally shortened forms of β-endorphin (details in text).

STABILITY

Once a defined ^{125}I-tracer has been prepared, it is important to extend the useful life of that tracer for as long as possible. We have studied several aspects of the long-term (up to 8 weeks) storage of ^{125}I-labelled peptides, and we describe some features of these studies using ^{125}I-calcitonin gene-related peptide (CGRP) as an example.

The storage conditions can have profound effects on the stability of an iodinated peptide. Table 2 shows the radiochemical purity (RCP) of ^{125}I-CGRP after 4 and 8 weeks' storage under three different conditions: lyophilized at +4°; in solution at +4°; in solution at -20°. Evidently degradation in terms of RCP as measured by analytical RP-HPLC is minimal when ^{125}I-CGRP is stored lyophilized at +4° or frozen at -20°. However, storage in solution at +4° leads to considerable degradation and consequently poor performance in RIA. In our hands, ^{125}I-peptides are consistently more stable when stored lyophilized.

Table 2. Stability of ^{125}I-CGRP on storage (± S.D.).

Condition	RCP after 4 weeks, %	RCP after 8 weeks, %
Lyophilized, at +4°	97.5 ±0.5	94.5 ±0.5
In aqueous solution at +4°	61.0 ±1.0	37.0 ±3.0
In aqueous solution at -20°	95.5 ±1.5	95.5 ±0.5
Starting RCP = 98.0 ±0		

DISCUSSION

We have drawn attention above to some of the potential advantages to be gained in RIA's and RRA's by using ^{125}I peptides which are homogeneous, stable and mono-iodinated at specific residues. Our results with different isomers of labelled human insulin clearly show that the position of labelling can significantly affect basal binding (zero standard), apparently by altering the affinity of the antiserum for the label. Improvements in assay performance may therefore be gained by selecting the labelled isomer with the highest apparent affinity.

Observations with ^{125}I-(Tyr27) β-endorphin demonstrated that this isomer was superior to ^{125}I-(Tyr1) β-endorphin in binding to the specific β-endorphin binding site in rat brain cortex membranes. Indeed, experiments with the non-radioactive ^{127}I-(Tyr27) β-endorphin showed that the receptor seemed not to distinguish the peptide labelled at Tyr27 from unlabelled β-endorphin 1-31. Heterogeneous preparations of labelled peptide can give multiphasic Scatchard plots arising from the same receptor having different affinities for the individual components of the mixture; this could readily, but erroneously, be interpreted as multiple populations of receptor. The use of homogeneous defined tracers can avoid this confusion. Altogether our results show that there are major advantages in using well-defined peptides, ^{125}I-labelled at specific residues, in assays for peptide receptors.

Methionine residues are often present in the receptor-binding regions of peptides, and oxidation of these residues can lead to a loss of receptor-binding activity [7]. Reduced immunoreactivity may also result from oxidation, exemplified above for oxidized ^{125}I-glucagon. Such effects depend, of course, on the particular Ab used, as evident from the apparently identical performance of oxidized and non-oxidized ^{125}I-α-ANP tracers in the assay of human α-ANP. It was also demonstrated that di-iodination of tyrosine residues can lead to reduced immunoreactivity which, coupled with stability problems, makes it essential to remove di-iodo peptides from the tracer preparation.

References

1. Greenwood, F.C., Hunter, W.M. & Glover, J.S. (1963) *Biochem. J.*
    89, 114-123.
2. Bolton, A.E. & Hunter, W.M. (1973) *Biochem. J. 133*, 529-538.
3. Schmidt, J. (1984) *J. Biol. Chem. 259*, 1160-1116.
4. Frank, B.H., Beckage, M.J. & Willey, K.A. (1983) *J. Chromatog.*
    266, 239-248.
5. Marie, J-C., Hui Bon Hoa, D., Jackson, R.H., Hejblum, G. &
    Rosselin, G. (1985) *Regul. Peptides 12*, 113-123.
6. Toogood, C.I.A., McFarthing, K.G., Hulme, E.C. & Smyth, D.G.
    (1986) *Neuroendocrinol.*, in press.
7. Mantyh, P.W., Hunt, S.P. & Maggio, J.E. (1984) *Brain Res. 307*,
    147-165.

#A-8

THE USE OF RADIOIMMUNOASSAYS FOR CRYPTIC REGIONS OF PEPTIDE PRECURSORS, IN THE STUDY OF BIOSYNTHETIC MECHANISMS

R. Dimaline[‡], H. Desmond, A-C. Jonsson[*], S. Pauwels[†],
H. Raybould, A. Varro, L. Vowles and G.J. Dockray

MRC Secretory Control Group
Physiological Laboratory
University of Liverpool
Brownlow Hill, P.O. Box 147
Liverpool L69 3BX, U.K.

Elucidation of gene sequences encoding peptide hormones and neurotransmitters has allowed prediction of the primary amino acid sequences of all the peptides that are likely to be produced by biosynthetic processing of the precursors for these substances. Thus, in addition to the known biologically active sequences, the precursors demonstrably contain sequences of peptides ('cryptic peptides') whose identity and function are so far unknown. We have raised Ab's[‡] to all the peptides expected to arise during biosynthesis of progastrin and proVIP, and to the C-terminal flanking peptide of CCK. All the Ab's were produced by immunizing rabbits with small fragments or analogues of the precursor sequences, coupled to carrier protein in such a way as to leave the appropriate sequence free to promote Ab formation. We have used these Ab's. in RIA to identify and characterize some novel peptides produced during gastrin and VIP biosynthesis, and to identify the cellular origins of the peptides by immunohistochemistry. The results have allowed elucidation of biosynthetic pathways and identification of cell-specific processing patterns. For progastrin at least, pathological changes in biosynthetic mechanisms have been identified.

[‡] Author to whom any correspondence should be addressed.
[*] Present address: Dept. of Zoophysiology, University of Göteborg, Box 250 59, S-400 Göteborg, Sweden.
[†] Present address: Centre de Médécine Nucléaire, Medical School, UCL 5480, Ave. Hippocrate 54, B-1200 Brussels, Belgium.
[≠] Abbreviations: Ab, antibody; CCK, cholecystokinin; VIP, vasoactive intestinal peptide; RIA, radioimmunoassay; PHI, peptide having N-terminal His and C-terminal Iln.

Recent advances in molecular biology have led to the elucidation of gene sequences encoding the precursors of various peptide hormones and neurotransmitters. This information allows prediction of the primary amino acid sequences of all the peptides that are likely to be produced by biosynthetic processing of the precursor. However, the precise identity of the peptides produced during biosynthesis needs to be confirmed by their identification and chemical characterization using conventional techniques. This is important, not only to identify sites of cleavage, but also other post-translational modifications, e.g. sulphation, acylation and glycosylation, that may not be predictable from the primary amino acid sequence. Moreover, it seems that the patterns of processing vary between different cells expressing the same gene, so that different biologically active products are found.

We have used information on the gene sequences encoding preprogastrin, preproVIP and preproCCK to study the biosynthesis of these substances. We describe here the experimental approaches that have been used, and discuss some of the problems encountered in these studies.

EXPERIMENTAL APPROACH

It is well established that regulatory peptides are produced first as large precursors that are then cleaved to form the final active products. By analogy with well studied systems such as insulin biosynthesis in the pancreatic β cell, cleavage of precursors may be assumed to occur at pairs of basic residues (or occasionally single basic residues) by two enzymes: a trypsin-like enzyme that cleaves to the C-terminus of basic residues, and a carboxypeptidase B-like enzyme that then removes the C-terminal basic residue [1]. We have sought to raise Ab's that would be expected to react with all of the major predicted products of progastrin and proVIP biosynthesis, and with the C-terminal flanking peptide of proCCK.

The Ab's have been used in immunohistochemistry to identify the cellular origins of the naturally occurring peptides; they have also been used in RIA to (a) identify and quantify these peptides in tissue extracts, (b) monitor their purification preparatory to structural characterization, and (c) study the pathways of metabolism, both in their cells of origin and after release. In addition, a start has been made with the identification of pathological changes in biosynthetic pathways, with particular regard to progastrin.

STRATEGY

The organization of porcine preprogastrin [2] is illustrated in Fig. 1. As with all other secretory peptides, the signal sequence is believed to be rapidly removed. The product, progastrin, contains a 34-residue sequence corresponding to big gastrin (or G34) that is

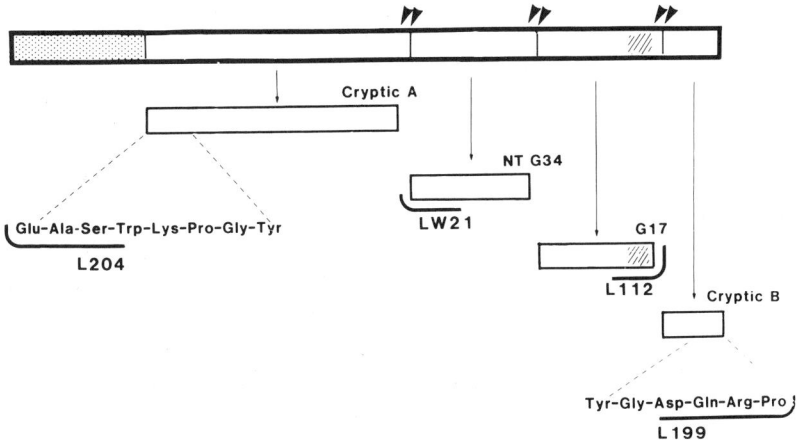

Fig. 1. Organization of porcine preprogastrin. The 34-residue biologically active gastrin sequence (G34) is flanked N-terminally by cryptic A and C-terminally by cryptic B. *Arrows* above the precursor indicate putative cleavage sites (pairs of basic residues); cleavage may occur within G34 to form biologically active G17 and an N-terminal fragment (NTG34). *Indicated schematically* below the appropriate sequences: region specificity of the antisera raised against progastrin. *Stippled area:* signal peptide; *cross-hatching:* the sequence of gastrin required for biological activity.

flanked N- and C-terminally by sequences of 37 and 9 residues, designated cryptic peptides A and B respectively. The latter sequences have no known biological activity, and prior to the present studies their natural occurrence was unknown (hence the name 'cryptic'). The cryptic peptides A and B are connected to G34 by pairs of basic residues; a further pair of basic residues occurs within the sequence of G34, and cleavage here produces the 17-residue form of gastrin (G17) and an N-terminal heptadecapeptide (NT-G34).

Thus in progastrin there is only a single sequence giving rise to material with known biological activity. In contrast, human preproVIP can give rise to two biologically active molecules, PHM and VIP (Fig. 2) [3]. (The name PHM connotes a peptide having N-terminal Histidine and C-terminal Methionine.) PHM is extended N-terminally by a sequence designated cryptic peptide 1; PHM and VIP are separated by a bridging peptide, cryptic peptide 2, and VIP is extended C-terminally by cryptic peptide 3. The PHM sequence is generally regarded as being the human equivalent of porcine PHI, originally discovered, isolated and characterized by Tatemoto & Mutt [4].

ANTIBODY PRODUCTION

In developing Ab's for RIA and immunohistochemistry, the initial choice of antigen is of great importance. Small synthetic peptides

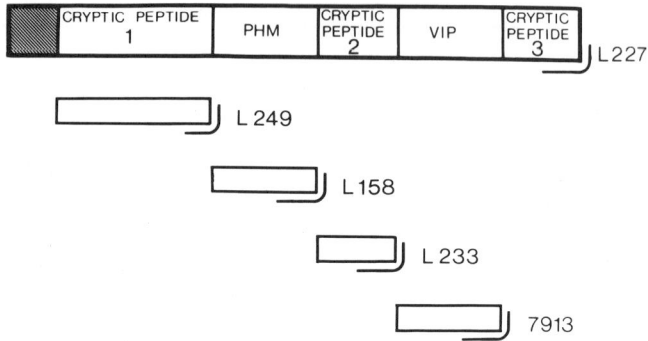

Fig. 2. Organization of human preproVIP. Beyond the signal peptide *(cross-hatched area)* is a sequence of unknown function, designated cryptic peptide 1, followed by the biologically active peptide
PHM (the human counterpart of PHI). A second cryptic peptide
precedes the biologically active VIP, and the precursor terminates
with a third cryptic peptide. *Illustrated schematically* below the
appropriate sequences: the specificities of antisera raised against
the various regions of preproVIP.

conjugated to thyroglobulin have invariably been used. Standard
protocols were used for conjugation, immunization, iodinations and
RIA; the methods have been published in detail for the cryptic or
related peptides [5-7]. In the present context the crucial question
is how to select the appropriate antigen.

Progastrin.- We reasoned that antisera to the C-terminus of
porcine progastrin cryptic peptide B might be of particular interest
and value because they would be expected to react with intact progastrin as well as the cryptic sequence itself. The appropriate Ab's
were obtained by immunizing with Tyr-Gly-Asp-Gln-Arg-Pro, a synthetic
analogue which corresponds to Tyr^{99}-preprogastrin 99-104 conjugated
to carrier protein through its N-terminus by glutaraldehyde. This
would be expected to leave the C-terminus free for Ab formation. The
Tyr residue was substituted to allow radiolabelling, and was positioned
as far as possible from the site expected to react with Ab's (Fig. 1).

To get Ab's to the N-terminus of cryptic peptide A we used the
synthetic analogue Glu-Ala-Ser-Trp-Lys-Pro-Gly-Tyr; triazine conjugation [8] was used in the hope of coupling through the phenolic
function of the C-terminal Tyr and so leaving the N-terminus free
for Ab formation.

Pro-VIP.- Antisera to the cryptic peptides of preproVIP were
raised by immunization with the three synthetic fragments or analogues
illustrated in Fig. 3, coupled by glutaraldehyde to thyroglobulin.
The rationale for selecting these peptides was similar to that descri-

Fig. 3. Amino acid sequences of preproVIP cryptic peptides 1, 2 and 3. In using synthetic fragments or analogues (**BOLD TYPE**) to raise antisera, a Tyr residue was incorporated at the N-terminus of the synthetic peptide and coupled to carrier protein, thus leaving the C-terminus free to promote Ab formation. It is assumed that the basic residues at each peptide's C-terminus have the normal susceptibility to removal by trypsin and carboxypeptidase B-type enzymes.

CRYPTIC PEPTIDE 1 (PreproVIP 22-80)

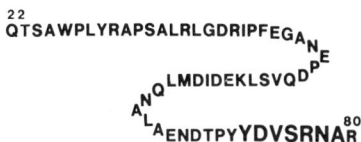

$$^{22}\text{QTSAWPLYRAPSALRLGDRIPFEGA}_{\text{N}}$$

LMDIDEKLSVQD, ANQ, E, P, D

$$_{\text{L}}^{\text{A}}\text{ENDTPY}\underline{\textbf{YDVSRNA}}^{80}_{\text{R}}$$

CRYPTIC PEPTIDE 2 (PreproVIP 111-124)

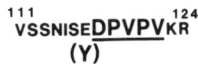

$$^{111}\text{VSSNISE}\underline{\textbf{DPVPV}}\text{KR}^{124}$$
$$\underline{(\textbf{Y})}$$

CRYPTIC PEPTIDE 3 (PreproVIP 156-170)

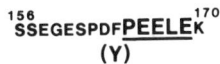

$$^{156}\text{SSEGESPDF}\underline{\textbf{PEELE}}\text{K}^{170}$$
$$\underline{(\textbf{Y})}$$

bed above for the progastrin-derived peptides. The conjoint use of Ab's obtained to the proVIP cryptic peptides and of VIP and PHI antisera already available enabled detection of all the predicted biosynthetic products of proVIP besides the intact precursor itself. ['PHI' connotes PHM too.-*Ed.*] For each cryptic peptide, C-terminal specific Ab's were expected.

ProCCK.- Antisera were raised to the C-terminus of preproCCK by immunization with the synthetic fragment Tyr-Glu-Tyr-Pro-Ser corresponding to rat preproCCK 111-115 (Fig. 4)[9]. As Tyr already occurs in the native sequence it was unnecessary to substitute Tyr for radiolabelling.

SOME PRACTICAL EXPERIENCES

Each of the peptides mentioned above has been successfully used to raise Ab's that are adequate for immunohistochemical or RIA studies. These Ab's have been used together with a range of region-specific Ab's to G17, G34 and VIP that have already been well characterized [6, 7, 10-13]. During the course of these studies, a number of practical issues have emerged that deserve further consideration and are discussed below.

Peptide heterogeneity

RIA's developed using synthetic fragments or analogues do not in themselves provide structural information on the naturally occurring immunoreactive sequences. We routinely use gel filtration, ion-exchange chromatography and reversed-phase HPLC of tissue extracts to provide information on the size, overall charge and hydrophobicity

| Porcine
Preprogastrin | 88
-Gly-Trp-Met-Asp-Phe | Gly-Arg-Arg-<u>Ser-Ala-Glu</u>-Glu-Gly-Asp-Gln-Arg-Pro | 82 |

(Figure boxed region)

Porcine Preprogastrin
88
-Gly-Trp-Met-Asp-Phe⎤Gly-Arg-Arg-<u>Ser-Ala-Glu</u>-Glu-Gly-Asp-Gln-Arg-Pro   82

Human Preprogastrin
88
-Gly-Trp-Met-Asp-Phe⎤Gly-Arg-Arg-<u>Ser-Ala-Glu</u>-Asp-Glu-Asn   100

Rat Prepro C C K
99
-Gly-Trp-Met-Asp-Phe⎤Gly-Arg-Arg-<u>Ser-Ala-Glu</u>-Asp-Tyr-Glu-Tyr-Glu-Tyr-Pro-Ser   110

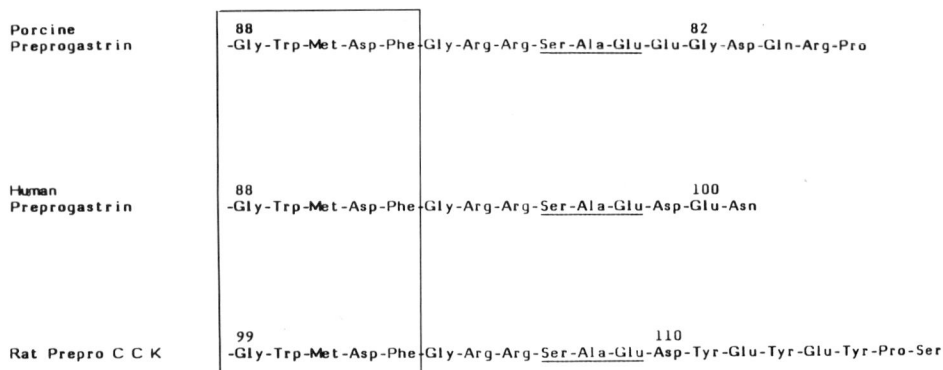

Fig. 4. Amino acid sequences of the C-terminal regions of human
and porcine preprogastrin and rat preproCCK. *Boxed:* C-terminal
pentapeptide common to gastrin and CCK, followed by Gly providing
the C-terminal amide group of the biologically active peptides.
The cryptic B regions of CCK and gastrin are similar only in the
shared sequence Ser-Ala-Glu *(underlined)*. The differences between
preprogastrin and preproCCK at the extreme C-terminus can be
exploited to raise antisera that will distinguish between gastrin-
containing and CCK-containing cells.

of any novel peptide detected.   Clearly, however, isolation and
full characterization of the naturally occurring   immunoreactive
material is an early requirement.

   This point is exemplified by our work on cryptic peptide B of
porcine progastrin.   Using antiserum L199 raised to the synthetic
analogue Tyr[99]-porcine preprogastrin 99-104, parallel dilution curves
were obtained with standard peptide and with extracts made from hog
antral mucosa by boiling with water (Fig. 5).   Moreover, the concentrations of cryptic B-like and (biologically active) gastrin-like
immunoreactivities were virtually identical, consistent with the idea
that in hog antral mucosa there is virtually complete cleavage of the
gastrin precursor at the appropriate point.

   However, when hog antral extracts were subjected to ion-exchange
chromatography or RP-HPLC there were two peaks of cryptic B immunoreactivity that were not separated by gel filtration and are therefore of
similar molecular size (Fig. 6) [5].   Both peaks have been purified
to homogeneity and sequenced by Dr. H. Gregory (ICI Pharmaceuticals),
whose unpublished results point in both cases to the primary amino acid
sequence Ser-Ala-Glu-Glu-Gly-Asp-Gln-Arg-Pro; these peptides are thus
the result of tryptic cleavage of preprogastrin between residues
95 and 96 (Fig. 4).   The reason for the different chromatographic
properties of the two forms is unclear; conceivably one may be generated
from the other as an artifact during isolation.   Alternatively there

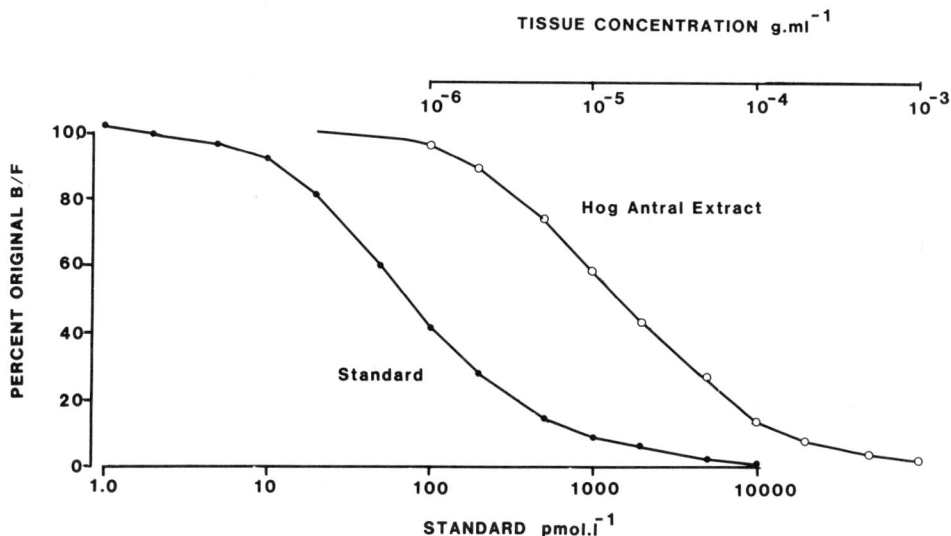

Fig. 5. Inhibition of binding of radiolabelled synthetic Tyr[99]-porcine preprogastrin 99-104, to cryptic B antiserum L199 (see Fig. 1) by standard synthetic hexapeptide and by extracts of porcine antral mucosa. *From Desmond et al. [5], by permission.*

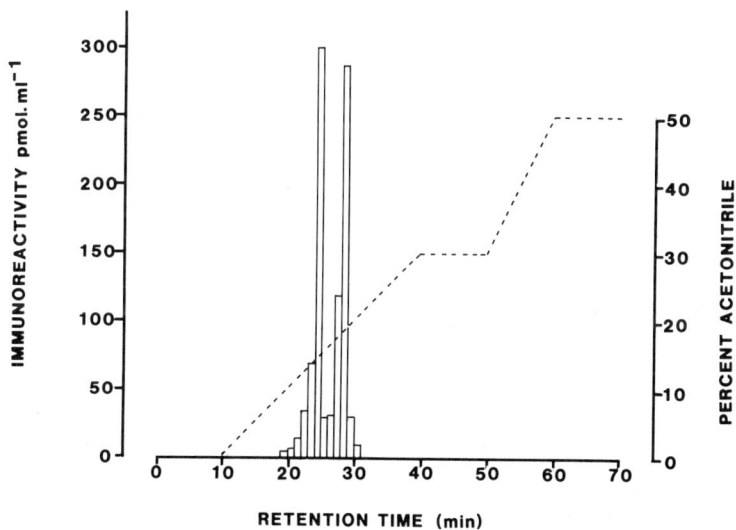

Fig. 6. HPLC elution profiles of purified extracts of hog antral mucosa. Techsil 5 μm C-18 column, 250×4.5 mm i.d.. equilibrated with 0.05% TFA; gradient *(broken line)* to 50% acetonitrile, 1 ml/min. Immunoreactivity in the eluate was estimated using antiserum L199 (see Fig. 1) and the synthetic standard Tyr[99]-porcine preprograstrin 99-104. *Acknowledgement as for Fig. 5.*

might be a post-translational modification of one of the forms. In any event, this finding illustrates the importance of characterization of natural material in the validation of this type of assay. It is also evident that this type of diversity could not be predicted from the sequence of preprogastrin and underlines the importance of combining conventional immunochemical, chromatographic and chemical techniques in the interpretation of information furnished by gene sequencing.

Species specificity

The Ab's to porcine cryptic peptides A and B described above have been successfully used in RIA and immunohistochemical studies of hog progastrin [5, 14]. However, neither Ab reacted with human material. The reason emerged with the elucidation of the gene sequence encoding human gastrin (Fig. 4) [15]. Whilst porcine and human progastrin are organized in similar ways, the human precursor has three residues deleted at the extreme C-terminus compared with the hog precursor [2, 15]. In the cryptic A region of progastrin there are also 15 out of 37 substitutions between the hog and human peptides, so it is not surprising that antisera raised to hog cryptic A did not react with human material.

In order to extend to human tissue the studies made in hog it has therefore been necessary to develop a further panel of Ab's [16]. Evidently, then, for some peptide precursors separate antisera to the cyptic regions may be required for each species under study. However, for the C-terminus of VIP cryptic peptide 1, we found that Ab's to the human peptide will also detect material in rat and hog, and that extracts of rat intestine dilute in parallel to the human cryptic 1 standard (Fig. 7).

Purity of peptides for immunization

Custom-synthesized peptides can be purchased either as crude deprotected material or in purified form. The former preparations have the advantage of reducing costs by up to 50%. State-of-the-art solid-phase synthesis for hexa- or hepta-peptides generates a product that is ~85% pure without chromatography. However, if these unpurified peptides are used for immunization, antisera may be raised against contaminants.

This point is illustrated by our experience with the deprotected synthetic peptide Tyr-Ala-Glu-Asp-Glu-Asn (which corresponds to human Tyr[96]-preprogastrin 96-101). This was purchased, and purified by RP-HPLC, with absorbance monitored at 214 nm. The HPLC elution profile indicated several peaks; the work described here on the identification of human progastrin made use of material found in the major peak that was subsequently used for conjugation and immunization. In addition, however, rabbits were immunized with material from one of the other

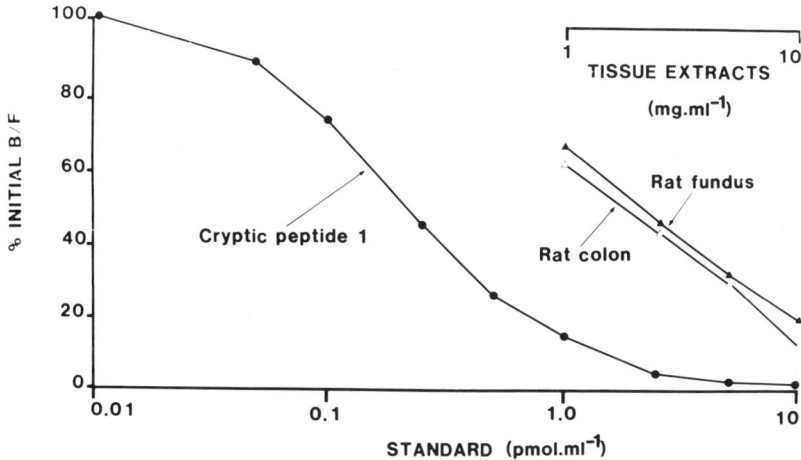

Fig. 7. Inhibition of binding of radiolabelled synthetic human preproVIP 73–79 with antiserum L249 (see Figs. 2 & 3) by synthetic human preproVIP 73–79 and by extracts of rat fundus and rat colon.

HPLC peaks: the resulting antisera bound the radiolabelled peptide, and binding was competitively inhibited by adding unlabelled standard peptide. However, the antisera failed to react with material in extracts of human antrum, which we know to contain ~5 nmol/g C-terminal progastrin-like (i.e. cryptic B-like) immunoreactivity.

Evidently Ab's were not specific for the authentic hexapeptide. Immunization with unpurified synthetic peptide can therefore give rise to antisera which will recognize the synthetic immunogen, but not naturally occurring material. To minimize this problem we routinely characterize and standardize all synthetic peptides by RP-HPLC and amino acid analysis. HPLC-purified peptides are hydrolyzed by HCl, and the hydrolysates reacted with phenyl isothiocyanate. The resulting phenylthiocarbamyl- (PTC-)derivatized amino acids are separated by RP-HPLC on a Waters 4 μm NovaPak C-18 column, detected at 254 nm and the peak areas integrated. The detection limit of this system is <100 pmol; besides providing information on the amino acid composition it allows accurate quantification of RIA standards.

Cell-specific pathways of processing

There are now good examples of patterns of processing of a particular precursor that vary between different cell types expressing the same gene. Thus, in the human antrum, >90% of the biologically active stored hormone is in the form of G17; in duodenal extracts, however, approximately equimolar concentrations of G17 and G34 are found [17–19]. It seems, then, that cleavage of G34 is less complete in duodenum than in antrum.

We have now extended these studies using an antiserum (L216) to the human progastrin cryptic B peptide, examining by gel filtration and HPLC the molecular forms of immunoreactive material in extracts of antrum, duodenum and gastrinomas. In antrum and duodenum the concentrations of cryptic B-like immunoreactivity were similar to those of G17, and on gel filtration 80-90% of this activity eluted in a position compatible with that expected for the C-terminal hexa-peptide. Accordingly, in both antrum and duodenum the cleavage to furnish the C-terminus of G17 is near-complete. In some gastrinomas, however, there was up to an 18-fold molar excess of cryptic B-like immunoreactivity compared with G17, and on gel filtration the cryptic B material appeared to be of high mol. wt. [16]. Digestion of this material with trypsin liberated peptides that reacted with antisera to cryptic B, the N-terminus of G17 and the N-terminus of G34.

Evidently in some gastrinomas the cryptic B immunoreactive peptide extends at its N-terminus beyond the N-terminal point of G34, and may include the entire prograstrin sequence [16]. This material does not react with conventional gastrin antisera, and so was discoverable only by the present approach. It is possible that this material occurs in plasma and might be a useful marker in the diagnosis of conditions characterized by abnormalities of gastrin biosynthesis.

Identification of cellular origins

RIA studies such as those described above do not provide detailed information on the events occurring at the level of individual cells. There is therefore a limitation to their use in the study of different populations of cells in the same tissue that express a common gene but process the peptide precursor differently. There are also problems where different populations of cells within a tissue express two separate genes encoding a common sequence. Two examples illustrate this.

First, in the case of VIP and PHI there are undoubtedly many cells containing both peptides. However, there are also other instances, e.g. fundus of the stomach and hypothalamus, where equimolar amounts of PHI/PHM and VIP do not occur [20, 21]. We have applied antisera to the proVIP cryptic peptides to study immunohistochemically the cellular aspects of this problem. In the myenteric plexus of rat fundus, nerve cell bodies that are 'stained' by VIP antisera are almost always also revealed by antisera to cryptic peptides 2 and 3. However, only about half the VIP-immunoreactive nerve cells are also stained by antisera to cryptic peptide 1 (unpublished observations). This raises the possibility that cleavage between cryptic peptide 1 and PHI may be incomplete in a population of gastric mucosa. Extension of this work to include chromatographic and RIA analysis of fundic extracts is now in progress, and might be expected to throw light on the biosynthetic mechanisms underlying the immunohistochemical findings. [See Vol. 15, this series, for cognate cell-type studies.-*Ed*.].

Secondly, it is well known that the peptides gastrin and CCK share a common C-terminal pentapeptide amide that includes the minimal fragment of both peptides with biological activity. Consequently, Ab's raised against the C-terminus of one molecule invariably cross-react to some extent with the other. Such Ab's cannot be used for the unequivocal immunohistochemical localization of the two peptides. This problem is particularly acute in those tissues that contain both gastrin and CCK, e.g. human duodenum, pig hypothalamus/posterior pituitary. However, as illustrated in Fig. 4, the extreme C-terminal sequence of preprogastrin differs from that of preproCCK. By using antisera to the respective cryptic peptides, we have been able to distinguish between individual gastrin and CCK cells even within heterogeneous populations. In antral mucosa, cells revealed by conventional C-terminal gastrin/CCK antisera are also stained by antisera to cryptic peptides A and B of progastrin, but not by antisera to the C-terminus of proCCK [15]. Conversely, the preproCCK antiserum reveals a population of cells in the duodenal mucosa that do not react with antisera to the gastrin cryptic peptides and so corresponds to CCK-producing cells (unpublished observations).

OVERVIEW

The present experimental approach has allowed the identification, isolation and localization of novel peptides whose existence was predicted from gene-sequence data but whose identity was not otherwise known. Amongst other benefits this approach has provided insight into cell-specific patterns of processing, and has helped illuminate possible abnormalities of peptide biosynthesis. By this approach it is also possible to identify cells that contain nascent precursor, but do not process it. The future application of these approaches may be valuable in reinforcing diagnostic methods for diseases associated with over- or under-production of peptide hormones and neurotransmitters.

Acknowledgements

We are grateful to Christine Williams for help in preparing the manuscript. The work described here was supported by the M.R.C. and N.A.T.O. We thank Carol Higgins, Geoffrey Williams and Ms. M. Lecroarp for technical assistance.

References

1. Kemmler, W., Peterson, J.D. & Steiner, D.F. (1971) *J. Biol. Chem. 246*, 6786-6791.
2. Yoo, O.J., Powell, C.T. & Agarwal, K.L. (1982) *Proc. Nat. Acad. Sci. 79*, 1049-1053.
3. Itoh, N., Obata, K., Yanaihara, N. & Okamoto, H. (1983) *Nature 304*, 547-549.
4. Tatemoto, K. & Mutt, V. (1981) *Proc. Nat. Acad. Sci. 78*, 6603-6607.

5. Desmond, H., Dockray, G.J. & Spurdens, M. (1985) *Regul.
    Peptides 11*, 133-142.
6. Dimaline, R. & Dockray, G.J. (1978) *Gastroenterology 75*, 387-
    392.
7. Dimaline, R., Vaillant, C. & Dockray, G.J. (1980) *Regul.
    Peptides 11*, 1-16.
8. Agarwal, K.L., Grudzinska, S., Kenner, G.W., Rodgers, N.H.,
    Shepperd, R.C. & McGuigan, J.C. (1971) *Experientia 17*, 514-515.
9. Deschenes, R.J., Lorenz, L.J., Huan, R.S., Roos, B.A.,
    Colliers, K.J. & Dixon, J.E. (1984) *Proc. Nat. Acad. Sci. 81*,
    726-730.
10. Dockray, G.J. & Walsh, J.H. (1975) *Gastroenterology 89*, 223-230.
11. Pauwels, S., Dockray, G.J., Walker, R. & Marcus, S. (1984)
    Gastroenterology 86, 86-92.
12. Pauwels, S., Dockray, G.J., Walker, R. & Marcus, S. (1985)
    Gastroenterology 89, 49-56.
13. Pauwels, S., Dockray, G.J., Walker, R. & Marcus, S. (1985)
    J. Clin. Invest. 75, 2006-2013.
14. Jonsson, A-C. & Dockray, G.J. (1984) *Regul. Peptides 8*, 183-
    190.
15. Boel, E., Vuust, J., Norris, F., Norris, K., Wind, A.,
    Rehfeld, J.F. & Marcker, K.A. (1983) *Proc. Nat. Acad. Sci.
    80*, 2866-2869.
16. Desmond, H.P., Pauwels, S., Dimaline, R. & Dockray, G.J. (1986)
    J. Clin. Invest., in press.
17. Berson, S.A. & Yalow, R.S. (1971) *Gastroenterology 60*, 215-222.
18. Malmstrom, J., Stadil, F. & Rehfeld, J.F. (1976) *Gastroenterology
    70*, 697-703.
19. Calam, J., Dockray, G.J., Walker, R., Tracy, H.J. & Owens, D.
    (1980) *Eur. J. Clin. Invest. 10*, 241-247.
20. Hokfelt, T., Fahrenkrug, J., Tatemoto, K., Mutt, V., Werner, S.,
    Hulting, A-L., Terenius, L. & Chang, K.J. (1983) *Proc. Nat.
    Acad. Sci. 60*, 895-898.
21. Hokfelt, T., Fahrenkrug, J., Tatemoto, K., Mutt, V. & Werner, S.
    (1982) *Acta Physiol. Scand. 116*, 469-471.

#A-9

CLINICAL ASSAY OF SOMATOMEDINS BY RIA

J.D. Teale and V. Marks

Clinical Biochemistry Laboratory
St. Luke's Hospital
Guildford, Surrey GU1 3NT, U.K.

The somatomedins (SM's) are a group of growth-hormone-dependent insulin-like growth factors (IGF's). The measurement of plasma concentrations of SM-C (IGF-I) in particular appears to have the greatest potential in clinical diagnosis, e.g. to assess growth hormone (GH) status in children; its level is more stable than that of GH, for reasons that are outlined.

The development of assay methodology has progressed from bioassay through receptor assay to immunoassay (IA) as sufficient amounts of purified hormone became available to permit the production of antibodies (Ab's). The purified hormone being scarce, there is an alternative approach to Ab production involving the use of synthetic fragments as immunogens. The resulting Ab's may exhibit sufficient cross-reaction with the whole peptide to permit the measurement of plasma SM-C levels in normal and acromegalic subjects. However, for adequate discrimination between normal and subnormal levels in young children, greater sensitivity is required. So far this has been achieved only with Ab's raised against the whole peptide. Variable interference by SM-binding proteins in IA methods may necessitate the initial extraction of samples in order to standardize procedures.

The SM's are a group of polypeptide growth factors showing a high degree of structural homology with proinsulin and therefore with insulin [1]. Before a specific RIA for insulin was available, one of the most sensitive methods for its measurement was a bioassay involving glucose oxidation in rat adipose tissue [2]. With the advent of RIA procedures, it became apparent that only ~10% of the total insulin-like activity in serum as measured by the bioassay could be attributed to insulin. This conclusion arose from the observation that only 10% of insulin-like activity in serum could be neutralized by specific anti-insulin Ab's. The remaining 90% was termed non-suppressible insulin-like activity (NSILA) [3]. The insulin-like properties of these preparations were, however, secondary to their growth-promoting activity.

The terminology of growth-factor preparations usually relates to the type of bioassay used to monitor the purification stages. Rationalization of the terminology was attempted in 1972 when the term somatomedin was proposed [4]. For a peptide to be classified as a somatomedin its serum concentrations must be GH-dependent, it must exert insulin-like actions on cells such as fat and muscle, it must promote sulphate incorporation into cartilage, and it must stimulate cell multiplication. Several preparations described in the literature meet these criteria: SM-A, SM-C, IGF's I and II, multiplication/sulphation activity (MSA). Although the separate designations have arisen, structural and immunological evidence has proved SM-C and IGF-I to be identical [5].

SM's differ from classical peptide hormones in that they are not synthesized in discrete glands but are widely distributed in most cell types. Most of the circulating hormone is, however, released from the liver under the influence of GH. SM's are also unique in that they circulate bound to high-mol. wt. carrier proteins. The relatively long half-life of SM-C in serum, reckoned to be between 2 and 4 h [6], may be attributable to the formation of these complexes. It appears probable that the binding of SM's to carrier proteins accounts for their relatively constant serum concentrations which are not therefore subject to the type of rapid fluctuation observed for GH. Single random measurements of SM-C appear to reflect overall GH output, and could be used as indicators of GH status in children, thus obviating the need for lengthy dynamic function test procedures currently required to assess GH status. In the diagnosis and treatment of acromegaly there are indications that plasma SM-C levels correlate more closely with the progress of the disease than to GH measurements.

Unlike steroid and thyroid hormones, of which only the free (non-protein-bound) fraction is regarded as biologically effective, no free SM has yet been identified in serum. It has therefore been suggested that the insulin-like effects are neutralized by the sequestration of SM's by carrier proteins [7]. Through these mechanisms the SM's exert their growth-promoting effects without undue influence on glucose homeostasis.

BIOASSAY

Assays based on biological activity have made use of the insulin-like and growth-promoting properties of SM's. The main methods have been: (1) sulphate incorporation into chondroitin sulphate by cartilage [8], or [^{3}H]thymidine incorporation into cartilage DNA [9]; (2) uptake and incorporation of radiolabelled glucose by adipose tissue [10]; and (3) stimulation of replication in cultured fibroblasts [11].

The importance of bioassay data is that they afford an assessment of the growth-stimulating activity in serum. Most of the reported bioassay systems are sufficiently sensitive but are non-specific: each growth factor has a different potency in any one assay system. Bioassays are also affected by SM-inhibitory substances in serum, the levels of which can change with varying metabolic requirements. Nevertheless this type of assay has made an important contribution, especially as a means of monitoring SM purification procedures. For clinical use, however, bioassays are time-consuming, tedious and fraught with variable quality of performance, making them impractical for extensive routine use.

RADIORECEPTOR ASSAY (RRA)

The displacement of radio-labelled insulin from insulin receptors on fat cells and liver membranes by partially purified SM is an early example of this type of system [12]. Thereby sufficient purified SM was made available for iodination [13]. Use of such a tracer allowed specific receptors to be located on placental membranes [14]. These receptors were distinct from insulin receptors, and the much higher affinity of the specific SM receptors permitted the establishment of an assay system capable of discriminating between the plasma SM-C levels encountered in GH-deficient, normal and acromegalic patients [15].

Although the specific receptors bind only SM's, the different degrees of cross-reactivity exhibited by the individual growth factors can complicate data interpretation. For example, normal serum IGF-II concentrations are usually 3-fold greater than for IGF-I, but IGF-II is only 50% as potent as IGF-I in decreasing IGF-I tracer binding to receptors [16].

The major problem to be overcome in the use of tissue receptors as binding agents is interference from carrier proteins. The affinity of SM's for these is of similar magnitude to that for receptors and some low-avidity Ab's [16]. The carrier proteins are only partially saturated [17] and therefore have spare capacity for binding the small amounts of SM tracer added to assay systems. Untreated serum therefore represents a multi-component system of analyte and binding proteins. Extraction of samples circumvents this type of interference, as discussed below.

Nevertheless RRA's, although less specific, sensitive and convenient than RIA systems, are still useful in determining biological activity, e.g. in cases of growth retardation secondary to circulating biologically inactive SM's [18]. [Vol. 14, this series, has articles on RRA approaches and scope, e.g. compared with RIA, and also touches on growth factors; Vol. 15, on Ab-binding sites, is also pertinent. - *Ed.*]

COMPETITIVE PROTEIN-BINDING ASSAY (CPBA)

Attempts have been made to measure SM levels using the SM-binding proteins that exist in serum, as in the development of CPBA's for cortisol using transcortin as the binding reagent. The endogenous SM's must be removed from the binding proteins, usually by chromatography under acidic conditions, but this is a relatively simple procedure and provides stable preparations [19]. Radiolabelled SM has been shown to bind to carrier protein preparations with sufficiently high avidity and to be displaceable by SM's, thereby providing a system sensitive enough to demonstrate differences between sera from normal, hypopituitary and acromegalic subjects [19].

It is the total SM of a sample that CPBA's measure, although different binding-protein preparations may have different affinities for individual SM's. For example, carrier protein from human serum binds IGF-II with greater affinity than IGF-I and when used with IGF-II tracer produces a system which measures mainly IGF-II [20]. However, carrier protein from rat liver has a higher affinity for IGF-I [21]. Comparison of data from different CPBA's is therefore complicated by such variations in reagent properties.

RADIOIMMUNOASSAY (RIA)

Since there are no discrete storage glands, serum has to be the main source of material for purifying SM's. A typical procedure [22] yielded 250 μg of pure IGF-I from 1200 l of pooled serum. Even these laborious efforts may not provide antigen for more than a short immunization schedule using only a few animals of moderate size, in seeking high-avidity Ab's for RIA use. The recent availability of biosynthetic material produced by genetic engineering should render such tedious and time-consuming procedures unnecessary.

Alternatively, Ab's have been raised in animals immunized with synthetic fragments of hormone [23, 24]; synthetic C- and D-regions of IGF-I and IGF-II were conjugated to a large carrier molecule (bovine thyroglobulin) in order to enhance the immune response to the comparatively small peptides. Ab's to the C-region proved to be of high avidity and showed sufficient cross-reaction with the whole IGF molecule to permit the measurement of normal serum concentrations [23] and to distinguish the supranormal levels found in acromegalic sera. However, the use of such systems is restricted to these higher concentration ranges; the low levels in GH-deficient patients, in young children or in malnutrition cases, for example, are below the detection limits of such RIA systems. Reported sensitivity limits, defined as amount per assay tube required to inhibit label binding by 50%, are as follows for SM-C/IGF-I.- **Whole-molecule RIA:** 60 pg [25], 60 pg [27], 100 pg [26], 1 ng [16]; **C-** or **D-region RIA:** each 80 ng/ml (incubation vol. unstated) [23, 24]; cf. **RRA:** 600 pg [27], 5 ng [26], 8 ng/ml (incubation vol. unstated) [24].

From these representative values (not an exhaustive survey) it is evident that RRA's [24, 26, 27] display greater sensitivities than the RIA's based on synthetic fragments, albeit RRA's are less selective in measuring individual IGF's. The most highly selective and sensitive assays are those RIA's that employ Ab's raised against the whole SM-C molecule [16, 25, 26, 27].

One point of controversy is whether it is necessary to remove binding proteins from samples to permit accurate measurement of plasma SM [28]. The carrier proteins, whilst contributing to the relative constancy of plasma SM levels, may in fact interfere in the assay of untreated samples, leading to erroneous estimates. Direct analysis of untreated samples may be possible with the availability of an antiserum whose avidity for a specific SM sufficiently exceeds that of the carrier protein. However, such antisera are not always immediately available; hence in order to circumvent potential interferences a simple extraction procedure has been devised [29], giving quantitative recovery of SM's and thereby improving the ability of assays to distinguish subnormal values.

In the following assay procedure adopted in our laboratory, the RIA is essentially identical with that of Baxter et al. [27] and has similar performance characteristics.
Sample preparation [29].- To the 200 µl sample, add 800 µl of acid/ ethanol (2 M HCl/ethanol, 1:7 by vol.).
- Centrifuge, and to 500 µl supernatant add 200 µl of a 10% solution of Tris; centrifuge.
RIA.- To 100 µl supernatant add 200 µl antiserum and 200 µl label, viz. iodinated SM-C.
- Incubate at 4°, overnight, and   then add 200 µl of the second Ab in 7.5% PEG solution.
-Incubate at 4° for 2 h, then centrifuge, aspirate the supernatant, count the pellet, and calculate the results.

A serum pool from normal adults is used as the standard reference preparation, assigned the value 1 Unit/ml. The assay limit of detection (sensitivity) was calculated to be 0.04 U/ml. In terms of age and sex (**M** or **F**), the reference ranges (and mean, with no. of observations), for SM-C/IGF-I as U/ml plasma, were as follows.-

<3 yrs.: **M**, 0.05-0.70 (0.20; 38); **F**, 0.08-0.70 (0.24; 29).
4-6:   **M**, 0.10-0.90 (0.31; 35); **F**, 0.12-1.20 (0.37; 24).
7-9:   **M**, 0.25-1.40 (0.60; 32); **F**, 0.36-1.40 (0.70; 17).
10-12: **M**, 0.30-2.00 (0.80; 65); **F**, 0.50-2.00 (0.95; 34).
13-15: **M**, 0.47-0.30 (1.20; 119); **F**, 0.60-3.00 (1.30; 45).
16-18: **M**, 0.56-0.30 (1.25; 27); **F**, 0.60-3.00 (1.30; 11).
20-40: **M** & **F**, 0.40-2.00 (0.90; 31).
41-60: **M** & **F**, 0.32-1.30 (0.65; 36).
>60:   **M** & **F**, 0.20-1.30 (0.50; 36).

The reference ranges imply that the assay system can detect sub-normal SM-C levels in even very young children. However, improvement in sensitivity would enhance the diagnostic value of the assay for this particular purpose. Currently the interpretation of plasma SM-C levels in young children is problematical because of the restricted availability of samples from normal healthy subjects and the poor sensitivity of most assay systems that have been reported.

APPLICATIONS

With the availability of methods for measuring individual SM's in serum, there is scope for improvement in the understanding of growth disorders. In particular, the ability to distinguish between GH and SM deficiency now exists and will influence future therapy. The use of SM measurements during therapy with GH [30] or GH-releasing factor [31] could help in the assessment of such treatment.

Being largely of hepatic origin, SM output reflects metabolic status and although SM is mainly under GH control it has been observed that insulin and nutritional status are important in its regulation [32]. Several other areas of influence have been investigated including SM interaction with other hormones such as thyroxine, prolactin, placental lactogen, oestrogens, androgens and cortisol [33].

The role of SM in the aetiology of diabetes is being examined, one important aspect being the use of plasma SM-C measurements as early predictive indicators of diabetic retinopathy [34].

Acknowledgements

We are indebted to Dr. R.C. Baxter for the provision of reagents.

References

1. Blundell, T.L., Bedarkar, S., Rinderknecht, E. & Humbel, R.E. (1978) *Proc. Nat. Acad. Sci. 75*, 180-184.
2. Winegrad, A.J., Shaw, W.N., Lukens, F.D.W., Stadie, W.C. & Renold, A.E. (1959) *J. Biol. Chem. 234*, 1922-1928.
3. Froesch, E.R., Burgi, H., Ramseier, E.B., Bally, P. & Labhart, A. (1963) *J. Clin. Invest. 42*, 1816-1834.
4. Daughaday, W.H., Hall, K., Raben, M.S., Salmon, W.D., Van den Brande, J.L. & Van Wyk, J.J. (1972) *Nature 235,* 107.
5. Van Wyk, J.J., Svoboda, M.E. & Underwood, L.E. (1980) *J. Clin. Endocrinol. Metab. 50*, 206-208.
6. Underwood, L.E., D'Ercole, A.J. & Van Wyk, J.J. (1980) *Ped. Clin. N. Am. 27*, 771-782.
7. Zapf, J., Schmid, C. & Froesch, E.R. (1984) in *Clinics in Endocrinology and Metabolism*, Vol. 13, Part 1: *Tissue Growth Factors* (Daughaday, W.H., ed.), W.B. Saunders, London, pp. 3-30.

8. Salmon, W.D. & Daughaday, W.H. (1957) *J. Lab. Clin. Med. 49*, 825-836.
9. Daughaday, W.H. & Reeder, C. (1966) *J. Lab. Clin. Med. 68*, 357-368.
10. Hall, K. & Uthne, K. (1971) *Acta Med. Scand. 190*, 137-143.
11. Durlak, N.C. & Temin, H.M. (1973) *J. Cell Physiol. 81*, 153-160.
12. Hintz, R.L., Clemmons, D.R., Underwood, L.E. & Van Wyk, J.J. (1972) *Proc. Nat. Acad. Sci. 69*, 2351-2353.
13. D'Ercole, A.J., Underwood, L.E., Van Wyk, J.J., Decedue, C.J. & Foushee, D.B.(1976) in *Growth Hormone and Related Peptides* (Pecile, A. & Muller, E.E., eds.), Excerpta Medica, Amsterdam, pp.190-201.
14. Marshall, R.N., Underwood, L.E., Voina, S.J., Foushee, D.B. & Van Wyk, J.J. (1974) *J. Clin. Endocrinol. Metab. 39*, 283-292.
15. D'Ercole, A.J., Underwood, L.E. & Van Wyk, J.J. (1977) *J. Paed. 90*, 375-381.
16. Zapf, J., Walter, H. & Froesch, E.R. (1981) *J. Clin. Invest. 68*, 1321-1330.
17. Hintz, R.L. (1984) *as for* 7., pp. 31-42.
18. Rudman, D.J., Kutner, M.H., Blackston, D.R., Cushman, R.A., Bain, R.P. & Patterson, J.H. (1981) *New Engl. Med. J. 305*, 123-131.
19. Zapf, J., Kaufmann, V., Eigenmann, E.G. & Froesch, E.R. (1977) *Clin. Chem. 23*, 677-682.
20. Zapf, J., Waldvogel, M. & Froesch, E.R. (1975) *Arch. Biochem Biophys. 168*, 638-645.
21. Rieu, M., Girard, F., Bricaire, H., & Binoux, M. (1982) *J. Clin. Endocrinol. Metab. 55*, 147-153.
22. Svoboda, M.E., Van Wyk, J.J., Klapper, D.G., Fellows, R.E. & Grissom, F.E. (1980) *Biochemistry 19*, 790-797.
23. Hintz, R.L., Liu, F., Marshall, L.B. & Chang, D. (1980) *J. Clin. Endocrinol. Metab. 50*, 405-407.
24. Hintz, R.L., Liu, F. & Rinderknecht, E. (1980) *J. Clin. Endocrinol Metab. 51*, 672-673.
25. Bala, R.M. & Bhaumick, B. (1979) *J. Clin. Endocrinol. Metab. 49*, 770-777.
26. Van Wyk, J.J., Svoboda, M.E. & Underwood, L.E. (1980) *J. Clin. Endocrinol. Metab. 50*, 206-208.
27. Baxter, R.C., Brown, A.S. & Turtle, J.R.(1982) *Clin. Chem. 28*, 488-495.
28. Furlanetto, R.W. (1982) *J. Clin. Endocrinol. Metab. 54*, 1084-1086.
29. Daughaday, W.H., Mariz, I.K. & Blethen, S.L. (1980) *J. Clin. Endocrinol. Metab. 51*, 781-788.
30. Russo, L. & Moore, W.V. (1982) *J. Clin. Endocrinol. Metab. 55*, 1003-1006.
31. Borges, J.L.C., Blizzard, R.M., Evans, W.S., Furlanetto, R., Rogol, A.D., Kaiser, D.L., Rivier, J., Vale, W. & Thorner, M.O. (1984) *J. Clin. Endocrinol. Metab. 59*, 1-6.
32. Phillips, L.S. & Unterman, T.G. (1984) *as for* 7., pp. 145-189.
33. Clemmons, D.R. & Van Wyk, J.J. (1984) *as for* 7., pp. 113-143.
34. Ashton, I.K., Dornan, T.L., Pocock, A.E., Turner, R.C. & Bron, A.J. (1983) *Clin. Endocrinol. 19*, 105-110.

#A-10

IMMUNOMETRIC APPROACH TO PEPTIDE HORMONE ANALYSIS

J.G. Ratcliffe, A. White, S. Dobson,
A.D. Swift and S. Bruce

University of Manchester
Department of Chemical Pathology
Hope Hospital, Salford M6 8HD, U.K.

*Theoretically, reagent-excess assays employing labelled Ab's** *(immunometric assays) offer several advantages over limited-reagent labelled antigen assays (e.g. RIA) for peptide hormones, notably in respect of detection limits, specificity, working range, incubation time and ruggedness - as now explored. For ACTH we have developed and selected compatible mouse MAb's directed towards the near-N-terminal (residues 14-18) and C-terminal (residues 24-39) sequences. A two-step protocol is employed: incubation of standard or test sample with ^{125}I-labelled N-terminal Ab, then addition of excess solid-phase (Sephacryl S300) C-terminal Ab. There was marked benefit, vs. RIA using the same Ab's, to detection limit (2 ng/l), working range and assay time (<24 h). The assay detected intact 1-39 ACTH, large mol. wt. precursors of the proopiomelanocortin family but not ACTH fragments.*

For TSH we have compared 6 commercial two-site assays employing MAb's and either radioisotopic or non-isotopic labels. All had detection limits <0.2 (some 0.05) mU/l, wide working ranges and overall incubation times <24 h. All were more sensitive with wider working ranges than current RIA's, and consistently allowed thyrotoxic and euthyroid patients to be distinguished by TSH levels. We conclude that the IMA approach to peptide hormone analysis is an important technical advance with major clinical applications.

The assay of peptide hormones in biological fluids presents a formidable analytical challenge because of their low circulating concentrations (picomolar) and heterogeneous molecular forms (precursors, fragments, isohormones). Of the general approaches to hormone analysis (biological, physicochemical and binding assays), only

---

* Abbreviations: (M)Ab, (monoclonal) antibody; I(R)MA, immuno(radio)-metric assay; RIA, radioimmunoassay; s.a., specific activity.

immunoassays are widely used clinically though bioassays and HPLC have important applications for research and reference. Over the last 20 years RIA has been applied to all known peptide hormones but often with only partial success: e.g. RIA's for the pituitary hormones and hormones regulating calcium homeostasis have problems of sensitivity and/or specificity. A fundamental problem with limited-reagent assays is their susceptibility to factors in the incubation milieu which alter the equilibrium constant of the Ab as the limit of detection is approached. Thus RIA is vulnerable to non-specific matrix effects near the assay detection limit. Peptide hormone RIA's also often have disadvantages of prolonged incubation times since the requirement for high sensitivity dictates that reagents be used at low concentrations, and of limited working ranges, with acceptable precision extending over only one order of magnitude.

An alternative type of immunoassay - immunometric - employs labelled Ab's rather than labelled antigen. The principle of the IMA differs fundamentally from RIA in that labelled specific Ab's are used in excess to bind to the analyte, to allow its detection as a labelled complex (Fig. 1). The concentration of analyte is thus directly proportional to the amount of labelled complex formed. The immunometric approach, first described in 1968 [1], made little impact on peptide hormone analysis until recent years. Thus in 1980, only ~2% of laboratories participating in U.K. External Quality Assessment Schemes (EQAS) for the pituitary hormones GH, LH, FSH and PRL, and α-foetoprotein, used IMA's, and few laboratories use them even now. In contrast, there has been a radical shift in methods used for TSH assays in EQAS from predominantly RIA (82% in 1981) to IMA (53% in 1985), for reasons that will be discussed below.

The slow application of IMA's to peptide hormones is surprising at first sight in view of their theoretical advantages, e.g. improved sensitivity, specificity, enhanced working range, short incubation times and ruggedness [2]. In part this was due to practical disadvantages in the original formulation of IMA's in which excess labelled Ab (purified from polyclonal antisera) is reacted with analyte and then solid-phase analyte added at the end of the incubation period to precipitate unreacted labelled Ab. Such single-site labelled Ab assays do not allow full exploitation of the theoretical potential, since the presence of any immunologically unreactive labelled Ab in the supernatant sampled for end-point detection increases the background response, thereby diminishing sensitivity.

RECENT DEVELOPMENTS IN IMMUNOMETRIC ASSAYS

There have been two key developments, described below, which have overcome the problems associated with the early immunometric assays, and are transforming the clinical application of this assay principle.

ONE SITE

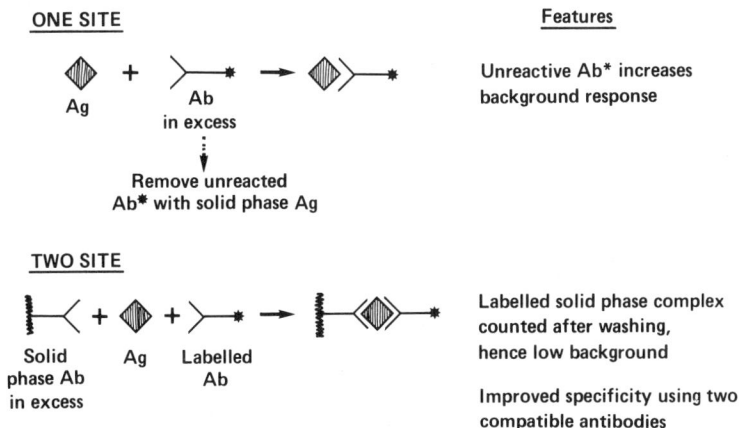

Ag   Ab
      in excess

Remove unreacted
Ab* with solid phase Ag

TWO SITE

Solid   Ag   Labelled
phase Ab   Ab
in excess

Features

Unreactive Ab* increases
background response

Labelled solid phase complex
counted after washing,
hence low background

Improved specificity using two
compatible antibodies

Fig. 1.   IMA principles.

(i) Two-site assays [3]

Instead of observing the response in the soluble antigen-labelled Ab complex as in the one-site assay, the labelled Ab-antigen complex is insolubilized by reaction with a second Ab (specific for the analyte) linked to solid phase. This enables the solid-phase-linked complex to be separated and washed thoroughly before measuring the response, thus minimizing background 'noise' and thereby enhancing sensitivity. Specificity is also improved since bcth labelled Ab and solid-phase Ab have to bind to analyte to generate the signal. Because reagents are in excess, the reaction times are short in comparison to RIA (hours *vs.* days) and the working range is wide (usually >1000-fold). The two-site assay also offers considerable flexibility in its design. Analyte can be reacted with solid-phase Ab followed by reaction of the product with labelled Ab, though this may reduce somewhat the extent of binding of labelled Ab. Alternatively, analyte can be reacted first with labelled Ab followed by reaction with excess solid-phase Ab. Or both Ab's can be reacted simultaneously with analyte, though this may to some extent involve competition between the two reactions with loss of sensitivity.

The ultimate sensitivity of any immunoassay is limited by four factors: Ab avidity, non-specific binding (misclassification), experimental imprecision and specific activity of label. With IMA's, Ab avidity is not so crucial as in limited-reagent assays, but non-specific binding and s.a. of label are critical. While it is possible to label Ab's to high s.a. with ^{125}I, the immunoactivity of such labels deteriorates rapidly, thus preventing realization of the high sensitivity of detection of ^{125}I ($\sim 10^{-18}$ moles). Non-isotopic labels offer improved stability, and chemiluminescent molecules can be detected with even greater sensitivity than ^{125}I or fluorescence [4].

Furthermore, the label signal can be amplified catalytically by enzymes to yield a colorimetric or luminescent signal (enzyme amplification, enhanced luminescence) [5, 6]. Full exploitation of the sensitivity potential of high s.a. labels depends on low non-specific background [7].

(ii) Monoclonal antibodies (MAb's)

A major factor in facilitating the practical implementation of IMA's is the increasing availability of MAb's, particularly for labelling. This approach allows easier production and selection of Ab's with defined specificities for defined peptide sequences. MAb's can be readily purified in large amounts from culture medium or ascitic fluid to provide a consistent reagent. Although specific Ab's can be prepared from polyclonal antisera by immunoselection with solid-phase antigen, the procedure requires large volumes of high-avidity antiserum, is complex and time-consuming, and the product is of variable quality. Because the Ab so prepared contains a mixture of immunoglobulins of varying specificities, non-specific binding is higher and more variable than with labelled MAb's. This impairs the signal-to-background ratio achieved at low analyte concentrations, thus decreasing the reliable sensitivity achieved.

For the solid-phase reagent, the clonality of the Ab is less critical, and both polyclonal and monoclonal Ab's are used successfully. Large volumes of either are required, as the solid-phase Ab must be present in excess to avoid reduced binding at high analyte concentrations (high-dose hook effect). In theory the use of MAb's for both label and solid phase may impose such unique specificity that the assay may recognize only a proportion of the molecular forms which it is desirable to measure. Careful selection of compatible Ab's is thus necessary to yield the desired specificity [8].

The requirements for a two-site IMA may thus be summarized:
(a) two Ab's with compatible specificities;
(b) pure Ab for labelling: preferably monoclonal for convenience, consistency and low non-specific binding;
(c) large supply of Ab for solid phase: this may be monoclonal or polyclonal;
(d) solid-phase support with high capacity to bind Ab, low non-specific binding and suitable physical characteristics - a variety of useful solid phases being available: walls of tubes or microtitre wells, single beads, particles which remain in suspension but are readily centrifuged, magnetizable particles, etc.

The following sections discuss these principles in relation to IMA's for ACTH and TSH. Current RIA's for both of these clinically important peptides have so far failed to meet the required criteria of sensitivity and/or specificity.

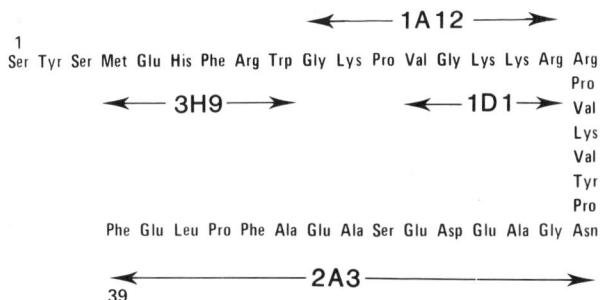

Fig. 2. Specificity of selected MAb's raised to ACTH or ACTH fragments as determined by peptide inhibition studies.

IMMUNOMETRIC ASSAY FOR ACTH

Clinical ACTH assays must have high sensitivity (1 pmol/l) and specificity for intact ACTH in the presence of structurally related peptides derived from its precursor (proopiomelanocortin) and ACTH fragments. The assay should also have a wide working range and be relatively unaffected by small technical variations. To this end the potential of a two-site IRMA for ACTH using MAb's has been investigated. ACTH is poorly immunogenic, and as we required Ab's to N- and C-terminal sequences a range of immunogens was employed. ACTH (1-24)-BSA was employed to raise mid N-terminal antisera, and ACTH (1-39)-IgG to raise extreme N- and C-terminal antisera. The latter immunogen was predicted to have two advantages - exposure of N- and C-terminal ACTH sequences by conjugation through ε-lysine residues at positions 11, 15, 16 and 21, and enhanced immunogenicity due to the carrier chicken IgG. The results of this strategy for raising MAb's and the selection and optimization of these Ab's for a two-site IRMA for ACTH have been fully described elsewhere [9, 10]. The following summarizes the main findings. Four MAb's were selected for further study, their respective specificities being towards the extreme N-terminal sequence (ACTH 4-10), mid N-terminal sequences (10-18 and 14-18) and C-terminal (24-29), as determined by classical fragment inhibition studies (Fig. 2).

Labelled Ab's were prepared by concentrating Ab's from culture media, followed by purification using protein A chromatography, and iodination by the chloramine T method. Solid-phase Ab's were prepared by purifying Ab from ascitic fluid on CM Affigel blue and coupling to activated Sephacryl S300. Combinations of labelled and solid-phase Ab's were then tested for compatibility and sensitivity. Separation was by the sucrose layering technique using a two-pass system, counting the bound fraction.

The results are shown in Table 1. Certain Ab combinations were incompatible (e.g. 1D1 and 1A12), suggesting that binding sites over-

Table 1. Compatibility of MAb's in a two-site ACTH IRMA.
Results are expressed as the assay detection limits (ng ACTH/1)
as defined by the 99% confidence interval of the zero standard.

Labelled Ab	Binding site in ACTH (peptide sequence)	Solid-phase Ab		
		3H9	1A12	2A3
3H9	4-10	–	2400	200
1A12	10-18	400	–	10
1D1	14-18	No binding	No binding	2
2A3	24-39	700	500	–

lap or are adjacent, resulting in severe steric inhibition. Other combinations gave a wide range of detection limits (2-2400 ng/1). One
striking finding was that all the IRMA's yielded more sensitive
assays than the corresponding individual Ab's in RIA. Fig. 3 shows an
example where the IRMA using labelled 1D1 and solid-phase 2A3 had a
detection limit ~500-fold lower than RIA with 1D1 and ~15,000-fold
lower than by RIA with 2A3. The lowest detection limit was found
using the highest-avidity Ab as label.

Using the most promising pair of Ab's, sensitivity was optimized
by varying incubation conditions and label and solid-phase concentrations. The lowest detection limit with greatest signal/background
ratio over the widest range of ACTH concentrations was achieved with
the two-step protocol where labelled Ab was incubated first with
analyte for 16 h followed by 2 h incubation with solid-phase Ab,
though the $2 + \frac{1}{2}$ h protocol was only marginally inferior. The single-
step protocols were less sensitive with lower signal/background
ratios over the entire standard curve. The formal detection limit of
the optimized system was 2 ng/1, and the within-assay precision
profile indicated a C.V. of <20% over the range 10-50,000 ng/1.

Assay specificity was highly interesting: as predicted, the
IMA did not cross-react with N- and C-terminal ACTH fragments, but
the precursor peptides containing the full ACTH sequence were detected
(Fig. 4). This feature is desirable for a clinical assay since
some of these peptides appear to have biological activity and circulate in patients with an ectopic source of ACTH.

It is concluded that a two-site IMA for ACTH using MAb's of
relatively low avidity offers potential for a sensitive and specific
assay without the need for preliminary extraction from plasma. Improved
sensitivity may be possible with non-isotopic labels and MAb's of
greater avidity.

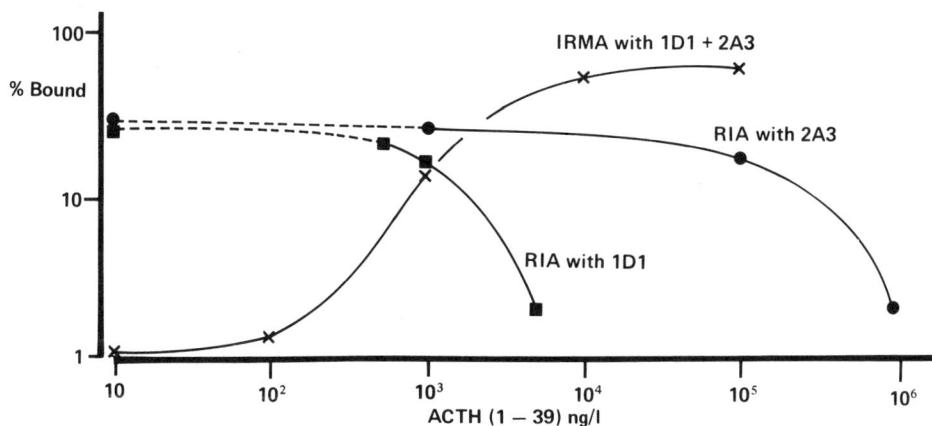

Fig. 3. Comparison of standard curves by two-site IRMA and by RIA using the same MAb's.

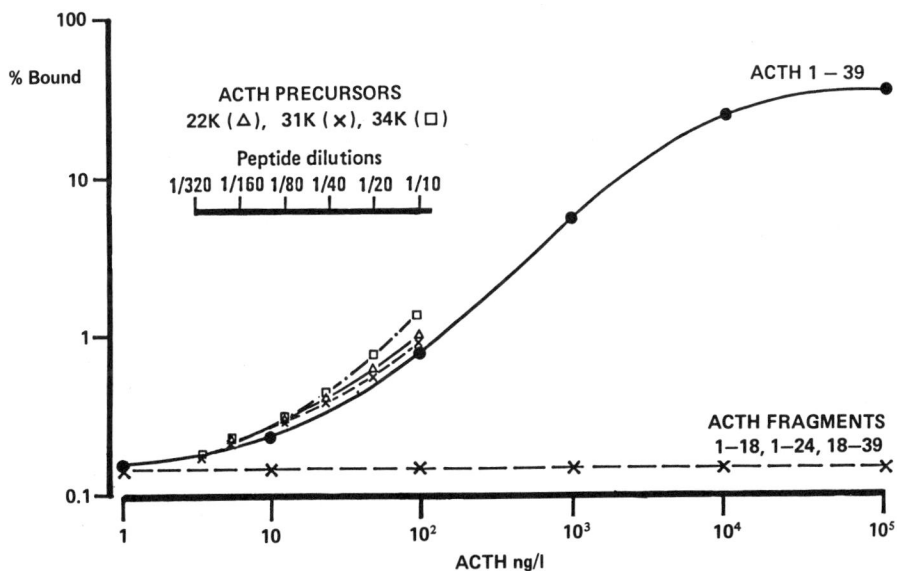

Fig. 4. Specificity of two-site IRMA for ACTH. Synthetic ACTH 1-39 (●), ACTH fragments as indicated (×), and ACTH precursor peptides 22K (Δ), 31K (×) and 34K (■) were tested. Human purified ACTH 1-39 was equipotent and parallel with the synthetic ACTH 1-39 curve (data not shown).

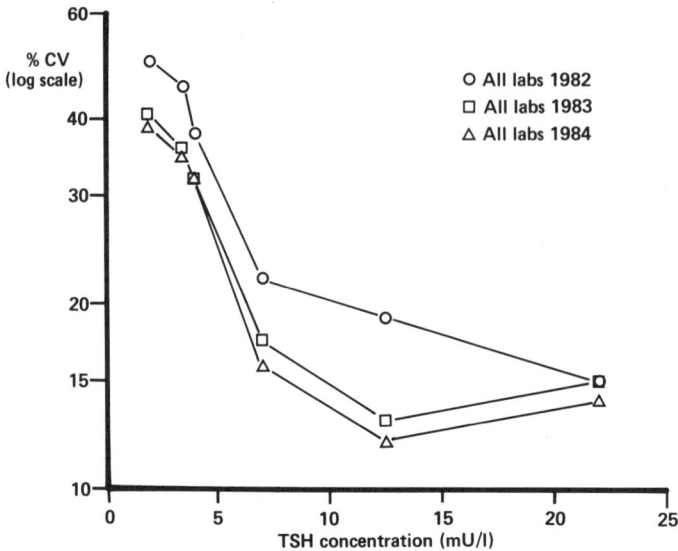

Fig. 5. Between-laboratory between-assay imprecision profiles for TSH assays from UK EQAS for TSH 1982-1984. Note the poor precision at euthyroid TSH levels (<5 mU/1).

IMMUNOMETRIC ASSAYS FOR TSH

TSH determination is among the most extensively applied endocrine assays ($>10^8$ tests per annum in the U.K. in 1983). It has a central role in the investigation of thyroid status; but current RIA's are in general only reliable for measuring high-normal and elevated concentrations whereas detection of subnormal levels is required in hyperthyroidism. Lack of sensitivity and baseline uncertainty has been highlighted recently for TSH in the above-mentioned EQAS: ~$\frac{1}{3}$ of the U.K. laboratories concerned have positive bias on T_3-suppressed or thyrotoxic sera, and some have gross bias-reporting levels (>3 mU/1; expected value <0.1 mU/1) on such sera. Between-laboratory between-assay imprecision profiles reflect this poor performance at normal and low levels (Fig. 5).

There has therefore been much interest in applying the immuno-metric approach, particularly with the development of MAb's and non-isotopic labels. A wide range of IMA's using MAb's has been developed, with variation in the following features.-

(i) **Label.**- Ab's have been labelled with radioisotopes (^{125}I) and non-radioactive moieties - e.g. chemiluminescent labels based on acridinium esters [4], fluorescent labels based on rare-earth chelates with delayed emission to overcome problems of non-specific fluorescence [11], enzyme amplification with either colorimetric or enhanced luminescence end-points.

(ii) **Solid phase.**- Ab's have been coupled to tubes, microtitre wells, single beads, or particles.

(iii) **Separation mode.**- Separation has been accomplished by simple washing of tubes, wells or beads, by magnetic precipitation or sucrose layering of particles [12, 13], or by centrifugation of particles with extensive washing.

(iv) **Incubation.**- The protocols have usually been sequential with either labelled Ab or solid-phase Ab incubated first. Occasionally simultaneous addition of both Ab's has given satisfactory sensitivity.

We have compared several of this new generation of highly sensitive IMA's based on variants of the above, to evaluate their analytical performance especially with respect to sensitivity, baseline certainty, working range, imprecision and ruggedness. The format of the experimental protocol and the detailed results of this evaluation are available elsewhere [14, 15]. From the clinical viewpoint we were especially interested in their ability to distinguish low TSH levels (in T_3-suppressed and thyrotoxic sera) from normal. Several of these IMA's performed well in respect of baseline certainty, sensitivity (detection limits between 0.005 and 0.2 mU/1) and imprecision profiles - considerably superior to RIA (Fig. 6) - and were able to distinguish euthyroid from thyrotoxic sera (Fig. 7). The working ranges (<10% C.V.) extended from low-normal to grossly elevated TSH levels in many cases, with no evidence of a high-dose hook effect at levels likely to occur clinically.

Preliminary evidence from clinical studies with both isotopic and non-isotopic IMA's confirms their superiority to RIA [16]. The improved performance of certain IMA's for TSH suggests that they may provide a valuable first-line test of thyroid function, reducing the need for further tests [17]. A normal TSH level, for example, may obviate the need for TRH tests. Moreover, sensitive IMA's will allow exploration of subtle abnormalities of TSH control not feasible by previous methods.

However, the exquisite specificity of MAb-based TSH assays raises its own potential problems. Thus they may distinguish between different molecular forms of TSH which could occur in pathophysiological situations, as well as between endogenous and exogenous TSH. Hence an assay could show quantitative recovery with exogenous TSH yet be biased either positively or negatively when applied to patient specimens, or *vice versa*. Discrepancies may then emerge between different IMA's and with RIA. The new technology may thus force a reappraisal of the question 'what is TSH?'. This emphasizes the need for reliable and sensitive bioassays for hormones such as TSH (and the other glycoproteins LH and FSH) which cannot be defined in precise chemical terms. Such assays would enable comparison of bio- and immuno-activity of the different molecular forms of peptides and furnish a reference point for IMA's.

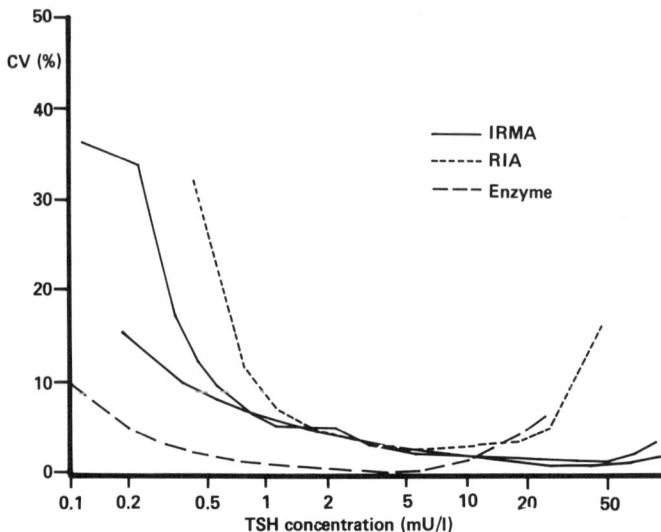

Fig. 6. Typical within-assay imprecision profiles for TSH of two IRMA's, one immunoenzymometric assay and one RIA. Note the improved sensitivity and working range potential of the IMA's.

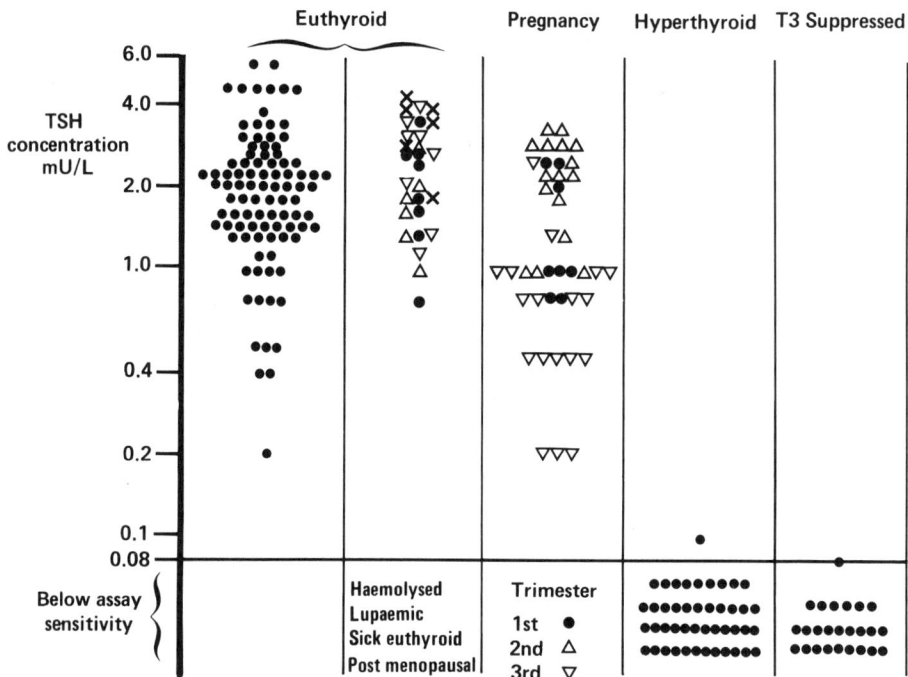

Fig. 7. TSH levels obtained by a sensitive two-side IRMA in various clinical conditions. Note the discrimination between hyperthyroid and euthyroid levels.

CONCLUDING COMMENTS

The immunometric approach, made practical by the use of MAb's in two-site assays, is transforming the sensitivity, specificity, speed and simplicity of peptide hormone analysis. This step change in technology is allowing the clinical biochemist to address pathophysiological problems hitherto inaccessible, of which the investigation of conditions with subnormal TSH levels is a striking example.

Acknowledgements

We acknowledge financial support from the North West Regional Health Authority, Boots-Celltech Ltd., and the Department of Health & Social Security, London. We thank Mrs. Pauline Bullock for expert secretarial assistance.

References

1. Miles, L.E.M. & Hales, C.N. (1968) *Nature 219*, 186-189.
2. Hunter, W.M. & Budd, P.S. (1981) *J. Immunol. Meths. 45*, 255-273.
3. Hunter, W.M., Bennie, J.G., Budd, P.S., Van Heyningen, V., James, K., Micklem, R.L. & Scott, A. (1983) in *Immunoassays for Clinical Chemistry* (Hunder, W.M. & Corrie, J.E.T., eds.), Churchill Livingstone, Edinburgh, pp. 531-544.
4. Weeks, I., Beheshti, I., McCapra, F., Campbell, A.K. & Woodhead, J.S. (1983) *Clin. Chem. 29*, 1474-1479.
5. Stanley, C.J., Paris, F., Plumb, A., Webb, A. & Johannson, A. (1985) *Int. Clin. Products Rev., July/Aug.*, 44-50.
6. Whitehead, T.P., Thorpe, G.H.G., Carter, T.J.N., Groucott, C. & Kricka, L.J. (1983) *Nature 305*, 158-159.
7. Ekins, R. (1980) *Nature 284*, 14-15.
8. Soos, M., Taylor, S.J., Gard, T. & Siddle, K. (1984) *J. Immunol. Meths. 73*, 237-249.
9. White, A., Gray, C. & Ratcliffe, J.G. (1985) *J. Immunol. Meths. 79*, 185-194.
10. Dobson, S.H., Gray, C., Smith, H., Baker, T., Ratcliffe, J.G. & White, A. (1986) *J. Immunol. Meths.*, in press.
11. Soini, E. & Hemmila, I. (1979) *Clin. Chem. 25*, 353-361.
12. Forrest, G.C. & Rattle, S.J. (1983) *as for* 3., 147-162.
13. Wright, J.F. & Hunter, W.M. (1983) *as for* 3., 170-177.
14. Dept. of Health & Social Security (1985) *Comparative evaluation of high sensitivity TSH kits*, Preliminary Report from Scientific Branch (February).
15. Dept. of Health & Social Security (1986) *Comparative evaluation of high sensitivity TSH kits*, Final Report from Scientific & Technical Branch, in press.

16. Weeks, I., Sturgess, M., Siddle, K., Jones, M.K. & Woodhead, J.S. (1984)   *Clin. Endocrinol.* *20*,489-495.
17. Caldwell, G., Kellett, H.A., Gow, S.M., Beckett, G.J., Sweeting, V.M., Seth, J. & Toft, A.D. (1985) *Lancet i*, 1117-1119.

#NC(A)

NOTES and COMMENTS relating to

PEPTIDES AND OTHER ENDOGENOUS-TYPE ANALYTES

Comments related to particular contributions

#A-3 & #A-4, p. 123
#A-5 & #A-6, p, 124
#A-7 -#A-9, p. 125
#A-10 & #NC(A)-2 to -4, p. 126

#NC(A)-1

A Note on

ENDOGENOUS MOLECULES IN RELATION TO DRUGS: COMMENTS PROMPTED BY THE FOCUS ON PEPTIDES

Stephen H. Curry

Division of Clinical Pharmacokinetics
College of Pharmacy, University of Florida
Gainesville, FL 32610, U.S.A.

Those of us who helped plan the Forum sessions on 'natural-type' analytes that feature in the foregoing articles had gained the impression that drug molecules increasingly resemble endogenous molecules. This is in sharp contrast to earlier years of biomedical drug analysis, when the drug molecules to be assayed were clearly exogenous; they were compounds which had emerged from the screening of large numbers of xenobiotics. These compounds were often highly lipophilic as compared with endogenous metabolites.

My own interests in recent years have taken me into a world of exogenous drugs being converted into endogenous metabolites, and into the interaction of drug metabolites with endogenous chemicals. Three examples are now given.

Dichloroacetic acid.- This drug is undergoing evaluation as a potential agent for therapy for lactic acidosis and familial hypercholesterolaemia [1]. It is a pyruvate dehydrogenase activator; hence it affects blood concentrations of alanine, cholesterol, glucose and lactate. Short-term use leads to virtually no side-effects, but long-term use in animals causes a quite severe neuropathy. This is thought to be caused by oxalic acid in particular, which is formed as a metabolite of dichloroacetic acid and is an endogenous chemical:

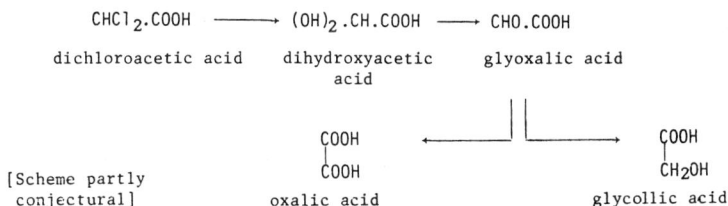

$$CHCl_2.COOH \longrightarrow (OH)_2.CH.COOH \longrightarrow CHO.COOH$$

dichloroacetic acid	dihydroxyacetic acid	glyoxalic acid

[Scheme partly conjectural]

$$\begin{array}{ccc} COOH & \longleftarrow \quad\quad\longrightarrow & COOH \\ COOH & & CH_2OH \end{array}$$

oxalic acid   glycollic acid

The analytical challenge is to find a method for analyzing dichloroacetic acid, oxalic acid and lactic acid in the same sample, so that the drug, its metabolite and the drug's biochemical effects can be evaluated in a single experiment. At present, dichloroacetic acid is assayed by GC-ECD, lactate is measured in clinical laboratories, and oxalate is measured following precipitation as its calcium salt from 24 h urine samples.   GC-MS approaches offer promise for solving this problem.

Cysteine, cystine and acetylcysteine.- Cysteine and cystine are, of course, normal constituents of the body. Acetylcysteine is a drug marketed as a mucolytic for various ear, nose and throat conditions.   It is, moreover, potentially valuable in a renal-stone condition where the stone is formed from cystine (which has low solubility) in patients with a genetically controlled tendency to convert cysteine to cystine excessively [2]; acetylcysteine breaks up cystine stones by an unknown chemical reaction.

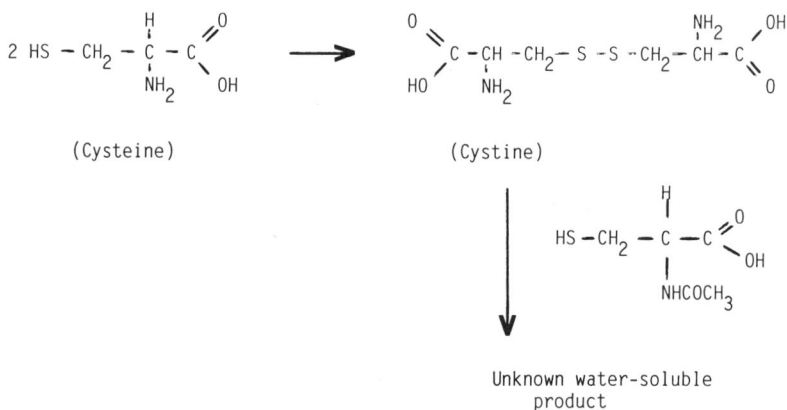

$$2\ HS-CH_2-\underset{NH_2}{\overset{H}{\underset{|}{\overset{|}{C}}}}-C\overset{O}{\underset{OH}{\lessgtr}} \longrightarrow \underset{HO}{\overset{O}{\gtrless}}C-\underset{NH_2}{\overset{|}{CH}}-CH_2-S-S-CH_2-\underset{}{\overset{NH_2}{\overset{|}{CH}}}-C\overset{OH}{\underset{O}{\lessgtr}}$$

(Cysteine)   (Cystine)

$$\downarrow$$

$$HS-CH_2-\underset{NHCOCH_3}{\overset{H}{\underset{|}{\overset{|}{C}}}}-C\overset{O}{\underset{OH}{\lessgtr}}$$

Unknown water-soluble
product

The analytical need is for a method whereby cysteine, cystine, acetylcysteine and the reaction product can be assayed in the same urine sample, so that both the kinetics of the drug and its effect could be monitored at the same time. HPLC has provided some partial answers to this problem.

Nitroglycerin.- As shown in the panel opposite, nitroglycerin is metabolized by denitration to two isomeric dinitroglycerols, glycerol itself, and inorganic nitrite and nitrate [3].   Glycerol itself is of no great importance in this context, as glycerol produced from nitroglycerin is unlikely to be important in mediating its effect.   However, glycerol formation provides a further example of drugs being metabolized to normal body constituents. Additionally, nitrite formed in the metabolism of nitroglycerin reacts with reduced glutathione (GSH) to form nitrate and oxidized glutathione (GSSG):

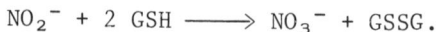

$$NO_2^- + 2\ GSH \longrightarrow NO_3^- + GSSG.$$

$$
\begin{array}{c}
CH_2ONO_2 \\
| \\
CHONO_2 \\
| \\
CH_2ONO_2 \\
\text{(Nitroglycerin)}
\end{array}
$$

$$
\begin{array}{c}
CH_2ONO_2 \\
| \quad + NO_2^- \\
CHONO_2 \\
| \\
CH_2OH
\end{array}
\qquad
\begin{array}{c}
CH_2ONO_2 \\
| \\
CHOH \\
| \\
CH_2ONO_2
\end{array}
\quad + NO_2^-
$$

$$
\begin{array}{c}
CH_2OH \\
| \\
CHONO_2 \quad + NO_2^- \\
| \\
CH_2OH
\end{array}
\qquad
\begin{array}{c}
CH_2ONO_2 \\
| \\
CHOH \\
| \\
CH_2OH
\end{array}
\quad + NO_2^-
$$

$$
\begin{array}{c}
CH_2OH \\
| \\
CHOH \\
| \\
CH_2OH \\
\text{(Glycerol)}
\end{array}
$$

$$
NO_2^- \longrightarrow NO_3^-
$$

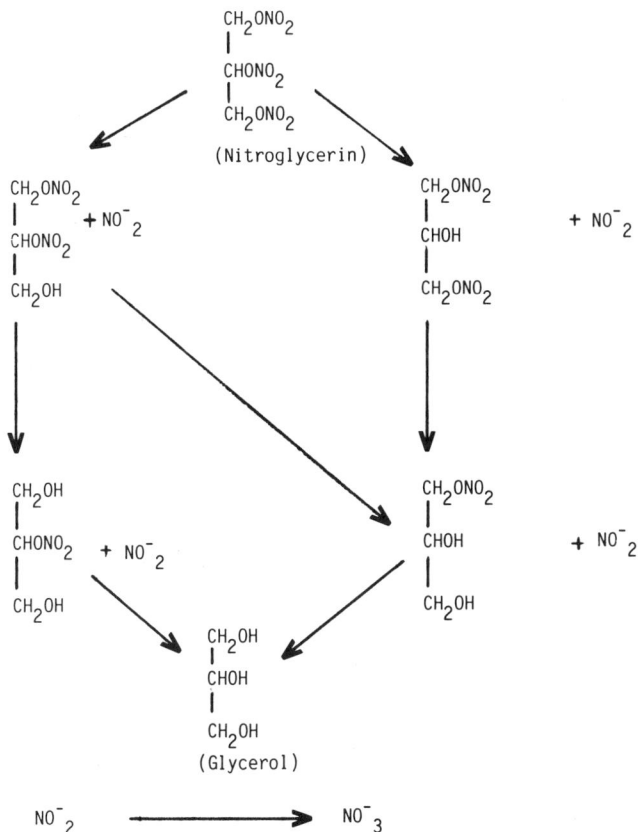

The analytical need here has been for a method to measure nitrite and nitrate, and GSH and GSSG, in the same sample [4].

CONCLUDING COMMENT

Two further examples of drugs and/or drug metabolites occurring endogenously concern fluphenazine, which probably gives rise to ethanol, and ethanol itself [4]. The foregoing examples are not directly in the area of this section, viz. peptides and prostaglandin-/endorphin-type molecules; but they do speak for the timeliness of considering compounds which are more 'endogenous' than 'exogenous'. It is from among synthetic peptides and prostaglandins, and other such compounds, that the next generation of new drugs will emerge, and hence new analytical problems. Perusal of the section should, therefore, relate to the question: "What can we learn from analyses of relevant types now being conducted?"

References

1. Curry, S.H., Chu, P.I., Baumgartner, T.G. & Stacpoole, P.W.
    (1985) *Clin. Pharmacol. Ther. 37*, 89-93.
2. Smith, A.D., Lange, P.H., Miller, R.P. & Reinke, D.B. (1979)
    Urology 13, 422-423.
3. Curry, S.H. & Aburawi, S. (1985) *Biopharmaceutics Drug Dispos.
    6*, 235-280.
4. Curry, S.H., Whelpton, R., de Schepper, P.J., Vranckx, S. &
    Schiff, A.A. (1979) *Br. J. Clin. Pharmacol. 7*, 325-331.

#NC(A)-2

A Note on

DETERMINATION OF 2-PYRROLIDONE IN PLASMA

D. Dell[*], G. Wendt, F. Bucheli and K-H. Trautmann

Biological Pharmaceutical Research Department
F. Hoffmann-La Roche Ltd.
CH-4002 Basel, Switzerland

2-Pyrrolidone (**I**)[⊗] is of considerable biochemical interest because of its possible role as an intermediate in neurotransmission. There is some MS evidence for its endogenous existence [1, 2]. Our aim was to obviate MS and develop a specific and sensitive HPLC method able to measure plasma **I** in the range 1-20 ng/ml, so that we could confirm its presence in blood. Possible approaches were considered in relation to foreseen difficulties besides those inherent in low mol. wt. compounds that are very water-soluble: **I** has a low UV absorption and fluorescence capability and is electrochemically unresponsive. It cannot readily be derivatized for GC; but in our laboratories a 2-step derivatization has been developed involving formation of *N*-TMS-pyrollidone followed immediately (the silyl derivative is unstable) by replacement of silyl by PFB, conferring negative-CI detectability [3].

Although **I** is very water-soluble, two successive extractions with 10 vol. of CH_2Cl_2 can give fair recovery (70%). Since **I** can be hydrolyzed to γ-aminobutyric acid (**II**), a key neurotransmitter much studied by analysts, we based our HPLC method on conversion of **II** to its highly fluorescent isoindole (**III**) by reaction with *o*-phthalde-hyde (OPA). Endogenous **II** cannot give false positives since **II** is not extracted under the conditions used for **I**.

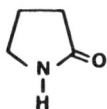
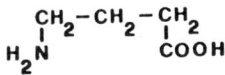
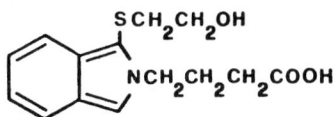

| I | II | III |

[*] Any correspondence to be addressed to this author, who agreed to editorial abridgement of details [cf. 4] in favour of 'rationale'.
[⊗] 2-Pyrrolidinone (more rigorous terminology)

METHODOLOGICAL POINTS AND PITFALLS (details in [4])

Extraction.- An improvement to the classical mechanical mixing approach was the adoption of solid-phase extraction using 'Extrelut' columns in cartridge form (Merck) [cf. R.D. McDowall et al., this vol., #C-2.-*Ed*.]. After applying 1 ml of plasma, **I** was eluted with 100% recovery by 3×5 ml CH_2Cl_2. Including the subsequent evaporation, the overall time for processing 16 samples was 1 h, compared with 2 h in the 'classical' method with its two extractions and centrifugatons. Other benefits were saving of solvent and glassware, and absence of emulsion formation. The Extrelut (kieselgur) cartridges showed no batch-to-batch variations, but did in initial work give a large interfering peak, corresponding to 10-20 ng/ml of **I**. This could be reduced to ~0.3 ng/ml by pre-washing the Extrelut with methanol and CH_2Cl_2 before use (Fig. 1).

Hydrolysis and derivatization.- Since 2 M NaOH gave complete conversion of **I** to **II** at 100° in 30 min, compared with 2.5 h for 2 M HCl, it was the preferred agent. The hydrolysate had to be adjusted finally to pH 9.5, the optimum for the very rapid reaction of **II** with OPA. A major problem was the instability of **III** (degradation 20%/h in the HPLC injection solution), necessitating injection within 10 min of the initiation of the derivatization. This precluded use of auto-injectors in their normal operating mode (but see later).

Chromatography.- For conditions see legend to Fig. 3; the mobile phase was methanol/phosphate buffer (pH 5). The composition of the injection medium is a compromise between chromatographic requirements and the stability of the isoindole. Generally, as has long been recognized, the greater the polarity difference between the injection solution and the mobile phase, the greater the danger of peak asymmetry, leading in the worst case to double peaking. For **III** this is a particularly acute problem, since the stability of the isoindole is maximized in the reaction mixture (little loss in 1 h) if the ratio of the organic component (alcohol) to aqueous component (borate buffer) is 3:1 by vol., whereas the losses are 15% and near 100% with ratios of 5:3 and 1:3 respectively. Similarly, when the organic/aqueous component ratio is kept constant (9:1) but the polarity of the organic component is altered, stability is affected (illustrated in [4]): thus, with a 3 h reaction time, the >15% loss with methanol as the sole organic component was minimized if almost half of the methanol were replaced by ethanol or, better, dioxan; pH 8.0 in place of pH 9.5 borate buffer aggravated the loss.

The actual injection solution finally adopted was a 1:1 mixture of methanol and neutralized hydrolysate, entailing sacrifice of stability in favour of good chromatography. If, for example, stability were maximized by using 4:5:1 methanol/ethanol/pH 9.5 aq. borate as injection solution, with methanol/phosphate buffer (pH 7.4) as mobile phase, double peaks were observed (Fig. 2).

Fig. 2. Incompatibility of injection solution with mobile phase: 2 peaks from III. RP-8 Lichrosorb column. See Fig. 3 legend; 1.0 ml/min.

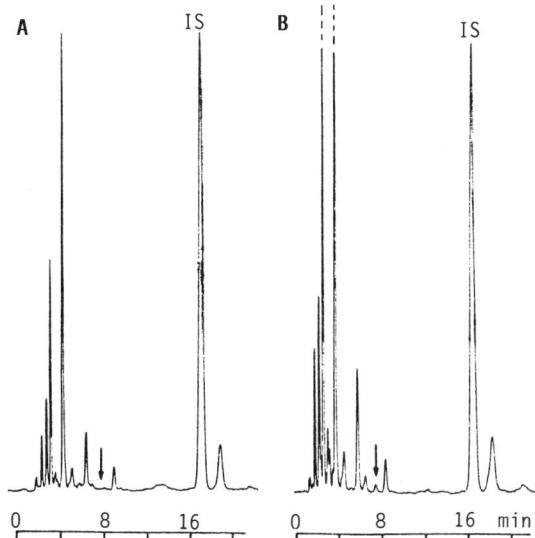

Fig. 1. **A:** Reagent blank chromatogram: residue from evaporation of the CH_2Cl_2 was subjected to the hydrolysis conditions and then the derivatization procedure. **B:** Extrelut blank chromatogram: 1 ml water applied to pre-washed Extrelute column, then elution with 3 × 5 ml CH_2Cl_2; thereafter as for **A.** *Arrows:* retention time of **III;** this peak in **B** is equivalent to 0.3 ng/ml of **I.** IS = internal std.
[Acknowledgement in Fig. 3 legend

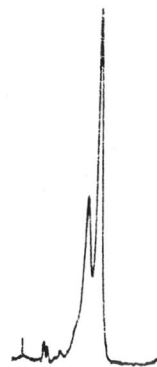

Quantification.- A rather large sample may be required if an endogenous component is determined by spiking standards into aliquots of the sample. Instead, we used aqueous standards for calibration – which is valid if the recovery from aqueous solutions is shown to be the same as from the biological matrix. With the two approaches we obtained virtually identical calibration curves, the respective mean intercepts corresponding to 9.4 and 9.7 ng/ml of plasma sample.

As no internal standard was found that could be taken through the whole procedure, the *N*-4-hydroxybutyl counterpart of **III** was added after the Extrelut extraction step, prior to hydrolysis. This compensated for any manipulative losses beyond the extraction stage, as well as for any variations during derivatization. Despite the lack of an internal standard during extraction, good precision and accuracy was observed over one month in assays with quality-control samples, spiked with **I** over the range 5-2000 ng/ml: the observed values (corrected for endogenous **I**) showed only small deviations from the spike values, e.g. -2%, -6% and +0.7% for 5, 100 and 2000 ng/ml respectively. The limit of detection (3 times blank value, for aqueous standards) was 1 ng/ml, and the limit was 2.5 ng/ml for satisfactory quantification.

Fig. 3. HPLC patterns:
A: blank human plasma;
B: blank dog plasma.
Arrows indicate the peak
corresponding to **III**,
equivalent to 5.0 ng/ml
in **A** and 2.5 ng/ml in **B**.
Standard conditions
(see text also): 250 ×
4 mm i.d. column, 5 μm
Hypersil ODS; mobile
phase methanol/0.1 M
pH 5 phosphate buffer
(45:50 by vol.); detec-
tion by fluorescence
(340/450 nm); flow-rate
1.0 ml/min.

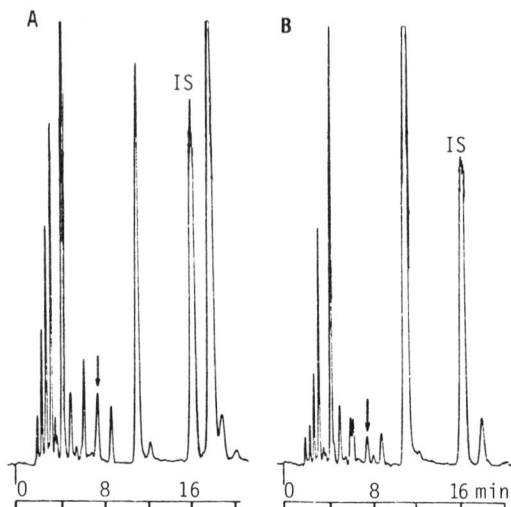

ASSAY APPLICATION AND POSSIBLE IMPROVEMENTS

For plasma samples from 12 different human subjects a mean
concentration of 8.3 ±2.3 ng/ml was found, as compared with 6.1±2.6
ng/ml obtained by GC-MS. Representative patterns are shown in Fig.
3 for human and dog plasma, with the HPLC conditions in the legend.

It would be helpful to use an autoinjector of a type now on
the market that allows automatic pre-mixing of reagents and substrate
for derivatization followed by immediate injection onto the HPLC
column, thus allowing unstable derivatives to be analyzed. Closer
investigation of the hydrolysis step is warranted, to avoid the need
for pH adjustment before derivatization. An internal standard which
could be carried through the whole method is desirable.

Acknowledgements

The authors thank Drs. Eric Bandle and Michael Wall for their
advice and helpful discussions.

References

1. Mori, A., Katayama, Y., Matsumoto,M. & Takeuchi, H. (1975) *IRCS
    Medical Science: Biochemistry, Neurobiology & Neurophysiology 3,* 590.
2. Callery, P.S., Geelhaar, L.A. & Stogniew, M. (1978) *Biochem.
    Pharmacol. 27,* 2061-2063.
3. Bandle, E.F., Wendt, G., Ranalder, U.B. & Trautmann, K-H. (1984)
    Life Sci. 5, 2205-2212.
4. Dell, D., Wendt, G., Bucheli, F. & Trautmann, K-H. (1985) *J.
    Chromatog. 344,* 125-136.

#NC(A)-3

A Note on

DETERMINATION OF PROSTAGLANDINS, PROSTAGLANDIN ANALOGUES AND LEUKOTRIENES IN BIOLOGICAL SAMPLES

M.V. Doig and J.A. Salmon

Wellcome Research Laboratories
Beckenham, Kent BR3 3BS, U.K.

Prostaglandins and leukotrienes are a family of biologically active compounds known as the eicosanoids. They are generated from unsaturated fatty acids, the main precursor being arachidonic acid (eicosa-5,8,11,14-tetraenoic acid). The eicosanoids are produced and found in most tissues of the body, and their diverse biological activities and possible role in human disease processes have received much attention within the pharmaceutical industry.

To define and elucidate their role in human disease and to investigate the role of various inhibitors, it is important to be able to detect and quantify these compounds in a variety of tissues. The normal physiological levels of the eicosanoids are ~3 pmol/g (~1 ng/ml); hence highly sensitive and specific assays are required. Examples are given below of the application of RIA, HPLC and GC-MS in the detection and quantification of these compounds.

Examples of products that arise from arachidonic acid are shown in Fig. 1. Bioassays were used initially for many of the metabolites. In fact, bioassays were crucial in the discovery of the prostaglandin endoperoxides (PGG_2 and PGH_2), thromboxane A_2 (TXA_2), PGI_2 and leukotrienes (LTB_4, LTC_4, LTD_4, LTE_4). Some of the bioassays are used for quantification, e.g. platelet aggregation/deaggregation for TXA_2 and PGI_2 [1] and leucocyte aggregation for LTB_4 [2]. Care must be taken when using these bioassays because biological samples usually contain a mixture of other biologically active components; these may modify the eicosanoid's response, and this lack of specificity can yield inaccurate results.

Another technique that is sensitive but may entail problems with specificity is RIA. RIA's for several PG's, PG metabolites, hydroxy acids and LT's have been described [3, 4]. The requisite

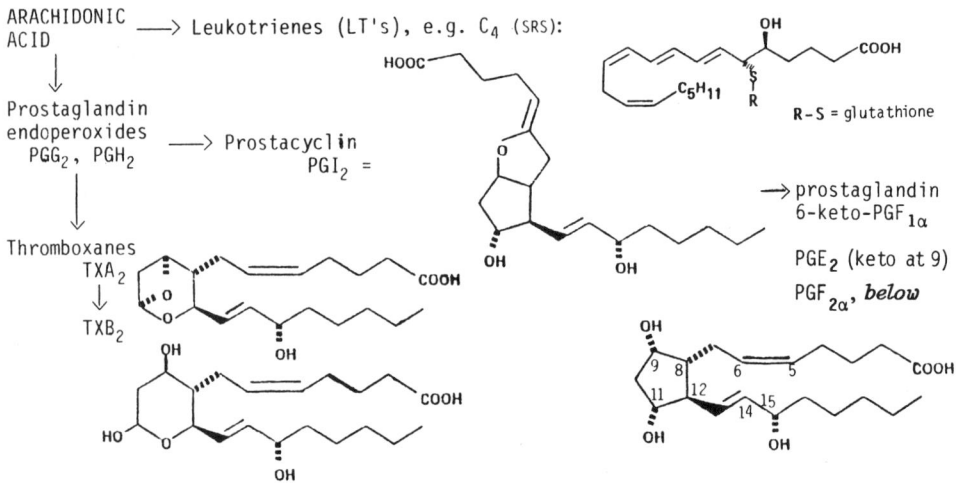

Fig. 1.   Some products that arise from arachidonic acid.

reagents are specific antibody (Ab), standard unlabelled eicosanoid and radiolabelled eicosanoid.

RIA OF EICOSANOIDS

Obtaining the Ab.- Eicosanoids are not antigenic and must first be coupled to an antigenic molecule, e.g. bovine serum albumin (BSA), γ-globulin or keyhole limpet haemocyanin. The conjugation of the eico-sanoid's free carboxyl group with the protein's free amino groups is done using either a water-soluble carbodiimide, e.g. 1-ethyl-3-(3-dimethylaminopropyl)carbodiimide, or a mixed anhydride reaction. The latter method is recommended for acid-labile compounds, e.g. PGE$_2$. With LT's that contain amino acids (C$_4$, D$_4$ and E$_4$) there is a choice of conjugation site. Conjugation via the carboxyl group yields Ab's that do not differentiate between these LT's; however, increased specificity has been achieved by coupling the free amino group to the protein.

The Ab's are produced by injecting into rabbits (weekly for 4 weeks, then monthly booster injections for 3-6 months) the conju-gates emulsified in Freund's complete adjuvant. Blood is collected from the marginal ear vein 7-12 days after booster injections, and is allowed to clot. The Ab-containing serum is kept frozen or freeze-dried.

Unlabelled eiconasoid.- In the past, investigators have had to biosynthesize eicosanoids or rely on the generosity of fellow-investi-gators (particularly the Upjohn Co.). However, most of the eicosanoids are now available from commercial sources (e.g. Sigma).

Radiolabelled eicosanoid.- Most of the RIA's utilize ³H-eicosan-
oids. Some are biosynthesized from [³H]arachidonic acid, and others
are available commercially from Amersham International or New England
Nuclear. A few investigators have used ¹²⁵I [5].

Assay procedure

The reagents are diluted in the RIA buffer, e.g. Tris-HCl or
phosphate-buffered saline (PBS), containing 0.1% gelatin and 0.1% Na
azide or 0.01% thiomersal; pH 7.4-8.6. Radiolabelled eicosanoid is
added to give ~10,000 dpm. The Ab is diluted so that ~50% of added
radiolabelled antigen is bound in the absence of unlabelled compound.
The antigen-Ab complexes are left to equilibrate overnight at 4°.
The free eicosanoid is removed by adding dextran-coated charcoal,
and the radioactivity in the clear supernatant containing the complexes is measured.

Validation.- The specificity of the antiserum is assessed by
comparing, on a weight basis, the amounts of the eicosanoid analyte
and of related compounds that cause 50% inhibition of the binding
of radiolabelled ligand. However, even a compound with low cross-
reactivity could affect an assay if present in a sample in great excess.
Consequently further validation should be performed by extraction
and chromatographic separation of the eicosanoid analyte before
RIA, to compare the data with those from direct assay. Direct RIA
results should also be compared with those from other types of assay
such as GC-MS.

GC-MS ASSAY

Prior to GC-MS assay, biological samples have to be purified.
Initially this was achieved by protein precipitation and solvent
extraction [4]. Recently these techniques have been superseded
by solid-phase extraction [6]. Once extracted, the samples must be
derivatized. The most robust procedures for the eicosanoids are to
form their methyl ester, methoxime, trimethylsilyl ethers [7].
These derivatives are stable for at least 6 weeks if stored desiccated
at room temperature. They have C-values within the range 23.5-25.0
and are normally chromatographed on a methyl silicone stationary
phase, with quantitation by selective ion monitoring. [In Vol. 7
of this series, T.A. Baillie discussed GC-MS assay of PGF-M, a urinary
metabolite whose extraction and clean-up is not easy.-*Ed*.]

HPLC ASSAY

HPLC is not normally used for assaying PG's and TX's since
they do not have a good natural chromophore. HPLC is, however,
applicable to LT's (example in Fig. 2) since the conjugated triene
in their structure gives strong UV absorption at 260, 270 and 280 nm.

Fig. 2. HPLC of LTB$_4$ and LTB$_5$, on a Spherisorb S5 ODS column. Mobile phase: methanol/water/acetic acid (65:35:0.01, v/v) adjusted to pH 5.7; 0.8 ml/min. Amount of LTB injected: 100 ng of each.

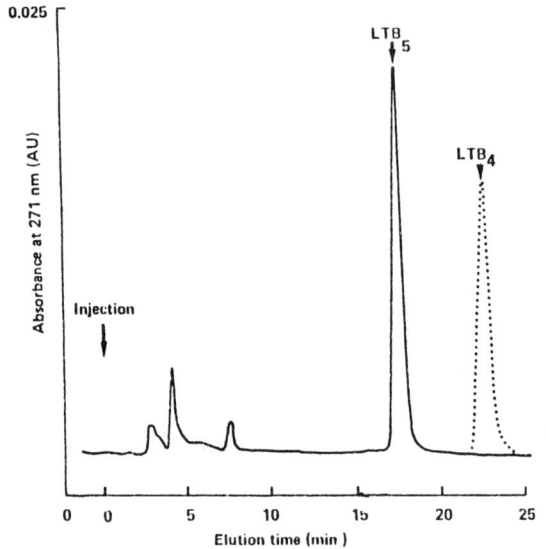

CONCLUDING REMARKS

Bioassays, RIA, HPLC and GC-MS can all provide valuable analytical data. In fact, since each approach has advantages and limitations, data from one assay should be used to complement the information provided by other assays. Thus, compounds of biological relevance can be detected by bioassays and their structures elucidated by GC-MS. Although bioassay, HPLC and GC-MS can be used for quantification, RIA's are probably the method of choice for routine measurements because of their sensitivity and convenience. However, development and validation of RIA's can be a lengthy process.

References

1. Moncada, S., Ferreira, S.H. & Vane, J.R. (1978) *Adv. Prostaglandin Thromboxane Res. 5*, 211-236.
2. Ford-Hutchison, A.W., Bray, M.A., Doig, M.V., Shipley, M.E. & Smith, M.J.H. (1980) *Nature 286*, 264-265.
3. Salmon, J.A., Simmons, P.M. & Palmer, R.M.J. (1982) *Prostaglandins 24*, 225-235.
4. Salmon, J.A. & Flower, R.J. (1983) in *Hormones in Blood*, 3rd edn., Vol. 3 (Gray, C.H. & James, V.H.T., eds.), Academic Press, New York, pp. 137-165.
5. Dray, F. (1982) *Metho. Enzymol. 86*, 297-306.
6. Powell, W.S. (1980) *Prostaglandins 20*, 947-957.
7. Cockerill, A.F., Mallen, D.N.B., Osborne, D.J., Boot, J.R. & Dawson, W. (1977) *Prostaglandins 13*, 1033-1042.

#NC(A)-4

A Note on

DYNORPHIN-(1-9) AND ENKEPHALIN STUDIES WITH VAS DEFERENS*

**Michael J. Rance, Lynne Miller, John S. Shaw
and ⊗John R. Traynor**

Bioscience Dept. II
ICI Pharmaceuticals
 Division, Alderley Park
Macclesfield SK10 4TG, U.K.

⊗Department of Chemistry
University of Technology
Loughborough
Leics. LE11 3TU, U.K.

Neuropeptides commonly occur in families of closely related sequences, possibly generated by the same gene product. Thus, with opioid peptides 3 distinct pro-hormones are processed to >20 peptides, all biologically active and containing the Tyr-Gly-Gly-Phe sequence. There are similar examples in the tachykinin and gastrin/CCK areas. Such structural similarities obviously complicate assay attempts, especially bioassay by a non-specific technique. Post-secretory processing can not only inactivate peptides in bioassay systems, giving an underestimate of potency, but can generate new bioactive peptides which may have substantially different properties. Caution is needed in neuropeptide bioassay, as in an organ assay now used (mouse vas deferens, electrically stimulated) for studying the inhibitory action of dynorphin-(1-9) (DYN) for which ICI 174864$^{\emptyset}$ is an antagonist: DYN (which is κ-selective) is converted *in vitro* to [Leu^5]-enkephalin (LE) which has little κ-affinity but shows δ-receptor selectivity [1]. The following amplification deals particularly with HPLC procedures used in the study.

The vas deferens slices were incubated at 37° in the presence of 100 nM ^{3}H-DYN and, in some experiments, 4 peptidase inhibitors [2]: 30 μM bestatin, 0.3 μM thiorphan, 10 μM captopril and 2 mM Leu-Leu. After 2.5 min a 400 μl aliquot was centrifuged (13,000 **g**, 1 min) and the supernatant quickly frozen in liquid N$_2$ and stored at 20°. For HPLC, marker peptides for which electrochemical (EC) detection furnished the peak positions were added to 100 μl aliquots as loaded. The null volume glassy-carbon EC detector cell was set at 1.0 V. Fractions (1 ml) were collected for scintillation counting. Other RP-HPLC conditions are stated in the legend to Fig. 1, which represents a typical primary run and the re-runs needed for two peaks.

---

* based on a Forum abstract and on ref. [1] as excerpted by Editor.
$\emptyset$ *N,N*-diallyl-Tyr-Aib-Aib-Phe-Leu-OH

Fig. 1. HPLC of products from ^{3}H-DYN, incubated without peptidase inhibitors. Column: 5 μm Ultrasphere ODS (Altex), 150 × i.d. 4.6 mm. Mobile phase, pH 2.7: 50 mM NaH$_2$PO$_4$ containing 1 mg/ml H$_3$PO$_4$, 5% (v/v) methanol, and acetonitrile; 1 ml/min. ^{3}H-recoveries ascertained on fractions.

A, primary run, with 17% acetonitrile. **B**, re-run of Peak 1 with 12% acetonitrile, to resolve the mixture. **C**, re-run of Peak 2 without acetonitrile, to resolve the mixture. Identifications were as follows, with % recoveries (and % in presence of inhibitors), the ^{3}H-DYN purity at zero time being 92%:
- present in peak **1**,
a: HTyrOH, 14; **b**, HTyrGlyGlyPheOH, 8.5 (10); **c**, HTyrGlyOH, no detectable ^{3}H; & *impurity*, 6;
- present in peak **2**,
d, HTyrGlyGlyPheOH, 9; **e**, LE-Arg^6-Arg^7, 10 (2 for **d** + **e**);
- peak **3**, LE-Arg^6, 9.5 (22);
- peak **4**, DYN, 16 (30);
- peak **5**, LE, 32 (36);
- peak **6**, dynorphin-(1-8), 0.3 (0.3).

For recovery S.E.M.'s see ref.[1], in which a similar Fig. appears.

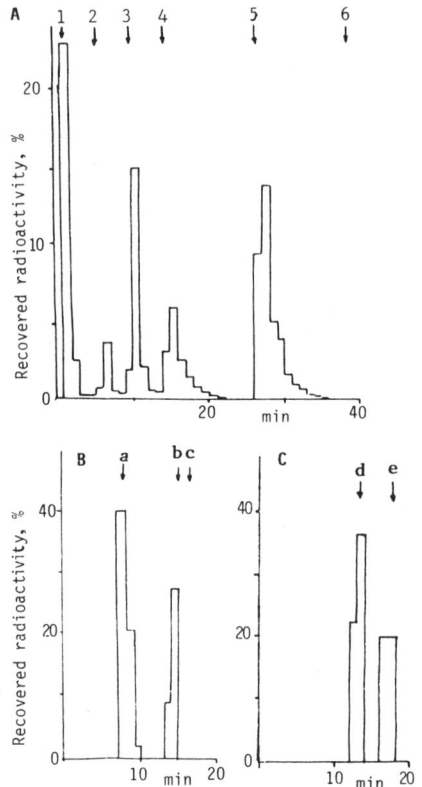

The major conclusion, for vas deferens at least, is that the inhibitory effects of DYN are largely mediated by degradation to LE, which in turn acts through δ-receptors [1]; LE was in fact the main degradation product (Fig. 1). Since peptidase inhibitors did not affect LE formation, possibly DYN is cleaved directly at the Leu^5-Arg^6 bond to yield LE and at the Arg^6-Arg^7 bond to yield LE-Arg^6; however, the amount of the latter was very small with the inhibitor 'cocktail' present, suggesting protection (by captopril and Leu-Leu) from attack at the C-terminus that may be attributable to non-specific endopeptidases. Reported differences in regional distribution between the dynorphin and enkephalin systems in brain indicate that generalizations would be unwise.

References

1. Miller, L., Rance, M.J., Shaw, J.C. & Traynor, J.R. (1985) *Eur. J. Pharmacol. 116*, 159-163.
2. McKnight, A.T., Corbett, A.D. & Kosterlitz, H.W. (1983) *Eur. J. Pharmacol. 86*, 393-402. *(The citation in 1. has minor errors.)*

Comments on material in #A

Comments on #**A-3**, J.A. Smith - HPLC OF GROWTH FACTORS

I.D. Wilson: do you 'pickle' the column and pumps in order to prevent salt corrosion by halides (chloride)? **Reply by J.A. Smith:** we pickle pumps annually with conc. nitric acid; columns seem reasonably resistant, but checking is warranted. **Query by S.H. Curry:** what is the origin and significance of your choice of highly halogenated ion-pairing agents? **Reply.-** Many years ago, TFA and TCA were (and still are) standard protein precipitants. When the protein was resuspended in water, residual TFA or TCA was present, and this, as it happened, made chromatography possible without adding an ion-pairing agent. When it was found that chromatography could not be performed in water/organic solvents alone, TFA or TCA was reintroduced. We chose to use the higher analogues, which were analogous and enabled us to examine the principles behind the ion-pair effect, besides being readily available. **Question by R.F. Venn.-** Is it necessary to clean up the ion-pair agents, e.g. HFBA, prior to use - especially with UV or fluorescence detection? **Answer.-** For steep but not shallow gradients it may indeed be necessary to clean up, suitably with C-18 BondElut and alumina; but with PDFOA no clean-up is needed. **Comment from A. Hulshoff** on choice of additives: fluorinated carboxylic acids are much stronger acids than the non-fluorinated analogues; therefore they can be used over a wider pH range as anionic ion-pairing agents. **Answer to query by J.G. Ratcliffe** on HPLC of glycoproteins and activity survival.- Glycoproteins can be chromatographed by any of the HPLC systems. Even with RP-HPLC, β-HCG and Ig have been run successfully. The limitations are that if the carbohydrate side-chains are heterogeneous, then the apparent efficiency of chromatography will be low and, as with any type of protein, some glycoproteins may be irreversibly denatured by the solvents used. This must be determined for each protein; but activity was in fact retained in the examples presented.

Comments on #**A-4**, G.W. Bennett - NEUROPEPTIDES BY HPLC-EC

G.W. Bennett, answering I.W. Wainer: where RP-HPLC of a single protein gave two peaks, we have no information on the nature of the difference; it could be conformational. **Suggestion by R. Whelpton.-** If you were to put the guard cell **post**-column [**response:** to be tried when we have a new gradient elution system and guard cell in operation], then you can have this cell at 0.4 V and the other two electrodes at 0.6 and 0.9 V for your ratio check of purity. Also, with both analytical electrodes at the same potential you might be able to use the difference mode and perform some simple gradient elution. **Question by K.G. McFarthing.-** Have you applied EC detection to the direct measurement of peptides such as ACTH and IGF-I which are associated with binding proteins in plasma? **Reply.-** ACTH fragments have indeed been measured, but the technique has mostly been applied to small peptides. Folding of large peptides may obscure tyrosine and tryptophan residues (**comment by McFarthing:** binding proteins will probably have the same effect).

G.W. Bennett, answering H. Frank.- We have not investigated whether the EC detector in the reductive mode is responsive to cystine; however, the sensitivity of the glassy-carbon EC detector is very low. **Comments from A. Hulshoff.-** Higher conversion of the analyte that is obtainable with the Coulochem detector does not necessarily mean that detector sensitivity is better than with other (non-coulo-metric) types; other factors, such as cell geometry, can play a very important role. Concerning peak homogeneity, it may be wrong to infer this from finding, with measurement at two potentials, the same ratio of signals for 'pure' standard and an analyte in a biological sample. Another protein with the same retention time and the same electroactive group (e.g. tyrosine) might be present without causing a shift in the signal ratio (similar voltammogram, the electroactive group being the same). **Remarks by R. Schmid.-** Working with the same EC detector (not for peptide measurements), we have found that the EC turnover is not near 99%, but is only ~40% or even lower. If one sets the two electrodes at the same potential, one can still measure with the second electrode.

R.D. McDowall, concerning the signal-to-noise ratios of EC detectors.- We find similar ratios for the BAS and Coulochem detectors, and therefore similar sensitivities for a particular analyte; but the Coulochem is a more robust instrument. In studying hot TFA hydrolysis of sulphated tyrosine, EC detection could have helped [**reply:** not tried]: with the first electrode set at +0.8 V to hydrolyze the conjugate and the second at 0.0 V, measuring the conversion back to tyrosine, the signal would be proportional to the amount of sulphated tyrosine originally present. **G.W. Bennett, answering Susan Fowles:** we have not ascertained what sensitivity decrease would result from using a normal C-18 column rather than the Waters radial compression type.

Comments on #**A-5,** J.M. Conlon - NEUROKININS BY HPLC/RIA
          & *on* #**A-6,** R.F. Venn - RIA OF PRECURSOR-PEPTIDE CRYPTIC REGIONS

Replying to a question, **J.M. Conlon** said that blister fluid does contain SPLI. **R.F. Venn, answering M.J. Rance:** we do not know the role of the unstable enkephalin peptides that are generated in the adrenal medulla. **Question by A. Electricwala:** does CSF or plasma contain any peptides, besides the opioid type, that are involved in pain regulation? **R.F. Venn's reply:** almost any neurotransmitter may be involved because of the complex nature of pain perception; plasma or even CSF may represent an overflow pool and not necessarily be relevant.

Comments on #A-7, K.G. McFarthing et al.- DEFINED TRACERS FOR RIA

   W.N. Jenner asked how indirect ^{125}I-labelling methods, e.g. Bolton & Hunter reagent, compared with direct oxidative methods. **K.G. McFarthing's reply.-** Direct methods can be used to specifically label lysine residues and N- and C-terminal amino acids, advantageously if there were several tyrosines in the peptide or if it was desirable to label the peptide in a specific position. **Comment by Jenner:** presumably in some cases the use of the indirect methods for iodination could reduce immunoreactivity because of the structural changes associated with the introduction of labelled moiety into the peptide structure.

   Remarks by R. Dimaline.- You have indeed been able to produce a range of HPLC-purified monoiodinated peptides of high s.a. and excellent stability. We usually use HPLC purification for our own radiolabels, but there are some instances where this may not be the method of choice. We purify radiolabelled gastrin (G17) by ion-exchange on aminoethylcellulose resin, gaining monoiodinated G17 of maximum theoretical s.a. and with full biological activity. The advantage of this chromatography is that we use a high-pH ammonium carbonate buffer that does not expose the highly acidic G17 molecule to the ion-pairing buffers of very low pH that are often used in RP-HPLC. **McFarthing's response.-** I agree that the acidic conditions produced by the type of ion-pairing reagents described by J.A. Smith [above] may be unsuitable for acidic peptides such as gastrin, and under these circumstances other techniques may have to be explored. Also, with larger peptides the secondary structure is very important, and HPLC conditions will disrupt it. Whether the peptide re-folds correctly should be ascertained empirically, with testing for the tracer's desired activity in RIA or RRA.

Comments on #A-8, R. Dimaline - RIA OF PRECURSOR-PEPTIDE CRYPTIC REGIONS
       & *#A-9*, J.D. Teale - SOMATOMEDIN RIA

   J.M. Conlon asked R. Dimaline whether use of his C-terminally directed antisera demonstrated that the pairs of basic residues flanking the cryptic sequences are completely removed in the tissues. **Reply.-** I think we can say that they are removed. The synthetic analogues of the cryptic peptides that we used as immunogens did not include these C-terminal basic residues. Since the antisera did not recognize natural cryptic peptide sequences in tissue extracts, then at least some of the natural material must have had the basic residues removed. **J.D. Teale, answering J.A. Smith:** our Ab's against IGF-I were polyclonal, and needed ~100 µg IGF-I to raise them although sometimes it suffices to use 10-20 µg, coupled to a carrier such as BSA or IgG.

Comments on #**A-10**, J.G. Ratcliffe - PEPTIDE HORMONES BY IMA

J. Tomašić asked about iodination procedures used for labelling Ab's and a possible effect of using chloramine T on the hapten-binding capacity of the Ab. **Reply by J.G. Ratcliffe.-** A wide range of iodination techniques can be used successfully for labelling Ab's. We have routinely used the chloramine T method, aiming with success to substitute no more than one iodine atom per molecule of Ab. Higher incorporations can lead to loss of immunoreactivity. **Replies to questions by R.F. Venn.-** The titres were indeed low in mouse MAb's, ~1:200 in mice prior to fusion. Concerning the smallest length of peptide assayable by 2-site IMA's, one would guess that a minimum of 10-12 amino acids is needed; theoreticians could tell us more.

M. Uihlein enquired concerning the definition of 'noise', in the context of the limit of detection being reckoned as 7 µg/ml whereas signal:noise = 2 at 10 µg/ml. **The reply** cited the IFCC recommendations on quality criteria, and **S.H. Curry added** that earlier vols. in the series are pertinent, particularly Vol. 10. **J.G. Ratcliffe further remarked** that the detection limit depends on precision of measurement as well as on the signal:background ratio.

Comments on #**NC(A)-2**, D. Dell - ASSAY OF 2-PYRROLIDONE (ENDOGENOUS)

Question by H. Frank.- Have you investigated whether, after the relatively simple work-up and the fairly complicated derivatization, a simple capillary-GC approach using an A-FID (NPD) might be preferable? **D. Dell's reply:** probably not feasible, since GC experts would predict poor sensitivity since the pyrrolidinone nitrogen is of amide type. **H. Frank also suggested** that, in relation to GC decomposition of the derivative, it would be preferable to find a GC system that could separate the GABA underivatized and perform on-line derivatization post-column. **Reply.-** Whereas our method entails the RP approach, amino acid separation would need anion-exchange separation, which is slower and gives poorer chromatography — and ~10 times poorer sensitivity (using OPA), as **R. Schmid remarked. Suggestion by A.A. Gulaid, agreed by D. Dell:** since the solid-phase extraction yield of the compound is 100%, column switching or back-flushing might be advantageous.

Comments on #**NC(A)-3**, M.V. Doig - PG's, LT's; & **-4**, M.J. Rance - PEPTIDES

J.E.H. Stafford asked M.V. Doig whether RIA specificity suffices for PG's assayed directly rather than pre-processed. **Reply:** some samples can be assayed direct, but if we encounter cross-reactivity problems during validation we purify the samples prior to RIA.

M.V. Doig's reply to a further question: although the BondElut column is washed with methanol/water and then with petroleum ether, we do not encounter immiscibility problems because the system is under vacuum and the column is 'sucked dry' between the two solvents. **Answer to query by A. Hulshoff** on the GC-MS assay: pre-GC derivatization of the carbamyl groups in the molecules is necessary because we have experienced thermal degradation and poor chromatography when analyzing eicosanoids with underivatized carbamyl groups. **R.F. Venn, to M.J. Rance.-** Do you think the various opioid receptors are biochemically different or are just pharmacological entities? **Reply:** there is good biochemical evidence for μ, δ and σ, but doubts about ε [Vol. 15, this series, is pertinent - *Ed.*].

SOME CITATIONS *contributed by* Senior Editor

Peptide separation and determination (*see also end of section*)

A useful sketch [1] of **hydrophobic interaction chromatography** (HIC), in the context of the Beckman-RIIC silica-based polyether matrix which, unlike a soft-gel matrix, is suitable for HPLC, alludes to guidance furnished by traditional salting-out methods when HIC conditions are being chosen for protein separation. A reverse salt gradient is typically used, and reduction of eluent polarity (e.g. by ethylene glycol) can have an advantageous influence on solute-to-matrix hydrophobic interactions.

HPLC separation of proteins on **alkyl-bonded packings** works well with a chain length of C-8 or lower, or with a C-18 packing having very wide pores [2]. Gradient elution with acetonitrile or propanol at acid pH is commonly the best approach. Some results with dynorphin and with forms of human GH are outlined.

Neuroendocrine studies concerned with, for example, oxytocin, vasopressin and neurophysins were performed with alkyl-bonded and ion-exchange HPLC columns [3]. M.T.W. Hearn's group publishes on **HPLC of hormonal peptides:** thus, their Part 47 (!) deals with anion-exchange separation of pituitary proteins [4].

With **three HPLC modes** - RP, cation-exchange and gel permeation; UV detection - vasoactive intestinal peptide (**VIP**) was investigated in guinea-pig enteric nerve [5].

C-peptide assay methodology, generally immunological, has been surveyed in the clinical context [6]. In an RIA procedure developed for **melatonin** ([7]; cf. procedures used in the laboratory of V. Marks), it was extracted by diethyl ether from the biological sample (plasma, urine, CSF, pineal gland) and assayed with a rabbit antiserum.

Exemplifying **MS assay of underivatized peptides,** the applicability of thermospray sample introduction [cf. #NC(D)-5, this vol.] has been demonstrated for a model mixture following RP-HPLC [8].

Opioid peptides

Compounds of this type, whose conformational features have been reviewed [9], can be grouped according to endogenous derivation as amplified in preceding articles:
- from proopiomelanocortin: α-, β- and γ-endorphins ('endogenous morphines');
- from proenkephalin A: leu^5- and met^5-enkephalins, metorphamide/ adrenorphin;
- from prodynorphin or proenkephalin B: dynorphin (1-17, 1-8), rimorphin.
The first 3 amino acids are Try-Gly-Gly in each group. *See also foot of next p. for another review, notably useful for orientation.*

For **β-endorphin, cation-exchange HPLC preceding RIA** improved the sensitivity and specificity of assays on plasma [10]. After deproteinization by acetonitrile, β-endorphin and β-lipotropin were separated by gradient elution with buffers which were removed by freeze-drying before RIA.

Enkephalin assay by MS on HPLC fractions was performed on brain regions, tooth pulp and CSF [11]. Deproteinization was with methanol, rather than acid, to obviate loss by back-exchange of the stable-isotope label (oxygen) in the internal standard added initially. In C-18 separations, preliminary (cartridge) and HPLC, an ion-pairing agent was added to ensure peptide retention. HPLC: the cartridge ethanol-rich eluate (pH 7.5) was chromatographed with the pH set at 3.2 by a volatile buffer (formic acid-triethylamine) with acetonitrile as modifier; detection was at a low UV wavelength. MS-SIM assay was by field desorption (FD) or, for most assays, by fast atom bombardment (FAB) as a gentler approach. The MS techniques on which the novel assay approach relies are well discussed.

References

1. England, E. (1986) *Lab. Pract.* January, 64-65.
2. Patience, R.L. (1985) *Anal. Proc. 22,* 296-297 [cf. *J. Chromatog. 324,* 385-393.
3. Chaiken, I.M., Kanmer, T., Sequeira, R.P. & Swaisgood, H.E. (1984) *J. Chromatog. 336,* 63-71.
4. Stanton, P.G., Simpson, R.J., Lambrou, F. & Hearn, M.T.W. (1983) *J. Chromatog. 266,* 273-276.
5. Murphy, R., Furness, J.B. & Costa, M. (1984) *J. Chromatog. 336,* 41-50.
6. Bonsner, A.M. & Garcia-Webb, P. (1981) *Ann. Clin. Biochem. 18,* 200-206.

7. Brun, J., Claustrat, B., Harthe, C., Vitte, P.A., Cohen, R. &
    Chazot, G. (1985) in *The Pineal Gland: Endocrine Aspects*
    (Brown, G.M. & Wainwright, S.D., eds.), Pergamon, Oxford,
    pp. 41-45.
8. Pilosof, D., Kim, H.Y., Dyckes, F.E. & Vestal, M.L. (1984)
    Anal. Chem. 56, 1236-1240.
9. Rapaka, R.S., Renugopalakrishnan, V. & Bhatnagar, R.S. (1985)
    Internat. Biotech. Lab., October, 10-24.
10. Stenman, U-H., Laatikainen, T., Salminen, K., Huhtala, M-L. &
    Leppäluoto, J. (1984) *J. Chromatog. 297*, 399-403.
11. Desiderio, D.M., Kai, M., Tanzer, F.S., Trimble, J. &
    Wakelyn, C. (1984) *J. Chromatog. 297*, 245-260.

Eicosanoids and various 'natural-type' analytes *(& see overleaf)*

Urinary PGE$_2$ was assayed in rats by eluting (isocratically) PGE$_2$
from a C-18 HPLC column, rendering alkaline, and detecting by absor-
ance at 278 nm [12]. Using model compounds, but envisaging eventual
application to plasma, Cox & Pullen [13] described procedures for
'automated heteromodal column switching' **HPLC of PGE$_2$ derivatives** –
(15R)-methyl-, (15S)-methyl- and 16,16-dimethyl-. Bonded-phase (CN)
and silica columns were used, and the compounds were run as panacyl
esters, with fluorescence detection.

Ion-pair RP-HPLC was used to assay **endogenous polyamines** [14] –
as found in HClO$_4$ extracts of tissues; the eluted analytes were
rendered fluorescent for detection. Ion-pairing was by use of octane
sulphonate.

To assay **N-acetyl-L-glutamate**, e.g. in liver (only 1 mg needed),
the analyte was freed from glutamate by a cation-exchange step
and then itself converted by acylase treatment to glutamate which,
with a fluorophore introduced, was subjected to RP-HPLC [15].

References *(including further citations on* **opioid** *peptides)*

12. Hansen, H.S. & Jensen, B. (1983) *Lipids 18*, 682-690.
13. Cox, J.W. & Pullen, R.H. (1984) *Anal. Chem. 56*, 1866-1870.
14. Seiler, N. & Knodgen, B. (1985) *J. Chromatog. 339*, 45-57.
15. Alonso, E. & Rubio, V. (1985) *Anal. Biochem. 146*, 252-259.

16a. Henderson, G. & McFadzean, I. (1985) *Chem. Brit. 21*, 1094-1097.
16b. Eybalin, M., Cupo, A. & Pujol, R. (1985) *Brain Res. 331*, 389-395.

In [16b], HPLC with RIA was used to investigate Met-enkephalin-Arg6-
Gly7-Leu8 in pig tissues (organ of Corti, cochlea). Immunoelectron
microscopy was also used in this study. Analgesics, e.g. naxolone, as
well as peptides are embraced in a recent outline [16a] of pharmacology (including 'receptor fit'), chemistry and derivation from precursors (pro-enkephalin, -dynorphin and -opiomelanocortin, POMC).

Further citations on **peptides** *and* **eicosanoids**

   RIA measurements on HPLC fractions were used in peptide isola-
tions from biological samples: **IGF-I** from lyophilized human serum,
with initial acetone/ethanol and Sephadex G-50 steps prior to 'FPLC'
[17], and various **neuropeptides** (including angiotensins and opioid
peptides) separated by RP-HPLC with acetonitrile/ammonium triflu-
oroacetate gradient elution [18].   **N-Acetylcysteine** in biological
fluids [cf. #NC(A)-1] was derivatized and assayed by RP-HPLC-UV [19].

   Leukotrienes and **prostaglandins**, with radiolabel derived from
^{14}C-arachidonic acid, were analyzed in lung extracts after solid-
phase (C-18) clean-up, by RP-HPLC with fraction collection for ^{14}C-
measurement and RIA [20].   The columns were C-18 for LT's and C-8 for
PG's, with different mobile phases. In humans given dazmegrel, an
inhibitor of thromboxane synthetase, **prostanoids** were assayed [21]:
TXB_2 was determined in plasma by RIA; 2,3-dinor-TXB_2 was measured in
urine by RIA after C-18 cartridge extraction and RP-HPLC separation;
and 2,3-dinor-6-keto-$PGF_{1\alpha}$ was measured in urine via solvent extraction, derivatization and GC-MS (with, for reference, a deuterated
derivative of the analyte as added to the urine).

   Assay procedures for **eicosanoids** used by M.V. Doig's colleagues
[cf. #NC(A)-3] have been outlined in the context of inflammatory
exudates in the rat as affected by feeding a lipoxygenase inhibitor
[22]. LTB_4, PGE_2 and TXB_2 were each determined directly by specific
RIA. With solid-phase extraction and then RP-HPLC (UV detection;
PGB_3 as i.s.), final RIA showed that LTB_5 - which cross-reacted
17% with LTB_4 - was present as a minor constituent. Triene PG's
were similarly extracted but examined by TLC, on plates impregnated
with AgNO$_3$; scrapings were eluted for RIA, which gave values for
PGE_2 and TXB_2; PGE_3 and TXB_3 were absent. **GC-MS** was the end-step
in determination of PGE_2, $PGF_{2\alpha}$, 6-keto$PGF_{1\alpha}$ and TXB_2, extracted from
plasma at acid pH and separated by NP-HPLC (then derivatized) [23].

References

17. Pfeifle, B., Maier, V. & Ditschuneit, H. (1985) *Prep. Biochem.*
    15, 291-307.
18. Hermann, K., Lang, R.E., Unger, Th., Bayer, C. & Ganten, D.
    (1984) *J. Chromatog. 312*, 273-284.
19. Frank, H., Thiel, D. & Langer, K. (1984) *J. Chromatog. 309*, 261-
    267.
20. Zijlstra, F.J. & Vincent, J.E. (1984) *J. Chromatog. 311*, 39-50.
21. Lorenz, R.L., Fischer, S., Wober, W., Wagner, H.A. & Weber, P.C.
    (1986) *Biochem. Pharmacol. 35*, 761-766.
22. Terano, T., Salmon, J.A., Higgs, G.A. & Moncada, S. (1986)
    Biochem. Pharmacol. 35, 779-785.
23. Schweer. H., Kammer, J. & Seyberth, H.W. (1985) *J. Chromatog.*
    338, 273-280.

Section #B

CNS-ACTIVE DRUGS AND THEIR METABOLITES

#B-1

THIRTY YEARS OF ANTIPSYCHOTIC DRUG ANALYSIS

Stephen H. Curry

Division of Clinical Pharmacokinetics
College of Pharmacy, University of Florida
Gainesville, FL 32610, U.S.A.

Interest in measurement of psychotropic drugs in biological fluids dates back to ~1955, soon after the introduction of chlorpromazine into psychiatry [1]. It was quickly realized that studies of chlorpromazine in regard to its disposition and metabolism, and detection in urine as a means of assessing compliance, would be useful [2]. Early attempts involved UV spectrophotometry and colorimetry, with or without prior derivatization [3]. However, it was not till GC-ECD was applied that sufficient sensitivity for plasma was achieved [4, 5]. Over the years, nitrogen detectors, mass spectrometry (MS) and liquid chromatography have been used [6-12]. Basically, the strategy has had to continuously evolve to keep up with knowledge about metabolites of the drugs concerned [13-20].

Benzodiazepine analysis has been relatively straightforward [21, 22]. Most benzodiazepines are amenable to GC-ECD, offsetting the relatively limited applicability of HPLC. Generally benzodiazepines are not so beset with the problems of non-separability of drugs from one another, and drugs from metabolites, as are phenothiazines and tricyclic antidepressants. Tricyclics were initially measured by isotope derivatization techniques [23], needing prior specific extraction of the drug. GC-NPD was later applied; but again, HPLC with UV-absorption or fluorescence detection has provided a solution to most problems.

Before 1960 most drug analyses involved selective solvent or column extraction and/or selective chemical reaction, and final spectroscopy [4]. Solvent extraction (see this Index entry in past vols. of this series) removed the drug of interest from the biological matrix, and selective reaction conferred colorimetric, spectrophotometric or fluorescent properties on the drug, facilitating detection and quantitation [1]. Although the concept of selective solvent extraction as exemplified in Fig. 1 is still important, the early approaches with a spectroscopic end-step were, in the main, unsuitable for

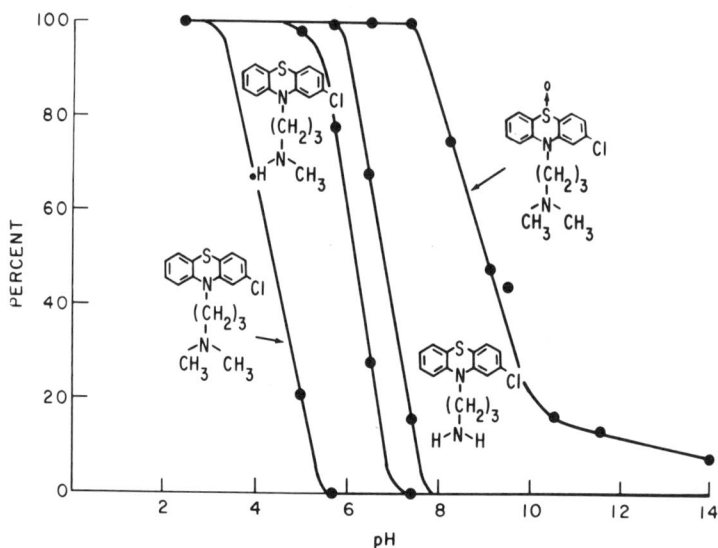

Fig. 1. Extraction of chlorpromazine and 3 of its heptane-extract-able metabolites as a function of pH, as % extracted from heptane containing 1.5% (v/v) isoamyl alcohol into an equal vol. of various buffer solutions. *From ref. [2], by permission.*

centrally-acting drugs of the phenothiazine, imipramine and diazepam types, with the notable exception of butaperazine and nitrazepam, which have been extensively studied with spectroscopic methods [24,25]. Centrally acting drugs are characterized by high lipophilicity and by conversion into numerous metabolites [5], with consequent analytical problems. High lipophilicity leads to tissue binding at the expense of plasma levels which are accordingly low, whilst the plethora of metabolites can cause specificity problems.

With revolutionary changes in analytical technology, systematic study of all three groups of drugs became possible between 1960 and 1970 through the application of isotope-derivative analysis [5], GC [5] and MS [26]. GC-FID was successful only with thioridazine, its dose being relatively high [27]. Moreover, numerous results have emerged from administration of radiolabelled drugs (especially fluphenazine) and from RIA [28, 29]. Such work was stimulated by interest amongst psychiatrists in the concept of psychotropic drug monitoring [8].

The first approach to tricyclic antidepressant assay involved isotope derivative formation (Fig. 2) [23], modelled to some extent on end-group analysis. Desipramine, a secondary-amine metabolite of imipramine marketed as a drug in its own right, was reacted with radio-labelled acetic anhydride as shown, and excess reagent removed; the radioactivity incorporated into the molecule indicated the quantity of drug originally present. A refinement of this was a double-isotope

$$\left.\begin{array}{l} \text{R–N–H} \\ \quad | \\ \quad \text{CH}_3 \\[4pt] plus \text{ trace } (<1\%) \\ \text{of } {}^{14}\text{C-drug} \\[6pt] (*)\text{R–N–H} \\ \quad\quad | \\ \quad\quad \text{CH}_3 \end{array}\right\} \begin{array}{c} (i)\ extract \\ and\ purify \\ \hline \longrightarrow \\ (ii)\ react \\ with\ {}^3H\text{-}acetic \\ anhydride \end{array} \quad \left.\begin{array}{l} \text{R–N–COCH}_3(*) \\ \quad\quad | \\ \quad\quad \text{CH}_3 \\[4pt] and \\[4pt] (*)\text{R–N–COCH}_3(*) \\ \quad\quad\quad | \\ \quad\quad\quad \text{CH}_3 \end{array}\right\} \begin{array}{l} Remove\ excess \\ reagent\ (*)\ by \\ solvent\ extr^n. \\ Separately \\ count\ {}^{14}C\ for \\ recovery\ cor\text{-} \\ rection\ and \\ {}^3H\ for\ assay \end{array}$$

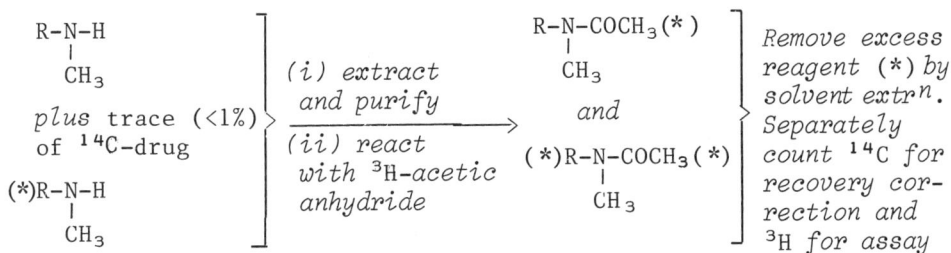

Fig. 2. Strategy for isotope derivative assay of secondary-amine antidepressants, with use of a radiolabelled internal standard (* denotes a labelled atom).

approach (Fig. 2) in which, as a recovery check, a trace of desipramine labelled with a different isotope was added to the biological sample, and extracted along with the unlabelled drug originally in the sample. This approach was very elegant; but it was limited to secondary amines, and most of the commonly prescribed psychotropic drugs are unreactive tertiary amines.

GC-ECD proved highly applicable to phenothiazine and benzodiazepine drugs [5, 21], due to the presence in many of the drugs of chlorine or other halogen atoms. These halogens had been introduced into the molecule during drug development to confer lipophilicity, but they also conferred ECD sensitivity. The same chemical properties led to successful use of packed GC columns from the SE and OV series.

Whilst GC-ECD has remained the method of choice for benzodiazepine analysis for some 15 years, it has waned somewhat in importance in other psychotropic drug assays [11]. This has been due to: (i) the method never having been applicable to non-halogenated, unreactive, tertiary-amine psychotropic drugs, e.g. most antidepressants and some phenothiazines; (ii) low sensitivity and unstable detector response to certain compounds; and (iii) chemical instability of some analytes in GC systems. Concerning (iii), whereas the parent drugs usually survived the high temperatures required for satisfactory chromatography, metabolites did not. In particular, *N*-oxides (tertiary amine oxides) undergo the Cope reaction when heated, decomposing to the parent drug and to the secondary-amine demethylation product. Thus, when present, the *N*-oxides could *inflate* values for the parent drug and for their monodemethylated metabolites; the assay then gave *reduced* values for the important *N*-oxides. For the parent drugs the problem could be overcome by using selective solvent extraction as the initial assay step, but difficulty remained in assaying metabolites. These also included hydroxylated compounds requiring prior derivatization under conditions which tended to decompose them [6].

Fig. 3. GC separation of
amitriptyline (AT), nortriptyline (NT) and chlorpromazine
(CPZ), using alkali-bead
detector (NPD). The drug
mixture was run on an OV-17
column at 250°.

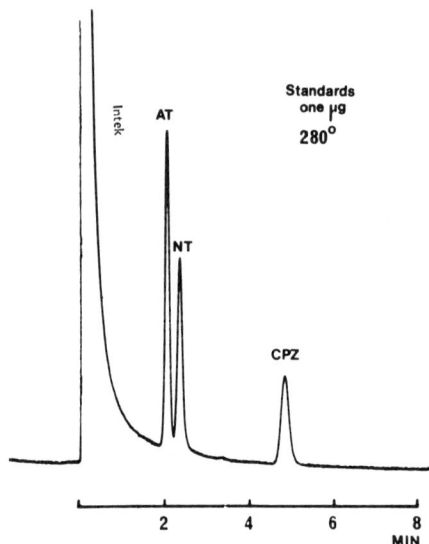

POWERFUL PRESENT-DAY APPROACHES

There was a vogue for use in psychotropic drug analysis of
GC with nitrogen detection (NPD, alkali bead), as illustrated in
Fig. 3. This afforded quite specific detection for non-halogenated
drugs, notably imipramine-type compounds. However, GC-NPD was ec-
lipsed by the remarkably powerful HPLC systems developed late in the 1970-80
decade [e.g. 11-17], as evidenced by articles in this book series.
For tricyclic antidepressants, excellent detection by UV or fluorescence is now obtainable after separation on silica (NP) or RP columns
(C.L. DeVane, #B-3, this vol.). For phenothiazines (cf. K.K. Midha,
#B-4, this vol.) the best separation has been achieved with nitrile-
bonded columns [11]; >10 ng/ml is detectable in a 1 ml sample with
almost any available detector, but lower levels appear to need electrochemical (EC) detection [19, 20].

The most significant aspect of the change from GC to HPLC has
been the minimization of drug decomposition problems. All of the
known and putative chlorpromazine metabolites can be separated from
each other using appropriate column conditions (Fig. 4) [15; cf. 18];
the hydroxylated metabolites can be chromatographed without derivatization. Chlorpromazine **N**-oxide seems not to revert to chlorpromazine
or decompose to demonomethylchlorpromazine in the system, so that in
this case at least, all compounds relevant to clinical monitoring
can be studied in a single extract [11], as now exemplified.

For a patient's sample, Figs. 5a and 5b illustrate the power of
the HPLC approach, tied to selective solvent extraction in the case of
the Fig. 5a chlorpromazine pattern. In contrast, Fig. 5b shows
chlorpromazine plus its important metabolites detected following non-
selective extraction, with a better recovery evident for 'F_2'.

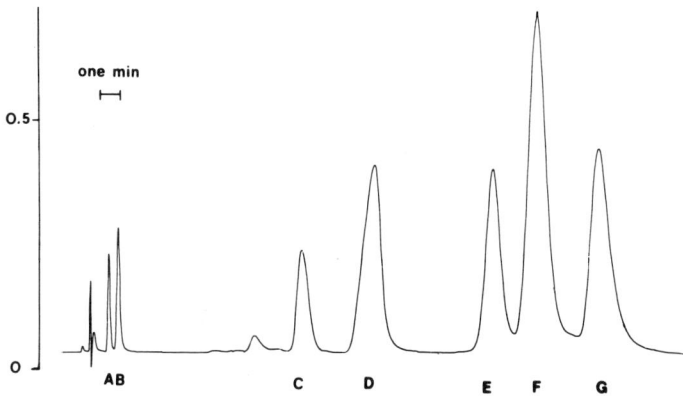

Fig. 4. HPLC separation of 8 chlorpromazine (CPZ) metabolites on a nitrile column. Mobile phase methanol/aq. ammonium acetate (9:1). A, CPZ-*N*-oxide-5-oxide; B, CPZ-*N*-oxide; C, 7-hydroxy-CPZ;   D, CPZ-5-oxide; E, dedimethyl-CPZ; F, dedimethyl-CPZ-5-oxide and (F₂) demonomethyl-CPZ, unresolved; G, demonomethyl-CPZ-5-oxide. UV detection, 254 nm. *Figs. 4-6 are from ref. [15], courtesy of Elsevier.*

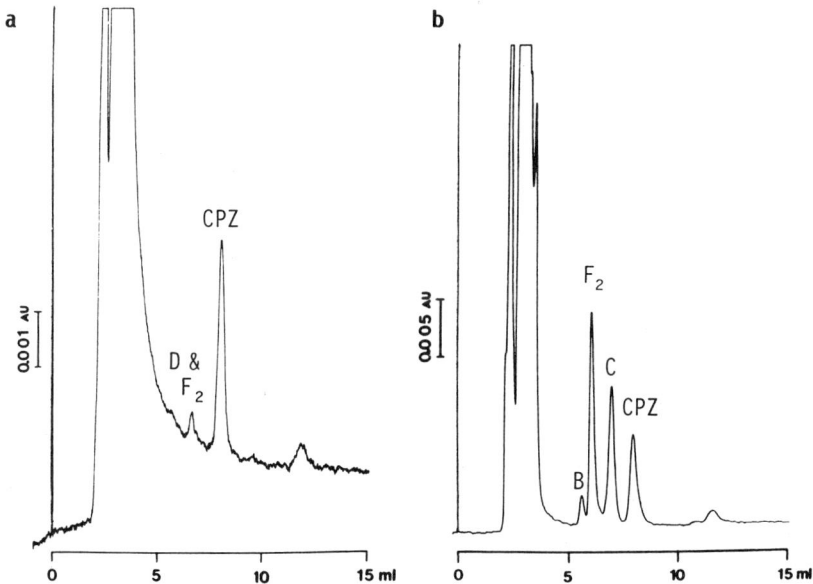

Fig. 5. HPLC separations as in Fig. 4, with same peak-identification letters: 2 ml of plasma from a patient receiving 3×100 mg CPZ/day, ~2 h post-dose. Analytes in a concentrated extract prepared from the plasma sample with (**a**) n-hexane, (**b**) diethyl ether.

Fig. 6.   Retention volume
of haloperidol as affected
by the ammonium acetate
molarity/pH in the mobile-
phase admixture (1:9) with
methanol, on a nitrile
bonded column.

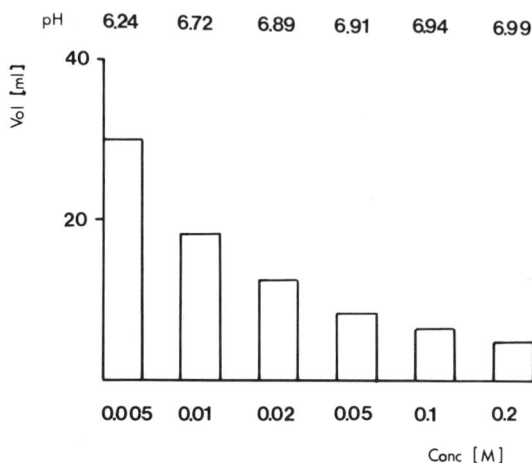

Fig. 6 shows the versatility of HPLC in that the retention
volume of haloperidol varies as a function of the concentration of
the ammonium acetate which, admixed with methanol (1:9), served as
the mobile phase.   One can choose a mobile phase which leads to
a convenient retention volume for any of the neuroleptics.

Mention should be made of the GC-MS combination, as first applied
by Holmstedt and his colleagues [26] in a study of chlorpromazine.
Selective ion monitoring was used, and the term mass fragmentography
was coined.   Excellent specificity and sensitivity were achieved.
More recently [10], trifluoperazine was studied by molecular ion
monitoring, using deuterated trifluoperazine as a cold carrier/MS
internal standard, and traces of radiolabelled trifluoperazine for
the purpose of recovery correction (Fig. 7).   While GC-MS is clearly
applicable to a wide range of research problems, it has not found
application in patient monitoring work [8].

The use of HPLC with EC detection has added considerably to the
sensitivity achievable in the field of antipsychotic drug research.
This is exemplified in Fig. 8 for the assay of a very low concentration
of trimeprazine, a hitherto undetectable drug.

In conclusion, this has been a necessarily brief overview of
the links between the strategy and techniques used during the last
20 years for psychotropic drug analysis.   The overview should be
considered in conjunction with relevant articles, especially CNS-drug
articles that follow, in this book and in preceding volumes of the
analytical subseries [listed opposite title p.- *Ed.*].

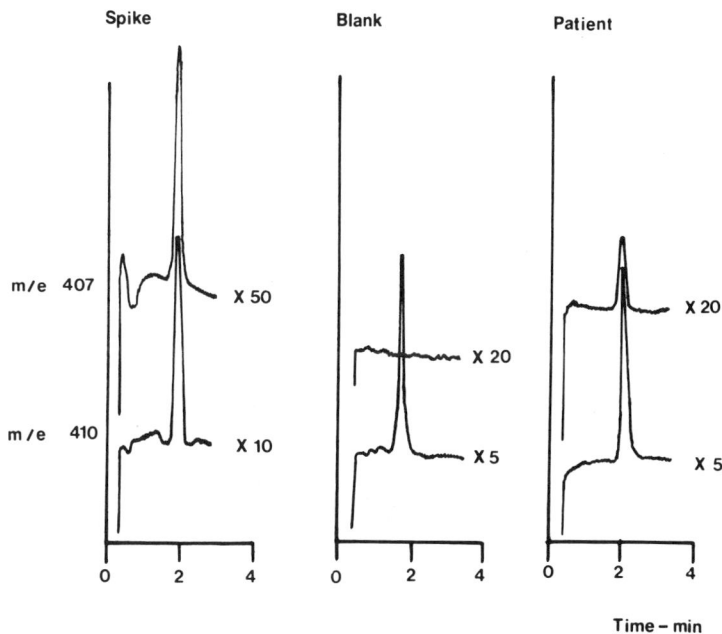

Fig. 7, *above.* GC-MS analysis of
trifluoperazine in plasma (spiked,
blank and post-dose), monitored at
m/z values of 407 (trifluoperazine)
and 410 (trifluoperazine-d_3). *From
ref. [10], courtesy of Elsevier.*

Fig. 8. HPLC with EC (amperometric)
detection: plasma from a patient given
5 mg trimeprazine, 5 h post-dose;
extract prepared with hexane/chloroform
was concentrated for HPLC. Nitrile-
bonded column; methanol/ammonium acetate
(9:1) mobile phase.
The peak at 4.5 min represents the drug,
0.8 ng/ml of plasma.
Imipramine (internal standard) gave a
peak at 6.5 min.
The EC detector was of BAS glassy-
carbon type [cf. D. Perrett's evaluation in Vol. 14, this series - *Ed.*].

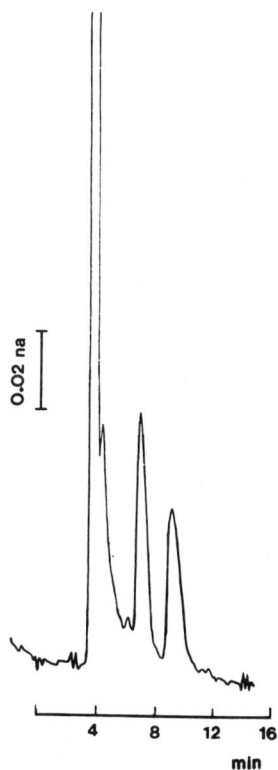

References

1. Salzman, N.P. & Brodie, B.B.(1956) *J. Pharmacol. Exp. Ther.* *118*, 46-54.
2. Forrest, F.M., Forrest, I.S. & Mason, A.S.(1961) *Am. J. Psychiat.* *118*, 300-307.
3. Usdin, E. (1971) *CRC Crit. Rev. Clin. Lab. Sci.* *2*, 347-391.
4. Brodie, B.B. (1967) *J. Am. Med. Assoc.* *202*, 600-609.
5. Curry, S.H. (1968) *Anal. Chem.* *40*, 1251-1255.
6. Curry, S.H. & Evans, S. (1975) *Psychpharm. Comm.* *1*, 481-490.
7. Curry, S.H. & Evans, S. (1976) *J. Pharm. Pharmacol.* *28*, 467-468.
8. Curry, S.H. (1985) *J. Clin. Psychpharmacol.* *1*, 263-271.
9. Javaid, J.I., Dekirmenjian, H., Liskevych, V., Lin, R-I.& Davis, J.M. (1981) *J. Chromatog. Sci.* *19*, 439-443.
10. Whelpton, R., Curry, S.H. & Watkins, G.M. (1982) *J. Chromatog.* *228*, 321-326.
11. Curry, S.H., Brown, E.A., Hu, O. Y-P. & Perrin, J.H. (1982) *J. Chromatog.* *231*, 361-376.
12. Midha, K.K., Loo, J.C.K., Hubbard, J.W., Rowe, M.L. & McGilveray, I.J. (1979) *Clin. Chem.* *25*, 166-168.
13. Butterfield, A.G. & Sears, R.W. (1977) *J. Pharm. Sci.* *66*, 1117-1119.
14. Heyes, W.F. & Salmon, J.R. (1978) *J. Chromatog.* *156*, 309-316.
15. Heyes, W.F., Salmon, J.R. & Marlow, W. (1980) *J. Chromatog.* *194*, 416-420.
16. Eggert-Hansen, C. (1976) *Br. J. Clin. Pharmacol.* *3*, 915-923.
17. Wallace, J.E., Shimek, E.L., Starcharsky, J. & Harris, S.C. (1981) *Anal. Chem.* *53*, 960-962.
18. Stevenson, D. & Reid, E. (1981) *Anal. Lett.* *14(B20)*, 1785-1805.
19. Kissinger, P. (1974) *Anal. Chem.* *46*, 15R-20R.
20. Koch, D. & Kissinger, P.T. (1980) *Anal. Chem.* *52*, 27-29.
21. Garratini, S., Mussini, E. & Randall, L.O., eds. (1973) *The Benzodiazepines*, Raven Press, New York, 685 pp.
22. de Silva, J.A.F. & Puglisi, C.V. (1970) *Anal. Chem.* *42*, 1725-1736.
23. Hammer, W. & Brodie, B.B. (1967) *J. Pharmacol. Exp. Ther.* *157*, 503-508.
24. Smith, R.C., Dekirmenjian, H., Davis, J.M., Crayton, J. & Evans, J. (1977) *Comm. Psychopharmacol.* *1*, 319-324.
25. Rieder, J. (1965) *Arzneim.-Forsch./Drug Res.* *15*, 1134-1148.
26. Hammar, C-G., Holmstedt, B. & Ryhage, R. (1968) *Anal. Biochem.* *25*, 533-543.
27. Curry, S.H. & Mould, G.P. (1969) *J. Pharm. Pharmacol.* *21*, 674-677.
28. Curry, S.H., Whelpton, R., de Schepper, P.J., Vranckx, S. & Schiff, A.A. (1979) *Br. J. Clin. Pharmacol.* *7*, 325-331.
29. Wiles, D.H., Kolakowska, T., McNeilly, A.S., Mandelbrote, B.M. & Gelder, M.G. (1976) *Psychol. Med.* *6*, 407-415.

#B-2

DETERMINATION OF BENZODIAZEPINES: THE PRESENT-DAY SCENE

M. Danhof, J. Dingemanse & D.D. Breimer

Center for Bio-Pharmaceutical Sciences
Division of Pharmacology
University of Leiden, P.O. Box 9503
2300 RA Leiden, The Netherlands

Methods that have been used for determining benzodiazepines in biological fluids include GC, HPLC, direct DPP, RIA and RRA methods*, of which GC, HPLC and RRA have proved the most valuable in clinical research on benzodiazepines. For low concentrations GC is particularly suitable, with ECD and possibly a SCOT column and a solids injector. Some hydroxylated benzodiazepines have to be derivatized. For thermally unstable compounds such as these, HPLC-UV is advantageous, although less sensitive than GC-ECD. HPLC with fluorescence detection is feasible but requires derivatization. HPLC with EC detection has so far been unpromising. HPLC could be useful for drug enantiomers.

RRA's can detect both parent drug and pharmacologically active metabolites, preferably with assay on the sample direct. Especial attention is needed to receptor quality (brain-membrane preparation).

Since their advent in 1960, benzodiazepines have proved valuable due to their anxiolytic, hypnotic, sedative, anticonvulsant, muscle-relaxant and amnestic properties. Whilst they have a common spectrum of pharmacological effects, pharmacokinetic behaviour shows remarkable differences that may be clinically important, and accordingly has been widely studied, with a range of assay procedures. This article discusses those that have been found most valuable in clinical research on benzodiazepines.

PHYSICOCHEMICAL AND PHARMACOLOGICAL PROPERTIES OF BENZODIAZEPINES

The 1,4-benzodiazepine nucleus is common to almost all the drugs concerned:

---

* DPP, differential pulse polarography; RRA, radioreceptor assay; EC, electrochemical.

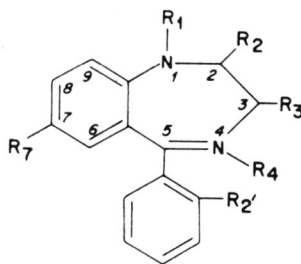

The various derivatives differ in the substituents at the 1, 2,
3, 4, 7 and 2' positions. Generally alkyl substituents are found at
1, hydroxy substituents at 2, 3 and 4, and halogen or nitro substituents at 7 and 2'. Analytically it is convenient to classify the
benzodiazepines into three groups. Class I contains what might be
considered the 'classical' benzodiazepines such as diazepam and
chloridazepoxide. Class II, e.g. oxazepam and temazepam, have a hydroxy
substituent in the 3 position. Class III are the so-called triazolo
and imidazolo(benzo)diazepines, distinctive in having a ring structure
attached to the diazepine moiety at 1 and 2; examples are triazolam
and midazolam.

    Analytically this classification is important for several reasons.
Firstly, the physicochemical properties of the three classes appear
to be somewhat different. Thus, class II compounds appear to be somewhat more polar and are rather unstable thermally, which may impose
constraints on the choice of analytical techniques. Pharmacologically
there are important differences, notably in potency: generally this
appears to be least for class II, the plasma concentrations needed to
get hypnotic action being in the range ~100-1000 ng/ml for oxazepam.
The class I benzodiazepines are of intermediate potency, the requisite
concentrations being ~20-100 ng/ml for nitrazepam, and class III are
the most potent, the concentrations being ~0.1-10 ng/ml for triazolam
and brotizolam. Obviously these potency differences affect the
detection limits needed in analysis and hence the selection of the
analytical method.

    Being lipophilic drugs, benzodiazepines are eliminated from
the body through metabolic conversion in the liver. In this respect
the three classes show notable differences that are analytically
relevant. Compounds of classes I and III are eliminated by metabolic
oxidation, which may result in pharmacologically active metabolites.
For example, diazepam gives rise to the active metabolites *N*-desmethyl-
diazepam (contributing notably to overall pharmacological activity),
oxazepam and temazepam. This emphasizes the need for selective
analytical procedures. On the other hand the class II benzodiazepines
are generally metabolized by conjugation reactions (in particular
glucuronidation), resulting in formation of inactive metabolites;
these do not cause significant analytical interference since they
are very different physicochemically from the parent compounds.

ASSAY TECHNIQUES FOR BENZODIAZEPINES IN BIOLOGICAL MATERIAL

    Techniques that have been used include GC, HPLC, TLC, direct DPP,
RIA, and RRA [1]. In clinical research, GC, HPLC and RRA have proved
especially valuable. [#B-1 by S.H. Curry, this vol., is pertinent.-*Ed*.]

GC assay

    GC-ECD procedures are the most widely used (e.g. [2-4], and
J.A.F. de Silva in Vol. 7, this series). The electronegative halogen or

nitro substituent at position 7 generally confers intrinsic ECD respon-
siveness, possibly improved by a carbonyl at 2 or a halogen at 2'.
Generally speaking, the GC-ECD methods are the most sensitive of
those currently available for benzodiazepines.

Derivatization to improve volatility is best avoided, as has often
proved possible through use of capillary columns. In the earlier
assay methods for underivatized benzodiazepines, support-coated open
tubular (SCOT) columns were used, for some class I and III benzodiazepines [3-5]. Recently, however, other types of capillary column,
e.g. with chemically bonded stationary phases, have been used successfully (unpublished work); hence a capillary column of polarity suitable
for the analyte can be chosen.

An important feature of many assay procedures has been use
of a solids injector, as developed by Driessen & Emonds [6] and
applied to benzodiazepines by de Boer et al. [3]. It consists of a
modified pyrolysis port through which the sample can be introduced
into the GC injection port on a glass-lined stainless steel needle
after evaporation of the solvent in which the residue was originally
dissolved. Such a system offers distinct advantages: a larger
fraction of the extract can be injected, thereby improving assay sensitivity; since the solvent is pre-evaporated the usual prominent
solvent peak is obviated with benefit to retention times and sensitivity; and the capillary-column life is improved since 'chromatography'
of large amounts of solvent is obviated.

Besides the foregoing solid-injection system, the 'falling needle'
solids injector [7] has also proved effective (unpublished work).
However, the 'ball valve' solids injector [8] cannot be used since it
contains teflon, which precludes ECD. Although solid injection
offers distinct advantages, it is not obligatory. Recently a method
for triazolam assay by capillary GC-ECD was described in which solvent
injection was used [9] – with, moreover, a 'retention gap' which was
claimed to greatly improve column life as compared to solid injection.

'Derivatization' for GC

Intactness during chromatography without derivatization is preserved with many benzodiazepines as confirmed by GC-MS [3, 4], but not
with all. Neither chlordiazepoxide nor class II diazepines can be
run underivatized. Different methods have been reported for the derivatization: acid hydrolysis to benzophenone 'derivatives'; methylation
with methyl iodide; and formation of a TMS (O-trimethylsilyl) product.

Conversion to O-aminobenzophenones (which are excellent electro-
phores) for GC-ECD was customary before capillary columns became
widely available, and so may be the oldest and best-known 'derivatization' procedure for benzodiazepines [10]. There is, however,
the major disadvantage of loss of selectivity, since the same product

can arise from different benzodiazepines and metabolites, e.g. from both diazepam and its metabolite temazepam. It has been argued that this may not matter where the parent drug is the main blood component, e.g. nitrazepam or flunitrazepam [1, 11]. However, inevitably there would be uncertainty, since the metabolic fate has not been fully elucidated for all benzodiazepines. Moreover, in special situations such as renal failure, there may be accumulation of metabolites which otherwise would be in low concentration. Conversion to benzophenones is, then, an obsolete approach, especially since there are now better alternative approaches of widespread availability.

There is only limited experience of methylation of benzodiazepines with methyl iodide as a derivatization procedure [2, 12]. As with the benzophenone approach there may be the problem of loss of specificity. Silylation is probably the method of choice for GC derivatization of class II benzodiazepines [12], and entails no loss of specificity. The TMS ethers of benzodiazepines are in general easily and quantitatively prepared, merely by adding a 40% solution of N,O-(trimethylsilyl)acetamide in acetone to the residue from the solvent extract and evaporating to dryness at 60°. The TMS derivatives can then be analyzed by capillary GC-ECD similarly to underivatized benzodiazepines of classes I and III, with the option of solid injection. Generally such methods have high sensitivity and acceptable reproducibility [4].

GC detection modes other than ECD

Few detection systems other than ECD are applicable. Chemical ionization mass spectrometry (CI-MS) is of both theoretical and practical interest [13, 14], and coupled with GC has high sensitivity and specificity, and so offer distinct advantages where the analyte has to be applied in low concentration or (e.g. paediatric specimens) sample size is small or, as in toxicological samples, identification of unknowns demands high specificity. However, instrumentation costs normally preclude GC-MS in the routine assay of benzodiazepines.

The nitrogen-detection mode (AFID, NPD) has been used in the GC assay of benzodiazepines [15-17], but is generally inferior to ECD in detection limits and thus is limited to assay of high metabolite concentrations in plasma and urine. It is rather unsuitable for pharmacokinetic studies, as levels may be low at late time points.

HPLC assay

One of the most attractive features of HPLC systems, as developed in several laboratories [18-24], is their versatility in discriminating amongst benzodiazepines. This often enables parent compound and metabolite(s) to be assayed in a single run; moreover, the thermally labile class II benzodiazepines (and chlordiazepoxide) need not be derivatized.

A major disadvantage of UV detection as generally practised for benzodiazepines (230-255 nm) is its relative insensitivity as compared to GC-ECD. This was nicely illustrated in a recent study by Puglisi et al. [25] on a pyrimido-benzazepine and its 5-hydroxy metabolite. Using HPLC with UV, the detection limits for both compounds were ~50 ng/ml plasma, whereas with GC-ECD 2 ng/ml could be detected. In our experience such differences in sensitivity between HPLC-UV and GC-ECD exist for many other benzodiazepines. Hence the main value of HPLC-UV procedures is for determining class II benzodiazepines, which cannot readily be run underivatized on capillary GC columns.

To improve sensitivity, other modes of detection have been examined. One option is fluorescence detection following conversion of the benzodiazepines into fluorescent derivatives. This involves a procedure originally introduced for TLC analysis of benzodiazepines [26], viz. hydrolysis to a benzophenone and then conversion to the fluorescent 9-acridone derivative with dimethylformamide and K_2CO_3. Sensitivity is thereby improved, but specificity suffers (see above). For amine metabolites fluorescamine is useful, with specificity [27].

EC detection has also been examined. Generally the detection limits using amperometric detection in the reduction mode vary with the type of electrode used (glassy carbon, carbon paste, Hg pool) and with the experimental conditions (reduction potential). Unfortunately the results to date have been rather disappointing in that the detection limits achievable under optimum conditions do not compare well with those of other modes including UV detection [28, 29].

Of considerable interest is the recent development, mentioned by I.W. Wainer elsewhere in this volume, of stereoselective HPLC assays for the optical isomers of benzodiazepine metabolites. Pirkle & Tsipouras [30] separated the optical isomers of 46 different 3-substituted diazepam analogues on stationary phases derived from (R)-phenylglycine or (S)-leucine, both preparatively and analytically. Separation of the diastereomeric glucuronides of oxazepam and other 3-hydroxy-benzodiazepine enantiomers by HPLC has also been described [31]. Whether these methods will be of great value in pharmacokinetic studies with numerous samples remains to be established.

RADIORECEPTOR ASSAYS (RRA's)

The discovery of specific binding sites (receptors) for benzodiazepine derivatives in brain membranes [32, 33] led to RRA's for their determination in biological fluids [34-38]. The methods are based on competition for the sites in a receptor preparation, obtained from rat or mouse brain, between a radiolabelled ligand (diazepam or flunitrazepam) and the compound to be measured. The binding of benzodiazepines to the receptor is highly specific in that there is no cross-reactivity with other drugs from a wide range of pharmacological classes. Yet there is also lack of specificity, since in

principle the RRA measures total benzodiazepine activity, i.e. all
the material with affinity for the receptor; thus RRA measures not only
the parent compound but also metabolites, active or inactive. By
comparing RRA results with those from specific procedures (GC, HPLC),
the presence of active metabolites in plasma may become manifest.
Hence RRA's are an invaluable research tool in pharmacological investigations with benzodiazepines where the relationship between pharmacokinetics and pharmacodynamics is studied. [Vol. 14, this series,
has a pertinent article by N. Ratnaraj et al., stressing that RRA can
help interpret therapeutic monitoring data for benzodiazepines.- *Ed.*]

Many publications have appeared on various aspects of the receptor
binding of benzodiazepines; but there is only limited experience
with RRA's *per se* and the optimal conditions are in fact poorly
defined. Factors to be considered, as now discussed briefly, include:
preparation of the receptor suspension; incubation conditions (duration,
temperature); and preparation of the sample to be analyzed. [In
Vol. 13 of this series, on membrane-located receptors, an article by
P. Laduron is particularly cogent on specificity etc.- *Ed.*]

The specific binding on which an RRA hinges cannot be determined
directly: it is the ascertained difference between total binding
(only the radiolabelled ligand added) and the non-specific binding
(a large excess of another benzodiazepine added as well). Accuracy
is therefore greatest when non-specific binding is low compared
with total binding. The ratio of specific to total binding may
depend on the technique used in preparing the receptor suspension
and especially on any purification procedure.

Recently we have studied [^{3}H]flunitrazepam binding in various
regions of the brain. In most regions (e.g. cerebral cortex, cerebel-
lum), non-specific binding was only ~5-10% of the total binding, but
in the brain stem it was much higher. It is, then, essential to
discard the brain stem; but otherwise the homogenate can be from total
brain, and purification by fractional centrifugation is unnecessary.

Very little is known about the influence of incubation conditions
on the reproducibility of benzodiazepine RRA's. Incubation is performed at 0° by some investigators [34] and at room temperature by others
[38], without justifying evidence for the choice. Assay at 0° might
improve sensitivity due to higher drug-receptor affinity. Another
uninvestigated factor is the optimal duration of incubation and in
particular of pre-incubation (before adding the radiolabelled ligand).

Benzodiazepines are commonly solvent-extracted by plasma prior to
RRA [34, 38]. In principle this is undesirable because it introduces
uncertainty about the recovery of any unknown active metabolite
that may have been present, and thus about its discovery. RRA is
best performed directly on plasma, if indeed feasible - as we have
recently investigated. When the amount of plasma in the incubation

mixture was varied, specific binding appeared to decrease with increasing amounts; typically it was halved with an increase to 20% (v/v) plasma.   There also appeared to be a considerable inter-individual variability amongst plasma samples in the degree of inhibition of [^{3}H]flunitrazepam binding. However, when serial samples were obtained within one individual, the degree of inhibition appeared to be quite reproducible.   Evidently a direct RRA for benzodiazepines may be feasible, provided that the blank plasma for obtaining the calibration curves is from the same individual. Whether this phenomenon applies to all benzodiazepines remains to be established.

CONCLUSION

Amongst the several methods developed for determining benzodiazepines in biological fluids, GC and HPLC have proved especially suitable in the elucidation of the pharmacokinetic properties of these drugs in man.   Current benzodiazepine research tends to be oriented towards the relationship between pharmacokinetics and pharmacological effects. This implies that from an analytical viewpoint further emphasis will be placed on the determination not only of the parent compound but also of active and inactive metabolites, and also of benzodiazepine enantiomers individually.   Taking into account the current developments in benzodiazepine bioanalysis, it is anticipated that a combined application of both chemical assay procedures (GC, HPLC) and 'biological' assay procedures (RRA) offers the greatest potential for future research. Of practical interest is the commercial availability of freeze-dried receptor preparations [38].

References

1.   de Silva, J.A.F. (1982) in *Pharmacology of Benzodiazepines* (Usdin, E., Skolnick, P., Tallmann, J.F., Greenblatt, D. & Paul, S.M., eds.), Macmillan, London, pp. 239-256.
2.   de Silva, J.A.F. & Bekersky, I.(1974) *J. Chromatog. 99*, 447-460 [see also 461-483].
3.   De Boer, A.G., Röst-Kaiser, J., Bracht, H. & Breimer, D.D. (1978) *J. Chromatog. 145*, 105-114.
4.   Jochemsen, R. & Breimer, D.D. (1982) *J. Chromatog. 227*, 199-206.
5.   Jochemsen, R., Van Rijn, P.A.,   Hazelzet, T.G.M. & Breimer, D.D. (1983) *Pharm. Weekbl. Sci. 5*, 308-312.
6.   Driessen, O. & Emonds, A. (1974) *Proc. Kon. Ned. Acad. Wetensch., Ser. C, 77*, 171-181.
7.   Van den Berg, P.M.J. & Cox, T.P.H. (1972) *Chromatographia 5*, 301-305.
8.   De Boer, A.G. (1979) *Ph.D. Thesis*, Leiden, pp. 21-38.
9.   Baktir, G. & Bircher, J. (1985) *J. Chromatog. 339*, 192-197.
10. de Silva, J.A.F. (1978) in *Antileptic Drugs: Quantitative Analysis and Interpretation* (Pippenger, C.E., Penry, J.K. & Kutt, H., eds.), Raven Press, New York, pp. 111-138.

11. Kangas, L. (1977) *J. Chromatog.* *136*, 259-270.

12. de Silva, J.A.F., Bekersky, I., Puglisi, C.V., Brody, M.A. & Weinfeld, R.E. (1976) *Anal. Chem.* *48*, 10-19.

13. Horning, E.C., Carroll, D.I., Dzidic, I., Lin, S-N., Stilwell, R.N. & Thenot, J.P. (1977) *J. Chromatog.* *142*, 481-495.

14. Garland, W.A. & Miwa, B.J. (1980) *Environ. Health Persp.* *36*, 69-76.

15. Bente, H.B. (1978) *as for* 10., pp. 139-145.

16. Kangas, L. (1979) *J. Chromatog.* *172*, 273-278.

17. Vasiliades, J. & Owens, C. (1980) *J. Chromatog.* *182*, 439-444.

18. Strojny, N., Puglisi, C.V. & de Silva, J.A.F. (1978) *Anal. Lett.* *B11*, 135-160.

19. Tjaden, U.R., Meeles, M.T.H.A., Thijs, C.P. & Van der Kaay, M. (1980) *J. Chromatog.* *181*, 227-241.

20. Vree, T.B., Baars, A.M., Hekster, Y.A. & Van der Kleyn, M. (1981) *J. Chromatog.* *224*, 519-525.

21. Vasiliades, J. & Sahawnez, T. (1982) *J. Chromatog.* *228*, 195-203.

22. Petters, I., Peng, D.R. & Rane, A. (1984) *J. Chromatog.* *306*, 241-248.

23. Heizmann, P., Geschke, R. & Zinapold, K. (1984) *J. Chromatog.* *224*, 129-137.

24. Kozu, T. (1984) *J. Chromatog.* *310*, 213-218.

25. Puglisi, C.V., Ferrara, F.J. & de Silva, J.A.F. (1983) *J. Chromatog.* *275*, 319-333.

26. de Silva, J.A.F., Bekersky, I. & Puglisi, C.V. (1974) *J. Pharm. Sci.* *63*, 1837-1841.

27. Sumirtapura, Y.C., Aubert, C., Coassolo, Ph. & Cano, J.P. (1982) *J. Chromatog.* *232*, 111-118.

28. Lund, W., Hannisdal, M. & Greibrokk, T. (1979) *J. Chromatog.* *173*, 249-261.

29. Hackmann, M.R. & Brooks, M.A. (1981) *J. Chromatog.* *222*, 179-190.

30. Pirkle, W.M. & Tsipouras, A. (1984) *J. Chromatog.* *291*, 291-298.

31. Mascher, M.A., Nitsche, V. & Schütz, H. (1984) *J. Chromatog.* *306*, 231-239.

32. Braestrup, C., Albrechtsen, A. & Squires, R.F. (1977) *Nature* *269*, 702-704.

33. Möhler, H. & Okada, T. (1977) *Science 198*, 849-851.

34. Hunt, P., Husson, J.M. & Raynaud, J.P. (1979) *J. Pharm. Pharmacol.* *31*, 448-451.

35. Skolnick, P., Goodwin, F.K. & Paul, S.M. (1979) *Arch. Gen. Psych. 36*, 78-90.

36. Lund, J. (1981) *Scand. J. Clin. Lab. Invest. 41*, 275-281.

37. Dorow, R.G., Seidler, J. & Schneider, H.H. (1982) *Br. J. Clin. Pharmacol. 13*, 561-565.

38. Jochemsen, R., Horbach, G.J.M.J. & Breimer, D.D. (1982) *Res. Comm. Chem. Pathol. Pharmacol. 35*, 259-273.

#B-3

ANALYTICAL PITFALLS WITH TRICYCLIC AND
NEWER ANTIDEPRESSANTS IN BIOLOGICAL SAMPLES

C. Lindsay DeVane

Division of Clinical Pharmacokinetics
College of Pharmacy, Box J-4
University of Florida
Gainesville, FL 32610, U.S.A.

With antidepressants and their active metabolites there are analytical complications: low concentrations; surface adsorptivity during extraction; chromatographic co-elution with other drugs and contaminants; and uncertainty about survival during storage and chromatography. Stability experience with the tricyclics does not hold for newer antidepressants. Thus, bupropion (but not its three major metabolites) showed temperature- and pH-dependent log-linear degradation in plasma. The importance of validating extraction techniques for each sample type is exemplified by trazodone, which was extractable from plasma by methyl-t-butyl ether but required isoamyl alcohol/hexane for brain tissue extraction to obviate emulsions and include an active metabolite. For cyclic antidepressants in general, sources of inaccuracy include the preparation of non-methanolic stock solutions, mode of rendering alkaline, standard-curve determination with homogenates of the tissue concerned, and HPLC validation with a converse-polarity system, e.g. NP instead of RP. Other points of practice are also discussed, e.g. sample collection, in the context of inter-laboratory differences in assay performance.

Soon after the prototype tricyclic antidepressant, imipramine, became available for clinical practice in the late 1950's, a 20- to 30-fold inter-patient variability in steady-state plasma concentrations was noted. This led to pharmacokinetic studies on tricyclics, aimed at improving the response and/or decreasing the incidence of side-effects through therapeutic monitoring. Whilst the results for some of the most popular tricyclics remain equivocal, it is agreed that routine monitoring is justified only for nortriptyline and for imipramine along with its secondary amine metabolite, desipramine.

Thus, unless newer antidepressants with fewer side-effects supplant tricyclics, it is likely that analytical methods for imipramine, desipramine and nortriptyline will continue to proliferate. By 1975 (as reviewed [1,2]) most types of analytical method had been applied to the tricyclics, including TLC, GC-NPD, GC-MS and HPLC. Immunological methods have been handicapped by formidable specificity problems due to metabolite multiplicity.

There is also the problem that methods suitable for measuring steady-state levels (~30-300 ng/ml) may be useless for research applications where 1 ng/ml may have to be measured. No single analytical method best serves all applications; the choice depends on equipment availability and envisaged applications. Our laboratory has emphasized HPLC, in either normal-phase mode (NP; Fig. 1) or reversed phase (RP; Fig. 2). Some of our experiences will illustrate common pitfalls encountered in tricyclic analysis.

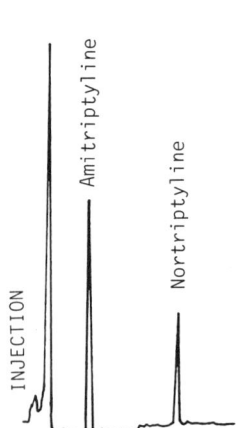

Fig. 1. NP-HPLC assay approach for tricyclic antidepressants. Column: 5 µm silica, 25 cm long. Mobile phase: acetonitrile/ methanol/NH$_4$OH/n-butyl- amine (93:6.6:0.4:0.12 by vol.). Detection at 254 nm. Amitriptyline elutes at 7 min, imipramine (not shown) at 8.5 min, and nortriptyline at 16 min.

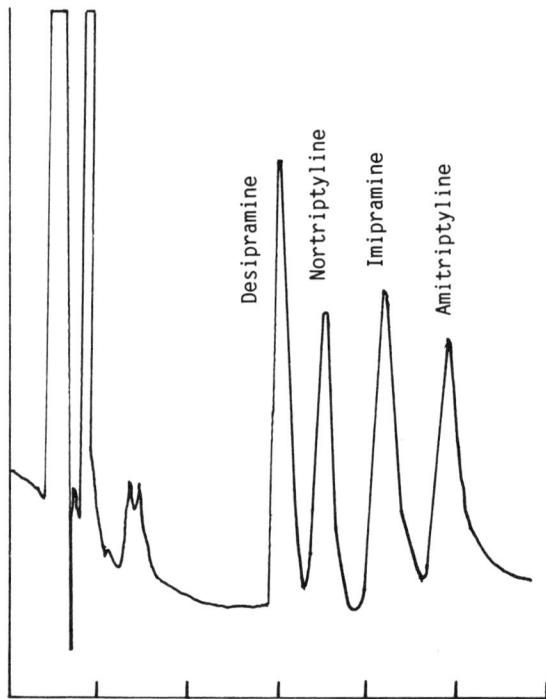

Fig. 2. RP-HPLC approach for tricyclic antidepressants. C-18 7 µm column, 25 cm long. Mobile phase: acetonitrile/10 mM phosphoric acid (48:52) with 50 mM tri- ethylamine. Detection at 202 nm. Peaks at 6,7, 8.5 and 10 min (axis spikes 2 min apart).

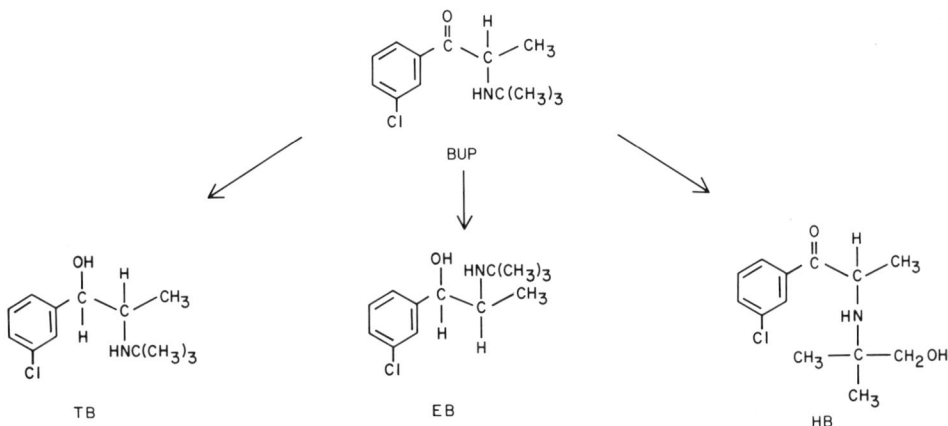

Fig. 3. Chemical structures and metabolic pathways of bupropion (BUP) and its three major metabolites in man: the threo-amino alcohol (TB), the erythro-amino alcohol (EB) and the hydroxy metabolite (HB).

SAMPLE COLLECTION AND STABILITY

The 'Vacutainer effect', not publicized till 1978, concerns plasticizer that leaches from the rubber stoppers of some brands of collection tubes upon contact with blood and displaces highly bound basic compounds from their binding sites on α_1-acid glycoprotein [see arts. in Vol. 10, this series, for accounts of this and other problems, *below*; also this vol., e.g. #B-4 (K.K. Midha) – *Ed.*]. The outcome is a re-equilibration with erythrocytes and a lower measurable drug concentration after plasma is separated. The problem is obviated by using tubes warranted not to cause spurious reduction in plasma level, or else all-glass apparatus in obtaining blood samples.

Following collection and separation of plasma or serum, tricyclics remain stable for months when kept at -17° or lower, and possibly up to a week at room temperatures up to 22° - such that plasma samples may be safely shipped by post to distant laboratories without dry-ice preservation. Such stability is not possessed by some of the newer cyclic antidepressants, as found in our laboratory for bupropion (BUP), a second-generation antidepressant. During assay development we got frozen samples collected elsewhere during a pharmacokinetic study, intending to compare RIA as already performed with our own HPLC assay. All three of the major, basic metabolites that firstly arise from BUP in humans (Fig. 3) were found by HPLC in substantial amount, but not BUP itself. This observation led us to question drug stability [3].

Human plasma was spiked with BUP and the three metabolites, and incubated under varying conditions of temperature and pH – both of which affected the observed log-linear degradation (Fig. 4). BUP half-life in pH 7.4 plasma kept at 22° was 54.4 and at 37° was 11.4 h.

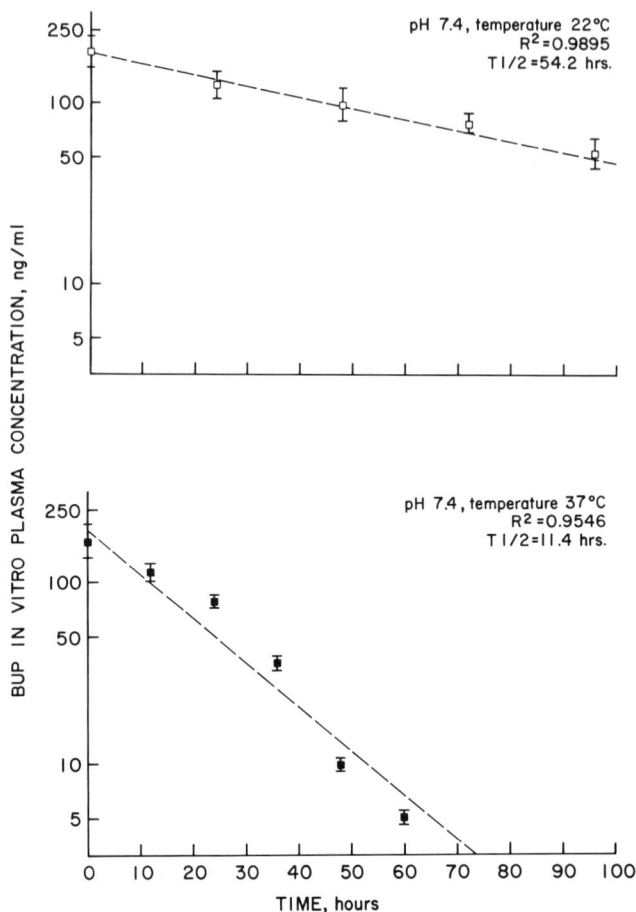

Fig. 4. Degradation of BUP in human plasma *in vitro* at pH 7.4. Each point is the mean (with S.D.) of 3 plasma aliquots. *From ref. [3], by permission.*

Metabolite concentrations hardly changed after 48 h at 37° in the pH range 2.5-10. When samples from subsequent studies were kept at -17° for as long as 8 months, then re-assayed, no change was found *vs.* the values from immediate assay, for BUP or any metabolite. Evidently some assumptions about drug stability in the tricyclics context may be inapplicable to the newer cyclic antidepressants. Each laboratory should check whether drug stability is affected by its procedures; one aspect is the temperature adopted for protein-binding studies. Nomifensine has similar instability [cf. #NC(B)-3, below.- *Ed.*]

EXTRACTION PROCEDURES

Another problem that plagues tricyclic analysis is loss during the extraction process. For the NP-HPLC approach shown in Fig. 1, plasma is brought with NH_4OH or NaOH to 2 pH units above the applicable pKa value, then extracted with between 1 and 3 vols. of isoamyl alcohol/ hexane (1-5% v/v of the former); the organic layer is concentrated in a N_2 stream.   Other common solvents such as diethyl ether also extract tricyclics well.   The alcohol supplement minimizes emulsion formation and is well known to decrease adsorption onto glass surfaces.   In the problematic evaporation step a relationship appears to exist between the tube's surface area and evaporative losses, which the use of small polypropylene tubes minimizes.   Near the end of the evaporation we have found it beneficial to wash the walls of the sample container with a small amount of methanol or mobile phase and continue N_2 flow to near dryness.   This step should be closely watched as continuation of N_2 after reaching dryness causes greater loss. [Points such as this have featured earlier in the series, e.g. Vols. 7 (p. 69), 10 (p. 360) & 12 (p. 263).-*Ed*.]   Whilst we find our work-up procedure satisfactory, it is particularly prone to variability when performed by different analysts.

An alternative to the procedure entailing one extraction and then concentration is back-extraction at pH <3 into water containing an organic acid.   This is advantageous for the RP-HPLC approach and may be necessary to eliminate interferences in tissue samples or plasma containing additional drugs and metabolites.   However, back-extraction may lower recovery because of incomplete partitioning and pipetting losses from additional sample manipulation.   Neither approach is con- sistently better than the other when rigorous attention is paid to technique. Use of both HPLC approaches (NP and RP) may be warranted on occasion, to help peak validation.

The   recovery of metabolites frequently differs from that of the parent drug and among different tissue types. This is illustrated by our experiences with a NP-HPLC assay for imipramine (IMI), developed for use in placental transfer studies in the rat [4, 5].   IMI and its demethylation product desipramine (DMI) each furnish the 2-OH metabol- ite, more polar than the parent compound and differing in extracta- bility.   Hexane or heptane containing 2% isoamyl alcohol extracted IMI and DMI nearly quantitatively (at pH 11) but only ~65% of 2-OH-IMI and hardly any 2-OH-DMI.

The best extraction solvent for tissues in general (homogenized in 20% v/v   perchloric acid) to encompass all compounds concerned was 20% (v/v) butan-1-ol in n-hexane; likewise for body fluids.   Yet for the hydroxylated metabolites the recovery was low, ~60% for whole blood; but the C.V.'s were <10%.   Several parameters of the extraction procedure were varied in attempts to increase recovery.   It was at least 15% better with an excess of solvent relative to sample (3 vols. instead of 1 vol.; no further increase with higher ratios). A re-extraction step gave only 4-6% improvement, yet is worth trying (despite the increased handling and evaporation time) if recoveries are unacceptably low. [In Vol. 10, p. 22 is pertinent.-*Ed*.]

There was no apparent increase in recovery with an increase
in shaking time beyond 15 min on a reciprocal shaker - which agitates
less thoroughly than vortex mixing but is less tedious and less
prone to operator variability.

PREPARATION OF STANDARD CURVES

The need for the spiking of blanks with standards to be done with
the same sample type as is to be analyzed is borne out for IMI and
its major metabolites by the data in Table 1. The difference in
extraction of 2-OH-IMI between whole blood and plasma is reflected in
a different calibration slope even though the reproducibility is
excellent. If, then, plasma standards were used in analyzing test
samples of a different type, there would be substantial under-estima-
tion. [Earlier vols. give other examples.- *Ed.*]

Another pitfall is the use of methanolic stock solutions of drug.
With such solutions used repeatedly during several months, changes
in calibration curves have been observed, probably due to non-obvious
evaporation of the methanol each time the container is opened.

SENSITIVITY

Exemplifying the importance of sensitivity for some samples,
administration of tricyclics may give plasma concentrations in the
low ng/ml range. HPLC peak symmetry and sensitivity may be improved
by adding modifiers to the mobile phase, giving reduced retentions and
saving operator time and solvent costs. As reflected in Fig. 5, n-butyl-
amine addition reduced from 20 to ~12 min the overall analysis time for
IMI and its metabolites, with ~2-fold gains in sensitivity [4].
Another approach to increasing sensitivity is to use a lower UV wavelength for detection; but potential interferences may be worse unless
the sample is cleanly extracted.

Where feasible, larger sample volumes may be used. Amitriptyline
and nortriptyline were extracted equally well from 5 ml of plasma
as from 1 ml, giving an effective sensitivity of 1 ng/ml for either [6].
This is applicable to patients, from whom it is customary to take
7-15 ml of blood regardless of the sample requirement.

DRUG METABOLITES, EXEMPLIFIED BY TRAZODONE

Most of the cyclic antidepressants have pharmacologically active
metabolite(s), which should also be determined. A single extraction
method may serve in some cases, e.g. IMI and metabolites (see above).
This is not always true. The antidepressant trazodone (TRAZ), a tri-
azolopyridine derivative, furnishes 1-*m*-chlorophenylpiperazine (m-CCP)
as its major active metabolite (Fig. 6). Because this metabolite is
a serotonin agonist whereas its precursor is an antagonist, pharmacolo-
gists benefit from the ability to analyze both compounds in plasma as

Table 1. Replicate slope determinations for imipramine (IMI) and its metabolites spiked into different drug-free biological samples (perchloric acid homogenates except for plasma and whole blood) from rats. Slope values are in arbitrary units based on peak areas. Each C.V. (S.D. as % of slope) was from N assays, on different days.

Sample type	N	IMI	Desipramine (DMI)	2-OH-IMI	2-OH-DMI
Plasma	4	3.94 (4.6%)	4.55 (3.2%)	9.49 (7.5%)	7.54 (5.4%)
Whole blood	5	3.81 (4.2%)	4.37 (1.8%)	7.18 (7.8%)	4.41 (11.1%)
Brain	9	3.61 (9.8%)	3.79 (6.6%)	7.68 (5.4%)	6.36 (6.3%)
Liver	5	3.22 (2.6%)	3.50 (4.1%)	7.16 (5.4%)	5.70 (4.0%)
Foetus	5	3.50 (4.9%)	3.87 (2.7%)	7.71 (5.6%)	5.60 (4.9%)

Data as in ref. [4].

Fig. 5. Effect of n-butyl-amine content of the mobile phase on the retentions of imipramine and its metabolites ($K' =$ capacity factor). The mobile phase was similar to that in Fig. 1.

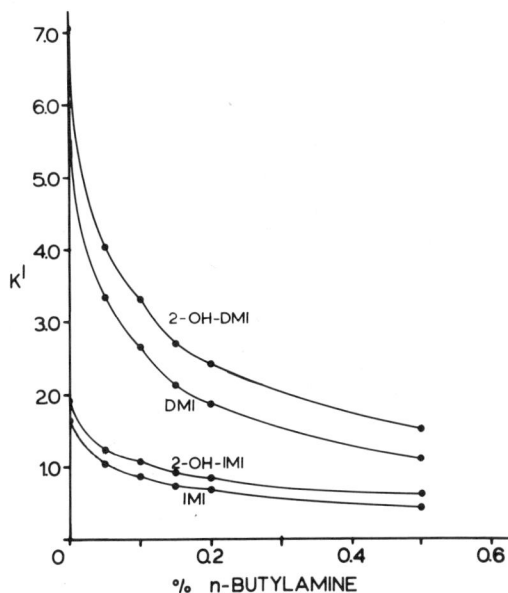

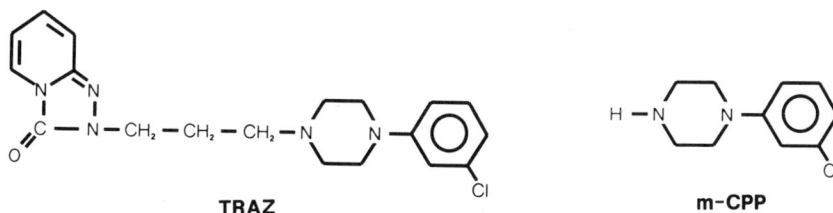

Fig. 6. Chemical structures of trazodone (TRAZ) and the major active metabolite named in the text (m-CPP).

well as brain tissue, the presumed site of antidepressant activity. The most frequently used solvents for TRAZ extraction from plasma have been diethyl ether, 2% isoamyl alcohol in hexane, and methyl t-butyl ether.   The latter has a higher flash point than diethyl ether, does not form peroxides, and extracts TRAZ better from plasma than isoamyl alcohol/hexane.   However, we found it unsuitable for brain tissue extraction, because emulsions often formed and TRAZ recovery was generally poor [7].   Isoamyl/hexane was more suitable for brain. There is the usual need to investigate quantitatively the specificity of extraction from each type of sample.

CONCLUDING COMMENTS

The analytical method is only one link in a chain of events between drug ingestion and accurate determination of plasma drug concentrations.   Areas which have often not received attention but may contribute to variability and error within and between laboratories include the following.-
(1) Changing haemodynamic influences, e.g. bed-rest or psychomotor activity just prior to sample collection.
(2) Temperature changes immediately after sample collection, i.e. the rate at which cooling of whole blood occurs, altering the distribution equilibrium of drug between erythrocytes and plasma.
(3) Atmospheric presssure in the analytical laboratory; altitude differences between laboratories influence the vapour pressure of aqueous mobile phases.
(4) The extent of variability in calibration results, e.g. how often the regression analyses show non-origin intercepts in standard curves.
(5) Differences among laboratories in the regression equations used, e.g. whether orthogonal least-squares or standard regression of x on y or y on x.
(6) Evaporation of mobile-phase modifiers during the course of analysis.
(7) Carry-over effects, e.g. failure to completely eliminate adsorbed drug from glass syringes from previous injections.
(8) The presence of shifting extraneous peaks in the chromatogram and of late peaks that elute during subsequent runs.
(9) Failure to account for variability in the extraction recoveries of internal standards.
(10) Changes in column performance due to non-eluted material remaining on the column.

Attention to these possible sources of error as well as to the ordinary pitfalls discussed above should improve the accuracy and reproducibility of assays for the tricyclic and newer cyclic anti-depressants.

Acknowledgements

The contributions of S.C. Laizure, R.L. Miller, S.S. Stout and S. Sunloff to antidepressant analysis in our laboratory have been especially valuable. Our work is supported in part by grant No. HD14075, National Institutes of Health, U.S.A.

References

1. Gupta, R. & Molnar, G. (1979) *Drug Metab. Rev. 9*, 79-97.
2. Scoggins, B.A., Maquire, K.P., Norman, T.R. & Burrows, G.D. (1980) *Clin. Chem. 26*, 5-17.
3. Laizure, S.C. & DeVane, C.L. (1986) *Ther. Drug Monit. 7*, 447-450.
4. Stout, S.A. & DeVane, C.L. (1984) *Psychopharmacology 84*, 39-41.
5. DeVane, C.L. & Simpkins, J.T. (1985) *Drug Metab. Dispos. 13*, 438-442.
6. Curry, S.H., DeVane, C.L. & Wolfe, M.M. (1985) *Eur. J. Clin. Pharmacol. 29*, 429-433.
7. Miller, R.L. & DeVane, C.L. (1985) *J. Chromatog. 374*, 388-393.

#B-4

DETERMINATION OF PHENOTHIAZINES: THE PRESENT-DAY SCENE

G. McKay, S.F. Cooper* and K.K. Midha[†]

College of Pharmacy, University of Saskatchewan
Saskatoon, Saskatchewan, Canada S7N 0W0

Patients given antipsychotic drugs differ widely in the plasma concentrations, complicated by the presence of various metabolites, some active and some unstable. With phenothiazines, analytical difficulties besides low concentrations include adsorptive losses. Chemical methods, based on GC or HPLC with appropriate detectors, are specific and often sensitive but are laborious. RIA methods are sensitive and quick, but often non-specific such that we routinely validate them with specific chemical assays. This article considers the quantitative methods that we have developed for chlorpromazine,[⊗] trifluoperazine, fluphenazine, trimethazine, proclorperazine and also their key metabolites.

Since the introduction of the phenothiazine antipsychotics in the early 1950's there have been innumerable publications on analysis, metabolism, mode of action, pharmacokinetics, toxicity, and correlations between blood levels and clinical response. [The background is also surveyed by S.H. Curry in a foregoing article.- *Ed.*] In a significant number of patients there is non-responsiveness, partly inborn. There are large individual variations, poorly understood, in the plasma levels attained. The study of inter-individual variation is complicated by the variety of competing metabolic transformations, giving both active metabolites and inactive ones which could impair drug response. Orally administered phenothiazines also undergo pronounced pre-systemic metabolism, in gut as well as liver. The apparent body-distribution volume may be as high as 40 1/kg, equally between central and tissue compartments. Since phenothiazines, and especially the piperazine derivatives, are psychotherapeutically so potent that their dosage is generally small, the problem of low plasma concentrations is accentuated.

*On sabbatical leave from INRS-Santé, Université du Québec, 245 Hymus Boulevard, Pointe-Claire, Québec, Canada.
[†]To whom correspondence should be addressed. ⊗Text abbreviation: CPZ.

ANALYTICAL APPROACHES

Besides the above-mentioned factors that contribute to low plasma concentrations, the phenothiazines and their metabolites are highly labile and are readily lost on glassware and glass columns during extraction, derivatization and analysis. Other complicating factors are artefactual interconversions of the metabolites to parent drugs and *vice versa* during extraction and analysis. Consequently the analysis of phenothiazines and metabolites is notoriously difficult.

We have approached the analysis of phenothiazines and their metabolites with a range of methods, both chemical - GC-NPD, GC-ECD, GC-MS and HPLC - and 'biological', mainly RIA based on both polyclonal antibodies and monoclonal antibodies (MAb's). The chemical methods are specific and often sensitive, but laborious and time-consuming, whereas RIA's are sensitive and apt for multi-sample throughput but often lack specificity, for which reason we routinely validate them with specific chemical methods. Here we describe the systematic approach used to develop methods for the various phenothiazines and metabolites.

Considerations that influence the choice of end-step and prior sample preparation have been surveyed in earlier books of this series; they include the physicochemical properties of the analytes and the metabolite picture. The context may vary from an overdose situation to a single-dose pharmacokinetic study. Amongst possible types of biological sample, plasma and serum are most commonly chosen.

Sample collection and storage

Sample handling is critical for meaningful results [as considered especially in Vol. 10, this series.-*Ed*.]. For example, the rubber stoppers of some Vacutainer tubes can affect the distribution of basic drugs, e.g. CPZ [1], fluphenazine, trifluoperazine and phenazine [2], between erythrocytes and plasma through leaching out of tris(2-butoxyethyl) phosphate. This or other neutral compounds may be extracted by organic solvents and give a peak coinciding with that for the drug, as in GC-NPD assay of trifluophenazine from blood collected in 'Venoject' evacuated tubes: the problem was obviated by using Vacutainer tubes and avoiding contact between blood and stopper [3].

If a specimen has to be stored, the risk of analyte decomposition [4] must be investigated, suitably by storing spiked samples along with the unknowns. Satisfactory stability has been shown for CPZ in blood or plasma (up to 84 days at -20°) [5] as earlier observed with biological fluids [6].

Artifacts in phenothiazine-containing samples

CPZ *N*-oxide can undergo time-dependent reduction to CPZ in plasma made alkaline with NaOH [7], distorting their relative levels.

With Na_2CO_3 in place of NaOH this reduction did not occur, and CPZ values were increased even >3-fold. Extraction time and amount of NaOH influence the extent of this reduction. With none of the conditions tested was there interconversion between CPZ or its *N*-oxide and CPZ sulphoxide [8]. That Na_2CO_3 is preferable to NaOH for achieving an alkaline pH before extraction was borne out by testing serum-albumin solutions of CPZ *N*-oxide; since no reduction occurred even with NaOH when protein-free solutions were tested, evidently the reduction arises from an action of NaOH on serum proteins.

In a further study with whole blood instead of plasma [9], it was found with either NaOH or Na_2CO_3 the CPZ was in part oxidized to CPZ sulphoxide and the CPZ *N*-oxide was converted completely into a mixture of CPZ and CPZ sulphoxide; CPZ sulphoxide itself was unaffected, and incubation time did not influence the interconversions. Thus it appears that conventional methods of analysis for CPZ are particularly prone to spurious results. Since we have found that CPZ *N*-oxide is actually plasma-located with <4% in the red cells, the facile reduction of CPZ *N*-oxide can be minimized by separating the red cells from plasma before extraction. It may be determined with appropriate extraction procedures in clinical plasma samples, which show a high content [4]. As CPZ itself [10] is largely in red cells, these must be separated off initially lest there be spurious oxidation of CPZ to CPZ sulphoxide, and alkaline extraction methods should be avoided in the analysis of red cells or whole blood for CPZ and CPZ sulphoxide.

In further studies with individual compounds under physiological conditions [8], incubation at 37° with whole blood in 0.1 M phosphate buffer (pH 7.4) showed remarkable stability: CPZ sulphoxide manifested no oxidation or reduction, and only ~1% of added CPZ was oxidized to CPZ sulphoxide. Since the latter conversion was much greater in previous reports [11-13], it indeed appears to be augmented when red cells come into contact with alkali [9].

At pH 7.4 as used for CPZ sulphoxide, conversion of CPZ *N*-oxide to CPZ is nil in plasma but ~1% in red cells, augmented to ~4% if a halogenated solvent such as dichloromethane is used. Therefore our approach to the solvent extraction of CPZ and CPZ sulphoxide from plasma entails no pH adjustment before performing direct extraction with n-pentane/2-propanol (97:3 by vol.).

CURRENT INSTRUMENTAL TECHNIQUES IN PHENOTHIAZINE ASSAY

GC with conventional detectors

Several investigators have used GC-FID, for butriptyline [14, 15], thioridazine and its metabolites [16, 17], methotrimeprazine and its sulphoxide metabolites [18], levomepromazine, propericiazine, dixyrazine, perazine, thioproperazine, trifluoperazine and prothipendyl [19], and perazine [20, 21] besides thioridazine and its metabolites [21]. The detection limit was typically 50 ng/ml of the biological fluid.

Since FID is rather non-specific, peak identity should be confirmed by an alternative technique such as GC-MS (cf. below).

The advent of NPD's, with selectivity for nitrogen, improved sensitivity and enabled therapeutic concentrations of CPZ and meta-bolites to be determined in 2 ml serum samples [22]: the amount/ml of serum that could be measured was as little as 5 ng for CPZ, 20 ng for CPZ sulphoxide or mono-*N*-desmethyl-CPZ and 10 ng for di-*N*-des-methyl-CPZ. GC-NPD was also used for butaperazine in rats (including liver and brain) and patients [23], and for trifluoperazine in humans (Fig. 1) [3]. The sample preparation entailed a simple one-step ext-raction of the drug and internal standard (prochlorperazine) from 2 ml of basified plasma into n-pentane/2-propanol (50:1 by vol.), fol-lowed by evaporation to dryness and reconstitution in 25 µl of meth-anol. The sensitivity, 0.5 ng/ml, was inadequate for single-dose pharmacokinetic or bioavailability studies but sufficed for steady-state plasma-level monitoring. The co-extracted important metabol-ites of trifluoperazine did not interfere with GC (Fig. 2). This GC-NPD procedure compared well with a GC-MS method (see below, also for RIA). It can readily be adapted for prochlorperazine assay with trifluophenazine as internal standard. Similarly, GC-NPD has been used, with adequate sensitivity, for fluphenazine [24, 25; cf. 26], promazine, CPZ, butaperazine and promethazine.

The GC-ECD approach, introduced for CPZ and metabolites nearly 20 years ago [27[⊗]], was sensitive down to 1 ng/ml in patients' serum [28]. GC-ECD techniques have been developed [29-33] for various piperazine- and piperidine-substituted phenothiazines and their meta-bolites. Perphenazine and its sulphoxide were measurable down to 0.2 ng/ml [29], and co-determination of 7-hydroxyperphenazine and the probable metabolites 8-hydroxy- and 7,8-dihydroxy-perphenazine has been described [31]. When perphenazine given along with amitriptyline was determined in 3 ml plasma samples, 5 ng/ml was detectable [32]. A sensitivity of 10 ng/ml has been obtained for pipotiazine [33].

In general, GC techniques for determining phenothiazines should be used with caution. Decomposition has been reported for *N*-oxides [34] and, with the injection port at >270°, for the sulphoxide meta-bolites of CPZ, prochlorperazine and trifluoperazine although decom-position rarely exceeded 2% with the port at 250-270° [35]. In the past, port temperatures for GC of CPZ and metabolites were in the range 275-310°. With phenothiazine ring-sulphoxide metabolites, which are thought to be relatively inactive therapeutically [12] but may be present in plasma at levels similar to or even exceeding that of the parent drugs [36, 37], the values for the latter may be artifac-tually elevated if the GC conditions are not such as to minimize decom-position. Evidently it is critical to carefully optimize the GC condi-tions prior to the analysis of phenothiazine sulphoxides.

[⊗] Other S.H. Curry refs. excised; in his own article (above) ref. [28] is particularly pertinent.- *Ed.*

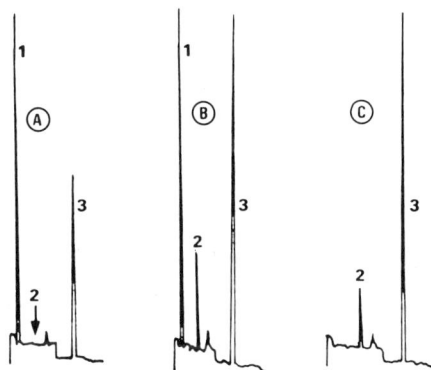

Fig. 1. GC-NPD patterns for extracts of
(A) blank human plasma; (B) human plasma
spiked with trifluoperazine (peak 2),
2.5 ng/ml; (C) plasma from a volunteer
2 h after receiving 5 mg trifluoperazine,
estimated to contain 1.45 ng/ml. Peak 1
= caffeine, 3 = prochlorperazine, added
to plasma as internal standard.
Column 1.8 m, i.d. 2 mm; 3% OV-17 on
acid-washed DMCS-treated high-performance
flux-calcined diatomite, 100-120 mesh.
Oven 310°, injection port and detector
300°; He, 30 ml/min. Peak 2 at ~8.3 min
from start of run.

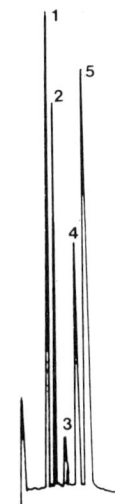

Fig. 2. As for B in
Fig. 1, but spiking
with trifluoperazine
(peak 1), N-desmethyl-
(2) and 7-hydroxy- (3)
trifluoperazine, pro-
chlorperazine (4) and
trifluoperazine sulph-
oxide (5); ~50 ng of
each on column.

GC-MS

The most sensitive and specific technique at present available is
GC combined with MS, whereby the intensities of diagnostic ions are
measured (mass fragmentography; selected ion monitoring, SIM). A mul-
tiple-ion detection system allows quantitation at the pg level,
e.g. when GC with EI-MS is performed on trifluoperazine (Fig. 3) extracted for the GC-NPD runs in Figs. 1 & 2.   Whereas GC-NPD allowed
0.5 ng/ml to be measured with C.V. 5.3% [3], GC-MS allowed assay down
to 78 pg/ml (same sample) with C.V. <7% [38], enabling plasma levels
to be measured as late as 24 h post-dose when, in a pharmacokinetic
study [39], volunteers took 5 mg of the drug orally.

In a GC-MS (SIM) procedure for fluphenazine [40], solvent-extracted from plasma and derivatized with N,O-bis(trimethylsilyl)acetamide,
as little as 78 pg/ml was measurable, with C.V. 4.6%. Specificity
and sensitivity were good enough to allow plasma levels to be followed
up to 32 h following a 5 mg oral dose. This sensitivity and reproducibility far surpassed what GC-NPD can furnish (see above).

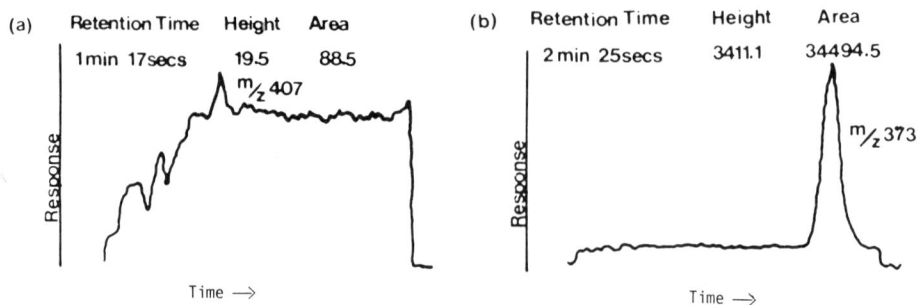

Fig. 3. GC-MS with SIM: **a**, trifluoperazine (85 pg/ml plasma; m/z 407) in a sample from a volunteer given 5 mg orally; **b**, prochlorperazine (50 ng/ml; m/z 373) as internal standard. Column 1.2 m, i.d. 2 mm; 3% OV-1 on high-performance GasChrom Q (100-200), 280°.

The greatest drawbacks to the use of GC-MS are its high purchase cost (including the computer) and the need for experienced, specialized personnel; yet the benefits to assay are dramatic. GC-MS serves also as a qualitative tool, e.g. to elucidate the ring-cleavage pathway for piperazine-type phenothiazines and the EI-MS fragmentation [41].

HPLC

An HPLC method with electrochemical (EC) detection enabled trimeprazine to be followed in volunteers' plasma for 24 h after a 5 mg oral dose, 0.25 ng/ml being measurable (0.125 ng/ml detectable) [42]. The limits were 0.25 (0.1) ng/ml for CPZ assayed by HPLC with EC detection, such that with 2 ml samples the levels up to 24 h after a 50 mg oral dose could be followed [43]. For thioridazine, however, oxidative EC detection was insufficiently sensitive and the detector response was non-linear over the wide range required. Fixed-wavelength UV detection at 254 nm provided the requisite sensitivity for the drug and its major active metabolites, mesoridazine and sulforidazine, and (1 ng of each being detectable) enabled plasma levels to be followed up to 72 h after a 50 mg dose [44].

RIA

Because sensitivity is high and sample preparation is minimal, RIA is especially useful for assaying the more potent antipsychotics such as trifluoperazine or fluphenazine where the plasma peak after an oral dose is only 1-2 ng/ml [39]. Having pioneered an RIA for CPZ [45], we now have a repertoire of RIA's (Table 1).

RIA for CPZ

Our RIA's for CPZ [45], CPZ sulphoxide and 7-hydroxy-CPZ [46], with a defined specificity, enable plasma levels to be monitored

Table 1.   Our drug and metabolite assays: approx. lower limit
of measurement, as ng/ml plasma (~twice the detection limit).

Class	Drug or metabolite	RIA[⊗]	GC	HPLC
Pheno-	Fluphenazine	0.25	0.08 (MS)	0.50 (EC)
thia-	Fluphenazine sulphoxide	0.30	–	–
zines	Prochlorperazine	0.25	0.13 (MS)	0.50 (EC)
	Perphenazine	0.25	–	0.10 (EC)
	Trimeprazine	0.31	–	0.25 (EC)
	Thioridazine	0.40	–	2.5 (UV)
	Trifluoperazine	0.15	0.08 (MS)	0.50 (EC)
	Trifluoperazine sulphoxide	0.30	–	–
	7-Hydroxytrifluoperazine	0.10	–	–
	Trifluoperazine N^4-oxide	0.10	–	–
	CPZ	0.15	0.25 (MS)	0.25 (EC)
	CPZ sulphoxide	0.20	–	–
	7-Hydroxy-CPZ	0.50	–	–
	CPZ-N-oxide	0.25	–	–
Tri-	Doxepin	⎤	–	2.5 (UV)
cyclic	N-Desmethyldoxepin	⎬ 0.25	–	2.5 (UV)
anti-	Trans-doxepin	⎦ 0.15	–	5.0 (UV)
depres-	Imimpramine/Desimipramine	0.10	2.0 (NPD)	–
sants	Amitriptyline	1.0	–	–
Miscel-	d-Ephedrine	2.5 ⎤		–
laneous	l-Ephedrine	2.5 ⎬ 5.0 (ECD)		–
	dl-Fenfluramine	0.30 ⎦	5.0 (ECD)	–
	Chlorphentramine	0.15	–	2.5 (UV)

[⊗] with ^{3}H-labelled ligands

for up to 24 h after a 50 mg dose.   The requisite antisera were
raised in New Zealand white rabbits with, for each compound, a
conjugate having $-N(CH_3).CH_2.CH_2.CO.NH.BSA$ in place of $-N(CH_3)_2$.
For 7-hydroxy-CPZ, mouse MAb's prepared with the same conjugate
[47] were adopted for routine use since specificity was far better
than for the polyclonal antiserum.   Some information on cross-
reactivities [46] is given in Table 2.   In all the RIA's there was
good sensitivity (Table 1).   However, assay of patients' plasma
for the three analytes gave inflated values, presumably due to an
unknown metabolite that cross-reacted.   Agreement with chemical
assays became closer with the routine adoption of differential extraction procedures (as already described for 7-hydroxy-CPZ [47]) before
the RIA determinations.   Obviously RIA's need searching evaluation.

RIA's for piperazine-type phenothiazines

Polyclonal antisera were raised in rabbits by immunizing
with conjugates appropriate for assay of trifluoperazine (TFZ) and 3
metabolites. The haptens to which BSA was covalently linked were,

Table 2. Antisera to CPZ and metabolites: profiles for cross-reactions (% values calculated by Abraham's method [48]). ND = not determined. SO = sulphoxide, 7-OH = 7-hydroxy, NO = N-oxide.

Compound	Antisera raised to:	CPZ [45]	CPZ-SO [46]	7-OH-CPZ [47] monoclonal	7-OH-CPZ [47] polyclonal
CPZ		(100%)	<1%	<1%	17%
7-HO-CPZ		<1%	<1%	(100%)	(100%)
CPZ-SO		<1%	(100%)	<1%	<1%
CPZ-NO		<1%	<1%	<1%	<1%
nor_1-CPZ		100%	<1%	<1%	<5%
nor_2-CPZ		7%	<10%	ND	ND
7-OH-nor_1-CPZ		ND	ND	37%	80%
8-OH-CPZ		ND	ND	<1%	<8%
6-OH-CPZ		<1%	ND	3%	3%

where **'X'** signifies 10-{[3-(4-(2-carboxyethyl)-1-piperazinyl)propyl]}2-trifluoromethyl-10H-phenothiazine:- N-(2-carboxyethyl)-desmethyl-TFZ for TFZ [49, 50], **X**-sulphoxide for TFZ sulphoxide [51], and 7-hydroxy-**X** for 7-hydroxy-TFZ [52]; also 7-(3-carboxypropionyl)prochlorperazine-$N^{4'}$-oxide   for TFZ $N^{4'}$-oxide (M. Aravagiri et al., in press*).

The above citations concerning antisera include data on cross-reactivities, now summarized for each.- TFZ: 26% towards N-desmethyl-TFZ, 24% towards 7-OH-TFZ. TFZ sulphoxide: 8% towards TFZ sulphone, 55% towards the N-desmethylsulphoxide metabolite of TFZ (not yet identified in man); also 39% towards prochlorperazine sulphoxide, 62% towards fluphenazine sulphoxide and 77% towards perphenazine sulphoxide.- Evidently there may be applicability to measuring sulphoxide metabolite levels of these other piperazine-type phenothiazines. 7-Hydroxy-TFZ: 27% towards N-desmethyl-7-hydroxy-TFZ, 16% towards 7-hydroxytrifluopromazine, also 76% towards 7-hydroxyfluphenazine, 52% towards 7-hydroxyprochlorperazine. Evidently there may be applicability to measuring these and possibly other 7-hydroxy metabolites of piperazine-type phenothiazines.

Attempts were made to prepare for TFZ $N^{4'}$-oxide assay a hapten having the carboxyl-terminated side-chain for conjugation with protein. However, the preliminary acylation of TFZ was unsuccessful even under strongly favourable conditions (M. Aravagiri et al., in press*), probably due to the strongly electronegative 2-trifluoromethyl group of the phenothiazine ring. The 2-chloro group in prochlorperazine is less electronegative, so it was successfully converted to a hapten for its $N^{4'}$-oxide; the protein was attached at position 7 on the ring system. The antiserum raised to this conjugate was used to measure TFZ $N^{4'}$-oxide: cross-reactivity was 90% with TFZ $N^{1'},N^{4'}$-dioxide (a probable metabolite not yet found in humans), but negligible with all other

* J. Pharmacol. Exp. Ther.

major metabolites of TFZ. Moreover, as expected, this antiserum cross-reacts strongly with prochlorperazine $N^{4'}$-oxide (100%) and flu-phenazine $N^{4'}$-oxide (67%), and so can serve to develop RIA's for these compounds and possibly the $N^{4'}$-oxide metabolites of other piperazine-type drugs.

The antisera raised for TFZ [49] were used for the RIA of prochlor-perazine in plasma [53]. There was cross-reaction with N-desmethyl-prochlorperazine but not any other of the available metabolites. For fluphenazine an immunogen was prepared by conjugating BSA to the hapten O-(3-carboxypropionyl)fluphenazine [54]. The resulting anti-sera had significant cross-reactivity (18%) towards one metabolite, 7-hydroxyfluphenazine. For perphenazine the analogous immunogen fur-nished an antiserum which did not cross-react with most of the major metabolites [55].

The above-mentioned antisera allow quantitation, on 200 μl of plasma, down to the levels shown in Table 1 for the various pheno-thiazines [49-55 & (TFZ N-oxide) in press],   usually with C.V. <10%. For each drug the RIA allows the plasma level to be measured as late as 48 h after ingestion of 5 mg by volunteers.

RIA for trimeprazine

Polyclonal antisera for trimeprazine was raised in rabbits to a conjugate of BSA with N-(2-carboxyethyl)desmethyltrimeprazine [56]. With a 200 μl plasma sample there was good sensitivity (Table 1; C.V. ~12%), allowing measurement up to 24 h after a 10 mg dose of trimeprazine tartrate. There was cross-reactivity to the supposedly active metabolite N-desmethyltrimeprazine (49%), but not to trimepra-zine sulphoxide (supposedly inactive).

RIA and stereoselectivity

Besides aiding monitoring in volunteers and patients, RIA's are just beginning to be exploited in studies involving stereospeci-ficity, e.g. a study on doxepin in our laboratories. Antisera obtained with a BSA conjugate of *trans-N*-(2-carboxyethyl)desmethyldoxepin mani-fested only 9% cross-reactivity with *cis*-doxepin and gave sensitivity (Table 1) adequate for doxepin plus N-desmethyldoxepin up to 72 h after a 25 mg oral dose (unpublished work). RIA is evidently a promising approach in investigation of the stereoselective metabolism of drugs and its therapeutic relevance.

VALIDATION OF ANALYTICAL PROCEDURES

RIA compared with HPLC.- Fig. 4 compares the two methods as applied to plasma samples from two healthy volunteers who had received an i.v. dose of 7 or 10 mg of CPZ [57]. There was good agreement (see Fig. 4 legend). With trimeprazine, however, the RIA [56] in

Fig. 4. Plasma levels of CPZ
in dosed volunteers: RIA values
compared with HPLC values.
Overall r = 0.993 (n = 26),
slope = 0.994.

Fig. 5, *below.* Plasma drug
levels *vs.* time in 4 volunteers
after ingestion of 10 mg of
trimeprazine tartrate: o, RIA;
●, HPLC. See text for comment
on the discrepancy.

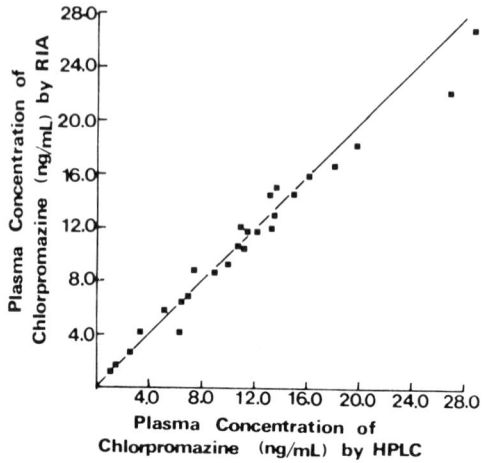

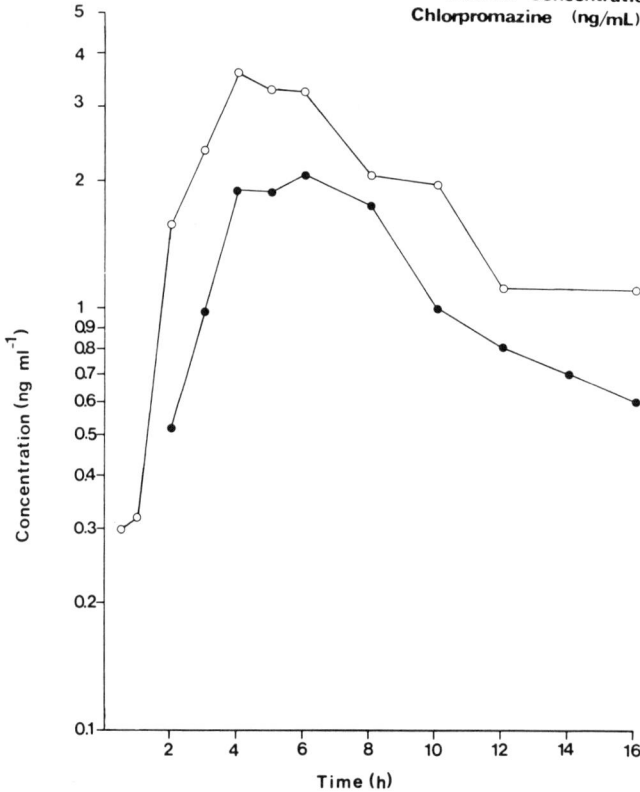

comparison with HPLC [42] gave much higher values (Fig. 5), attributable
to significant (49%) cross-reactivity of the trimeprazine antiserum
with the active metabolite *N*-desmethyltrimeprazine.

HPLC compared with GC–MS.- For CPZ in plasma from dosed volunteers,
these specific chemical procedures [43, 58] showed excellent agreement
(r = 0.962, slope = 0.971; 90 samples).

CONCLUSION

Improved analytical methods for measuring antipsychotic drugs in plasma are constantly being developed (as also noted by S.H. Curry, (this vol.), RIA's have the necessary sensitivity, which should improve further with the commercial availability of ^{125}I-labelled antipsychotics. Evidently, however, RIA's need to be checked for specificity against chemical methods such as GC-MS. HPLC may become a preliminary step in the analyses, both for clean-up and to concentrate the biological sample or extract before measurement by other procedures. The availability of sensitive and specific methods brings benefit to drug development, e.g. single-dose pharmacokinetic studies, and to assessment of patients. Correlation of plasma drug level with clinical response may hinge on measuring important metabolites.

Acknowledgements

The authors thank the Medical Research Council of Canada for support (MT 7838, PG-34), and the Institut National de la Recherche Scientifique - Santé, for sabbatical leave (S.F.C.; see foot of title page of this article).

References

1. Midha, K.K., Loo, J.C.K. & Rowe, M.L. (1979) *Res. Comm. Psychol. Psychiat. Behav. 4*, 193-203.
2. Midha, K.K., Cooper, J.K., Lapierre, Y.D. & Hubbard, J.W. (1981) *Canad. Med. Ass. J. 124*, 263.
3. Roscoe, R.M.H., Cooper, J.K., Hawes, E.M. & Midha, K.K. (1982) *J. Pharm. Sci. 71*, 625-627.
4. Craig, J.C., Gruenke, L.D., Hitzman, B.A., Holaday, J. & Loh, H.H. (1980) in *Phenothiazines and Structurally Related Drugs* (Usdin, E., Eckert, H. & Forrest, I.S., eds.), Raven Press, New York, pp. 129-132 (*Simultaneous determination of chlorpromazine and its major metabolites..... Clinical implications*).
5. McKay, G., Cooper, J.K. & Midha, K.K. (1984) *J. Pharmacol. Meths. 12*, 221-223.
6. Gupta, R.N., Bartolucci, G. & Molnar, G. (1981) *Clin. Chim. Acta 109*, 351-354.
7. Hubbard, J.W., Cooper, J.K., Hawes, E.M., Jenden, D.J., May, P.R.A., Martin, M., McKay, G., Van Putten, T. & Midha, K.K. (1985) *Ther. Drug Monit. 7*, 222-228.
8. Hawes, E.M., Hubbard, J.W., Martin, M., McKay, G., Yeung, P.K.F. & Midha, K.K. (1986) *Ther. Drug Monit.*, in press.
9. McKay, G., Cooper, J.K., Hawes, E.M., Hubbard, J.W., Martin, M. & Midha, K.K. (1985) *Ther. Drug Monit. 7*, 472-477.
10. Lund, A. (1980) *Acta Pharm. Toxicol. 47*, 300-304.
11. Minder, R., Schnetzer, F. & Bickel, M.H. (1971) *Nauyn-Schmied. Arch. Pharmak. 268*, 334-347.
12. Traficante, L.J., Sakalis, G., Siekierski, J., Rotrosen, J. & Gershon, S. (1979) *Life Sci. 24*, 337-345.

13. Kaul, P.N., Chopde, C.T. & Clark, M.L. (1980) *as for* 4.,
    pp. 159-162.
14. Bruderlein, H., Kraml, M. & Dvornik, D. (1977) *Clin. Biochem.*
    10, 3-7.
15. Norman, T.R., Maguire, K.P. & Burrows, G.M. (1977) *J. Chromatog.*
    134, 524-528.
16. Curry, S.H. & Mould, G.P. (1969) *J. Pharm. Pharmacol.21*, 674-677.
17. Dinovo, E.C., Gottschalk, L.A., Nandi, B.R. & Geddes, P.G. (1976)
    J. Pharm. Sci. 65, 667-669.
18. Dahl, S.G. & Jacobson, S. (1976) *J. Pharm. Sci. 65*, 1329-1333.
19. De Leenheer, A.P. (1974) *J. Pharm. Sci. 63*, 389-394.
20. Schley, J., Riedel, E. & Muller-Oerlinghausen, B. (1978)
    J. Clin. Chem. Clin. Biochem. 16, 307-311.
21. Vanderheeren, F.A.J., Theunis, D.J.C.J. & Rosseel, M.T. (1976)
    J. Chromatog. 120, 123-128.
22. Bailey, D.N. & Guba, J.J. (1979) *Clin. Chem. 25*, 1211-1215.
23. Javaid, J.I., Dekirmenjan, H., Liskevych, U. & Davis, J.M. (1979)
    J. Chromatog. Sci. 17, 666-670.
24. Javaid, J.I., Dekirmenjian, H., Liskevych, U., Lin, R.L. &
    Davis, J.M. (1981) *J. Chromatog. Sci. 19*, 439-443.
25. Dysken, M.W., Javaid, J.I., Chang, S.S., Schaffer, C. & Shahid, A.
    (1981) *Psychopharmacol. 73*, 325-331.
26. Midha, K.K., McKay, G., Edom, R., Korchinski, E.D., Hawes, E.M.
    & Hall, K. (1983) *Eur. J. Clin. Pharmacol. 25*, 709-711.
27. Curry, S.H. (1968) *Anal. Chem. 40*, 1251-1255.
28. Davis, C.M., Meyer, C.J. & Fenimore, D.C. (1977) *Clin. Chim.*
    Acta 78, 71-77.
29. Larsen, N.E. & Naestoft, J. (1975) *J. Chromatog. 109*, 259-264.
30. Hansen, C.E., Christensen, T.R., Elley, J., Hansen, L.B.,
    Kragh-Sorensen, P., Larsen, N.E., Naestoft, J. Hvidberg, E.F.
    (1976) *Br. J. Clin. Pharmacol. 3*, 915-923.
31. Cooper, S.F., Albert, J.M., Dugal, R. & Bertrand, M. (1978)
    J. Chromatog. 150, 263-265.
32. Cooper, S.F., Albert, J.M., Dugal, R. Bertrand, M. & Elie, R.
    (1979) *Arzneim.-Forsch./Drug Res. 29*, 158-161.
33. Cooper, S.F. & Lapierre, Y.D. (1981) *J. Chromatog. 222*,291-296.
34. Craig, J.C., Mary, N.Y. & Roy, S.K. (1964) *Anal. Chem. 36*, 1142-
    1146.
35. Hall, K., Yeung, P.K.F. & Midha, K.K. (1982) *J. Chromatog. 231*,
    200-204.
36. Philipson, O.T., McKeown, J.M., Baker,J. & Healy, A.F. (1977)
    Br. J. Psychiat. 131, 172-184.
37. MacKay, A.V.P., Healy, A.F. & Baker, J. (1974) *Br. J. Clin.*
    Pharmacol. 1, 425-430.
38. Midha, K.K., Roscoe, R.M.H., Hall, K., Hawes, E.M., Cooper, J.K.,
    McKay, G. & Shetty, U. (1982) *Biomed. Mass Spectrom. 9*, 186-190.
39. Midha, K.K., Korchinski, E.D., Verbeeck, R.K., Roscoe, R.M.H.,
    Hawes, E.M., Cooper, J.K. & McKay, G. (1983) *Br. J. Clin.*
    Pharmacol. 15, 380-382.

40. McKay, G., Hall, K., Edom, R., Hawes, E.M. & Midha, K.K.
    (1983) *Biomed. Mass Spectrom. 10*, 550-555.
41. Shetty, U.M., Hawes, E.M. & Midha, K.K.(1983) *Biomed. Mass
    Spectrom. 10*, 601-607.
42. McKay, G., Cooper, J.K., Midha, K.K., Hall, K. & Hawes, E.M.
    (1982) *J. Chromatog. 233*, 417-422.
43. Cooper, J.K., McKay, G. & Midha, K.K. (1983) *J. Pharm. Sci. 72*,
    1259-1262.
44. McKay, G., Cooper, J.K., Gurnsey, T. & Midha, K.K. (1985)
    LC Liq. Chromatog. HPLC Mag. 3, 256-258.
45. Midha, K.K., Loo, J.C.K., Hubbard, J.W., Rowe, M.L. &
    McGilveray, I.J. (1979) *Clin. Chem. 25*, 166-168.
46. Yeung, P.K.F., Hubbard, J.W., Cooper, J.K. & Midha, K.K. (1983)
    J. Pharmacol. Exp. Ther. 226, 833-838.
47. Yeung, P.K.F., McKay, G., Ramshaw, I.A., Hubbard, J.W. &
    Midha, K.K. (1985) *J. Pharmacol. Exp. Ther. 233*, 816-822.
48. Abraham, G.E. (1969) *J. Clin. Endocrinol. Metab. 29*, 866-870.
49. Midha, K.K., Hubbard, J.W., Cooper, J.K., Hawes, E.M.,
    Fournier, S. & Yeung, P.K.F. (1981) *Br. J. Clin. Pharmacol. 12*, 189-193.
50. Hawes, E.M., Shetty, H.U., Cooper, J.K., Rauw, G., McKay, G., &
    Midha, K.K. (1984) *J. Pharm. Sci. 73*, 247-250.
51. Aravagiri, M., Hawes, E.M. & Midha, K.K. (1984) *J. Pharm. Sci.
    73*, 1383-1387.
52. Aravagiri, M., Hawes, E.M. & Midha, K.K. (1985) *J. Pharm. Sci.
    74*, 1196-1202.
53. Midha, K.K., Hawes, E.M., Rauw, G., McVittie, J., McKay, G.,
    Cooper, J.K. & Shetty, H.U. (1983) *Ther. Drug Monit. 5*, 117-121.
54. Midha, K.K., Cooper, J.K. & Hubbard, J.W. (1980) *Comm.
    Psychopharmacol. 4*, 107-114.
55. Midha, K.K., Mackonka, C., Cooper, J.K., Hubbard, J.W. &
    Yeung, P.K.F. (1981) *Br. J. Clin. Pharmacol. 1*, 85-88.
56. McKay, G., Rauw, G.A.J., Stonkus, M.D., Dulos, R.A., Gedir, R.G.,
    Hawes, E.M. & Midha, K.K. (1984) *J. Pharmacol. Meths. 12*, 203-211.
57. Midha, K.K., Cooper, J.K., McGilveray, I.J., Butterfield, A.G.
    & Hubbard, J.W. (1981) *J. Pharm. Sci. 70*, 1043-1046.
58. McKay, G., Hall, K., Cooper, J.K., Hawes, E.M. & Midha, K.K.
    (1982) *J. Chromatog. 232*, 275-282.

#B-5

ANALYSIS OF THIOXANTHENES BY HPTLC, HPLC, CAPILLARY GC, AND RIA

A. Jørgensen, K. Fredricson Overø,
T. Aaes-Jørgensen and J.V. Christensen

H. Lundbeck A/S
Ottiliavej 7-9
DK-2500 Copenhagen-Valby, Denmark

Require-ment	*Assay methodology for several thioxanthenes (see Fig. 1), e.g. zuclopenthixol [the cis(Z)-isomer of clopenthixol], present in serum at levels down to 1 ng/ml or even less.*			
End-step	**HPTLC**	**HPLC**	**Capillary GC**	**RIA**
	Ascending mode; a purification run, then a separation run; acidified plate examined for fluorescent spots.	*Straight-phase (NP) HPLC with ammoniacal heptane/isoProH; detection by absorption at 254 or 229 nm.*	*Good peaks (N-P detection) on column with film of phenyl-methyl-silicone.*	*Incubate with antiserum and ³H-drug; charcoal to adsorb unbound drug, then count.*
Sample preparation	*Heptane extraction, alkaline pH.*	*Hexane extraction, alkaline pH; repeat after back-extraction.*	*Extraction procedure awaits development.*	*Clean-up by treating with petroleum-benzine.*
Comments	*Metabolite geometric isomers not separated.*	*Geometric isomers separated.*	*Potentially sensitive & specific.*	*Interferences from related drugs.*

The thioxanthene neuroleptics (Fig. 1) are closely related to the phenothiazines, the only difference being replacement of a nitrogen atom in the central ring by a carbon atom in the plane of the ring. The double-bond linkage of the side-chain to the ring structure allows the possibility of two geometric isomers, termed cis(Z) and trans(E). Neuroleptic activity has been shown pharmacologically and clinically only for the cis(Z) isomers. Of the four thioxan-

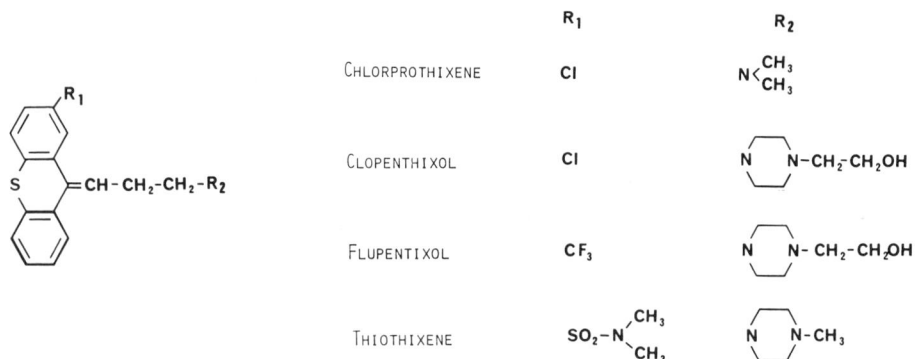

		R_1	R_2
CHLORPROTHIXENE		Cl	$N\begin{smallmatrix}CH_3\\CH_3\end{smallmatrix}$
CLOPENTHIXOL		Cl	$N\bigcirc N-CH_2-CH_2OH$
FLUPENTIXOL		CF_3	$N\bigcirc N-CH_2-CH_2OH$
THIOTHIXENE		$SO_2-N\begin{smallmatrix}CH_3\\CH_3\end{smallmatrix}$	$N\bigcirc N-CH_3$

Fig. 1. Chemical structures of the thioxanthene neuroleptics.

thenes that are on the market, for 3 only the active cis(Z)-isomer is used. Analytically the double bond can be advantageous since strongly acid conditions lead to formation of a thioxanthylium ion, which has a yellow fluorescence. Since the early 1960's, as the title of this article indicates, we have used different analytical techniques, each of which has advantages and disadvantages. Since these drugs have very high volumes of distribution, 10-20 l/kg, and are given in low dosage, an analytical method for serum or plasma has to have a limit of sensitivity as low as ~1 ng/ml (2.5-3 nM).

HPTLC APPROACH

The determination of thioxanthenes by TLC hinges on treatment with strong acids to form a fluorescent thioxanthylium ion:

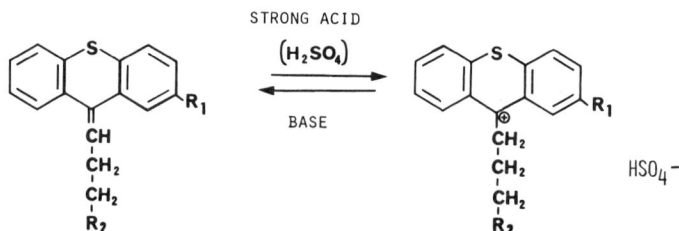

Ions with the same fluorescence characteristics arise from either isomer or from metabolites which differ from the parent drug only in the side-chain. Thus this principle can be used only if a separation precedes the acidification and fluorescence measurement. The procedure for zuclopenthixol is as follows. Plasma (up to 2 ml) is shaken to extract at alkaline pH with heptane containing 0.1% isopropylamine (NaOH used for the alkalinization). After centrifugation and freezing, the heptane layer is removed to a conical tube and taken to dryness (air

stream) at 40°. (The isopropylamine is added to counteract adsorption
onto glass surfaces.) The residue is redissolved in 100 μl chloroform
and the whole sample is applied to a HPTLC plate (Merck, Silica Gel 60)
using a Desaga Autospotter.   Ascending chromatography is performed
firstly with pure ethyl acetate, which removes impurities but does
not cause migration of the drug and metabolites. Then development is
performed with acetone/heptane/diethylamine (30:20:3.5   by vol.)
which gives a good separation of drug and metabolites. After drying,
the plate is acidified by immersion in 10% (v/v) conc. sulphuric acid
in ether for 1 min, and dried for 20 min at 80°.   The plate was
scanned using a Perkin-Elmer MPF-3L fluorescence spectrophotometer
(excitation, 388 nm; emission, 554 nm) equipped with a TLC scanning
device.

There is ~75% recovery of the parent drug and the *N*-dealkyl
metabolite through the extraction procedure. Standard curves obtained
from drug-free plasma spiked with zuclopenthixol and the metabolite are
linear up to ~25 ng on the plate. The C.V. is <10%, and the limit of
detection for the parent compound is ~2 ng per sample.

The HPTLC method has a relatively high throughput, one technician
being able to process ~20 samples in a working day. Specificity is
good, except that separation of cis(Z)- and trans(E)-isomers of
metabolites is incomplete. Sensitivity is quite good, and adequate
for most samples, but is inferior to that of HPLC.

HPLC APPROACH

Most problems faced by analysts during the first two decades with
the neuroleptic drugs were overcome with the advent of HPLC in the
late 1970's. We have developed a method for zuclopenthixol [1]
which with minor modification of the eluent can be used also for
flupentixol and chlorprothixene. The method gives values not only for
the drug but also a *N*-dealkyl metabolite and an internal standard
(i.s.) closely related chemically to the drug but without a double
bond - so escaping the complication of two isomers.

The sample treatment, somewhat complicated, entails extraction
of serum (up to 3 ml), with a 300 μl/ml ethanol addition, at alkaline
pH with heptane containing 0.1% isopropylamine; then back-extraction
into 0.1 M HCl or 0.05 M H_2SO_4, and re-extraction with heptane after
rendering the aqueous phase alkaline. The final heptane phase is
taken to dryness and the residue dissolved in 120 μl heptane, of
which 100 μl is chromatographed; the extraction recoveries of drug
and metabolite are ~50%.

HPLC is done with a Waters pump (#6000 A) and 254 nm detector
(#440), and a NP column (250×i.d. 4.6 mm) containing Spherisorb S5W
(spherical silica, 5 μm). The mobile phase is heptane/isopropanol/

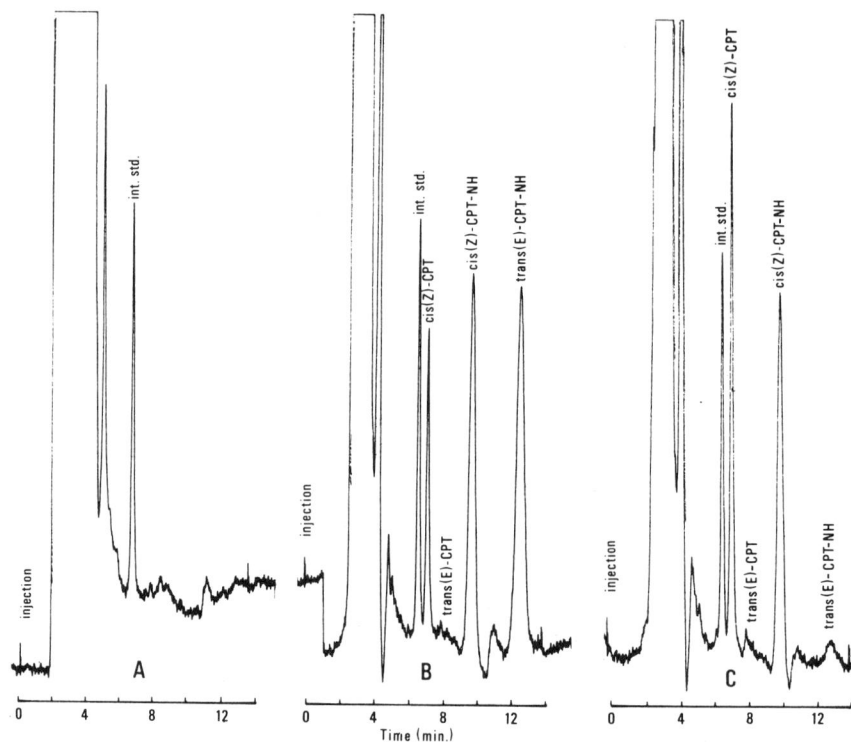

Fig. 2. HPLC patterns. A: Blank serum with added internal standard, 25 ng.   B: Blank serum with spiked-in internal standard
(as in A); zuclopenthixol [cis(Z)-CPT, 10 ng]; the dealkylated
metabolite cis(Z)-CPT-NH (clopenthixol minus R_2 chain, Fig. 1; 28 ng);
trans(E)-CPT-NH (22 ng). C: Serum sample from a patient given
daily doses of zuclopenthixol. *From ref. [1]©, by permission of
Elsevier Scientific Publishing Co.*

conc. NH_3/H_2O (85:15:0.4:0.2 by vol.); flow 1 ml/min. Fig. 2 illustrates
the chromatographic results.   Blank serum spiked with i.s. showed
no impurity peaks in the positions manifest in Fig. 2B for spiked-in
zuclopenthixol, trans(E)-clopenthixol, or the two isomers of the
N-dealkyl metabolite. The small peak observed for trans(E)-clopen-
thixol is due to a trace present in the zuclopenthixol standard
and small amounts formed during the extraction procedure. In serum
from a patient given zuclopenthixol orally (Fig. 2C), quite high concentrations of the drug and the cis(Z)-isomer of the metabolite
are seen, but only trace amounts of the trans(E)-isomers.

A standard curve was produced from blank serum spiked with
zuclopenthixol, with pooling of the very reproducible results from
several days to give a curve with a large number of data points.
The validity of this curve is checked for each batch of samples, by

inclusion of a sample containing 10 or 30 ng/ml of zuclopenthixol. From the standard curve and actual samples, the limit of sensitivity has been estimated as 1 ng/sample, hence <1 ng/ml is measurable using 2 or even 3 ml of serum. Based on the assay of identical standard samples the C.V. is 3-7%, independent of concentration in the range 3-90 ng/ml. A throughput of 16-20 samples in a working day is feasible. The use of shorter columns with smaller particles (e.g. 100×4 mm; 3 μm) somewhat improves sensitivity, also achievable by detecting at 229 nm. (Other wavelengths could help since neither 254 nor 229 nm represents a UV absorption maximum in the absorption spectrum of the thioxanthenes.)

RP-HPLC columns (e.g. CN or C-8) have also been investigated, but in general this type of column gives less distinct peaks and thus (by a factor of 2 or 3) lower sensitivity. For two of the drugs, cis(Z)-flupentixol and zuclopenthixol we have also worked with fatty acid esters which are used as pro-drugs (given intramuscularly as a solution in oil). The decanoate esters are eluted close to the solvent front on a NP column, and for these compounds we have accepted a lower sensitivity and used a RP column. For short-chain esters such as acetates a NP column may still be used but with a more polar mobile phase.

CAPILLARY GC APPROACH

GC analysis of neuroleptic drugs using packed columns has been rather beset with problems. For the simplest thioxanthene, chlorprothixene, we succeeded in developing a method and getting some values using an OV-17 packed column. However, we found that the results were too variable and stopped using this method. For flupentixol and clopenthixol, which both have a more complex side-chain, we attempted to use packed columns, with or without derivatization, but never succeeded in getting a reasonable sensitivity. This was possibly due to adsorption onto the column material or to breakdown due to the high temperature used. We concluded that GC with packed columns could not be used for estimation of thioxanthene neuroleptics. However, the development of cross-linked phases for capillary GC has provided new possibilities. On a 10 m column, i.d. 0.32 mm, with a 0.52 μm film of 5% phenylmethylsilicone we have obtained very sharp peaks for chlorprothixene, zuclopenthixol and cis(Z)-flupentixol by using on-column injection, temperature programming up to 300°, and a N-P detector (Fig. 3). So far we have not developed extraction procedures, but the chromatograms show that there may be great potential for the use of capillary GC.

RIA APPROACH

Our effort to develop an RIA for flupentixol began in 1973, before HPLC became commonly available and at a time when attempts to assay these drugs by GC had been unsuccessful. Today, with other

Fig. 3. Capillary GC
chromatogram of a standard
mixture of neuroleptic
drugs, 20 ng of each. The
time from injection to the
appearance of peak 5 was
11 min.

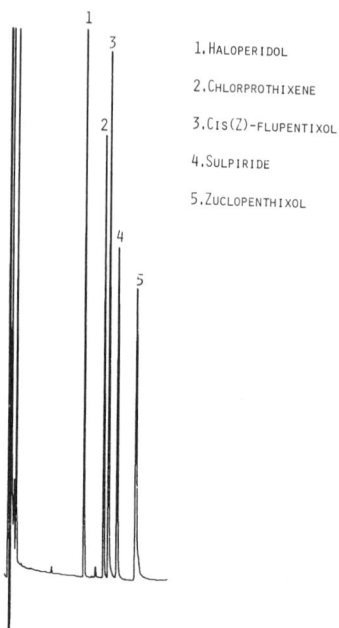

1. HALOPERIDOL
2. CHLORPROTHIXENE
3. CIS(Z)-FLUPENTIXOL
4. SULPIRIDE
5. ZUCLOPENTHIXOL

techniques available, I doubt whether we would feel it worth trying
to develop RIA's for these drugs. We did succeed in developing a
RIA for cis(Z)-flupentixol [2]. To enable it to be attached to
a protein we synthesized a 7-carboxy derivative of the drug (Fig. 4),
choosing position 7 as it is a reasonable distance from the three
positions of metabolic attack - the sulphur atom, the piperazine ring
and the OH-group. We confirmed the success of the coupling by subjecting the dialyzed end-product to hydrolysis followed by qualitative
detection of the 7-carboxy derivative by TLC. The coupled product
with Freund's adjuvant was given to animals by several i.m. and
s.c. injections, firstly with small animals - guinea pigs and rabbits.
Andibodies (Ab's) were indeed obtained, but they lacked specificity,
especially in respect of metabolites, which cross-reacted substantially.

Fig. 4. Immunogen
used to immunize
animals for production
of Ab's towards
cis(Z)-flupentixol.
A carbodiimide reac-
tion was used for
the coupling to
bovine serum albumin.

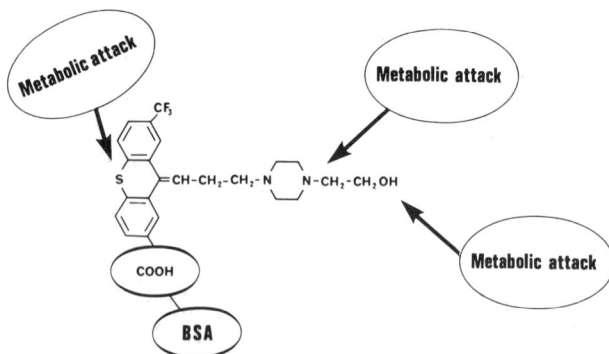

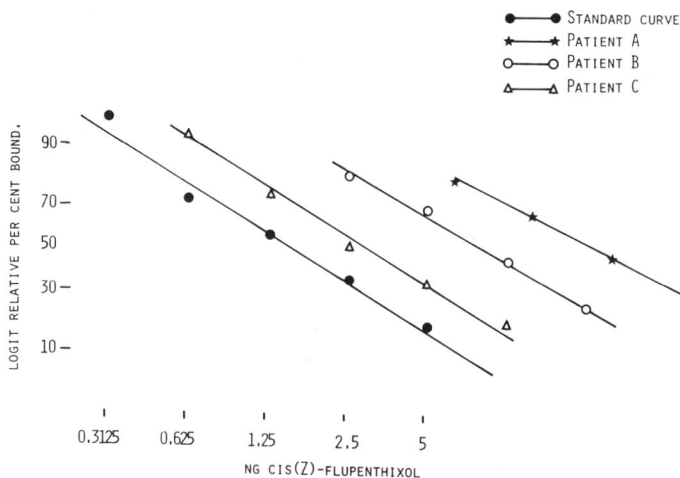

Fig. 5. Comparison of relative % binding after adding known amounts of cis(Z)-flupentixol to blank human serum (standard curve; the values represent ng/ml and the relative binding in three different patient sera diluted 1+1 with blank human serum. *From ref. [2]©, by permission of Pergamon Press.*

In order to obtain greater specificity, we turned to sheep, which did furnish the requisite Ab's. Based on Ab serum from the sheep and [^{3}H]cis(Z)-flupentixol of high specific activity (10-20 mCi/mg) a RIA was devised. To obtain high sensitivity, up to 250 μl of serum was used, and this caused some variability presumably due to interference from serum constituents. We therefore introduced an initial purification step. The serum is acidified with acetic acid and shaken with 2.5 ml of petroleum-benzene (40-60°). The organic phase is discarded. The aqueous phase neutralized with phosphate buffer, and labelled drug and diluted antiserum (1:100,000) are added. Incubation is done overnight, as with only 1-2 h specificity is poorer. Charcoal is added to adsorb unbound drug, followed by centrifugation, and 1 ml of supernatant is counted in a liquid scintillation counter with external quench correction.

The logit of relative binding plotted against the logarithm of drug content gives a straight line (Fig. 5). The standard curve is never used outside the 10-90% range, and we usually dilute high-level samples to obviate low binding values. The limit of sensitivity of the assay (concentration giving 90% relative binding) is 0.2-0.3 ng/ml when 0.25 ml of serum is used. Fig. 5 also shows results for three successively diluted sera from patients treated with cis(Z)-flupentixol decanoate. The fact that we have obtained straight lines, which are parallel to the standard curve, is a good indication that no other compound in the samples except the drug influences the binding to any appreciable degree. The precision of the assay, estimated by taking 8 identical samples from each of two pools of patient sera, was 6-7%, whereas the day-to-day variation in estimating identical samples was ~20%.

The specificity of the assay can be judged from the cross-reactivity of a number of related compounds including the metabolites. The pharmacologically inactive trans(*E*)-isomer gives 7% cross-reaction and has to be corrected for when flupentixol tablets containing a 1:1 mixture of the two isomers are administered; it is assumed that the two isomers behave identically after administration. The two most important metabolites, *N*-dealkyl flupentixol and flupentixol sulphoxide, show only 2% and 1% cross-reaction respectively. Since they are present in serum only to about the same extent as the parent drug isomer, this interference is of no practical importance. Cis(Z)-flupentixol decanoate which is the ester used in the depot formulation of cis(Z)-flupentixol cross-reacts 6%, but this ester has never been detected in serum.

Some other neuroleptic drugs may interfere with the assay. Zuclopenthixol, which differs in the ring substituent, shows 14% cross-reaction. The cis(Z)-isomer of fluprothixene, which has a different side-chain to cis(Z)-flupentixol, shows 5% cross-reaction. Chlorprothixene, differing from cis(Z)-flupentixol in substituents as well as side-chain, has only 1% cross-reactivity. Neuroleptics of the phenothiazine group may also cross-react. Fluphenazine, which is the phenothiazine corresponding to flupentixol, is 17% cross-reactive, whereas chlorpromazine, which differs in ring substituent and side-chain, has negligible cross-reactivity (0.1%).

The throughput of the RIA can be very high: one technician can handle 100-150 samples in one batch. As mentioned above, sensitivity is good: down to 0.2-0.3 ng/ml (0.5-0.8 nM).

CONCLUDING COMMENT

Whilst RIA could seem to be the method of choice, it is our opinion that one should rather work with chromatographic procedures, as RIA is more susceptible to interference from other drugs prescribed by the clinician or taken by the patient on his own initiative, and from other constituents of serum or plasma. The choice of chromatographic approach hinges on the sensitivity needed, whether inactive isomer is present, and whether metabolites are to be determined.

References

1. Aaes-Jørgensen, T. (1980) *J. Chromatog. 183*, 239-249.
2. Jørgensen, A. (1978) *Life Sci. 23*, 1533-1542.

#B-6

HPLC-EC DETERMINATION OF PHYSOSTIGMINE
IN BIOLOGICAL SAMPLES

Robin Whelpton and Peter Hurst

Department of Pharmacology and Therapeutics
London Hospital Medical College
Whitechapel, London E1 2AD, U.K.

Require- *An assay sensitive enough (<0.1 ng/ml) for pharmacokinetic*
ment   *studies after injected or oral doses of physostigmine in*
        man. Fluids to be assayed: plasma, blood, urine.

End-step *HPLC with dual electrode electrochemical (EC) detection;*
         3 μm silica column eluted with alkaline eluent.

Sample   *(1) Diethyl ether or benzene extraction of sample after*
prepar- *adding alkali; concentration by evaporation. Residue dissol-*
ation   *ved in methanol and transferred to autosampler for injection.*

         (2) Solid-phase extraction using CN BondElut columns. Drug
         eluted with methanol.

Comments *Stability problems due to (i) chemical hydrolysis in alkaline*
         media, and (ii) enzymatic hydrolysis in blood and plasma.

Physostigmine, an alkaloid from the Calabar bean, is a potent inhibitor of cholinesterase. Unlike the other carbamate anticholinesterases, neostigmine and pyridostigmine, it is a tertiary amine and enters the CNS. It is used for treating poisoning with anticholinergic drugs and is being evaluated for the treatment of the memory defects of Alzheimer's disease. (Its formula appears below Fig. 2.)

We became interested in assaying physostigmine in 1980 when a colleague desired pharmacokinetic data in order to plan behavioural studies with reference to predicted plasma concentrations. Pharmacokinetic data were lacking because there was not a sensitive enough assay. At the time we were assaying thioridazine by HPLC with UV detection, and as physostigmine is a lipophilic base with a molar extinction of ~13,000 $M^{-1}cm^{-1}$, at 252 nm, we attempted to assay it using the thioridazine system. In two days we achieved a calibration

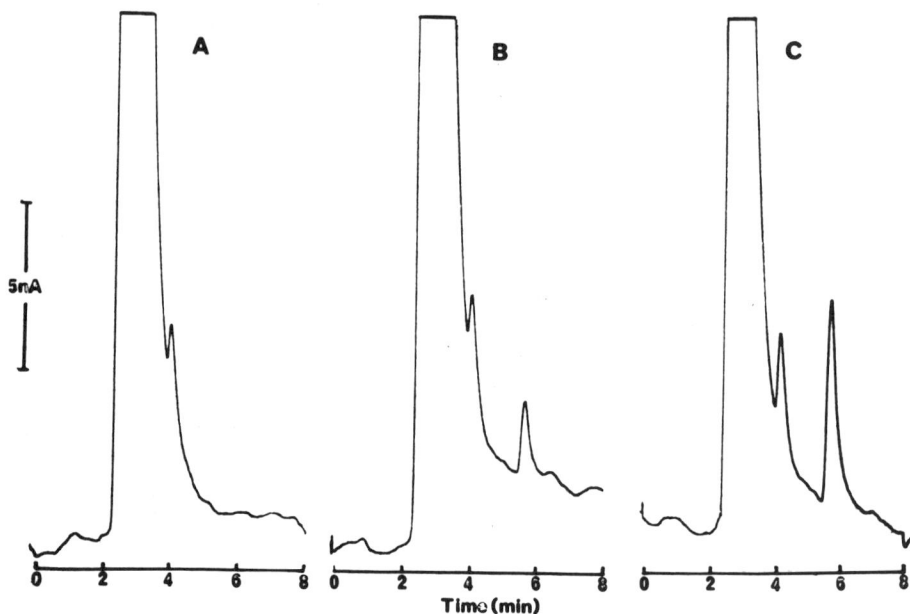

Fig. 1. Chromatograms of physostigmine with the EC detector at 0.8 V. **A:** pre-dose plasma; **B:** plasma from subject receiving 0.75 mg physostigmine s.c.; **C:** standard plasma containing 10 ng/ml.

curve for between 5 and 20 ng/ml plasma, better than the existing enzymatic method that was sensitive only down to 7 ng/ml [1].

Hexane and diethyl ether were tried as solvents for extracting physostigmine from alkalinized plasma. However, the higher extraction efficiency into diethyl ether was offset by the presence of many UV-absorbing materials that produced interfering peaks and prevented reliable quantification.

Electrochemical (EC) detection was attempted, initially without success but after more experience of the Bioanalytical Systems (BAS) detector we developed a method, extracting with diethyl ether (freshly distilled to remove electro-active antioxidants) and detecting amperimetrically, that was sensitive down to 0.5 ng/ml [2]. This enabled us to measure physostigmine concentrations in plasma after a low dose (0.75 mg) given subcutaneously (Fig. 1).

REFINEMENT OF HPLC ASSAY WITH ELECTROCHEMICAL DETECTION

To measure the lower plasma concentrations expected after oral doses, the above method was modified. As column packing, 5 µm was replaced by 3 µm silica; a dual-electrode coulometric detector was used instead of glassy carbon, and an internal standard (i.s.) was

Fig. 2. Per-cent physostigmine remaining in plasma as a fuction of time and temperature. The initial concentration was 5 ng/ml.

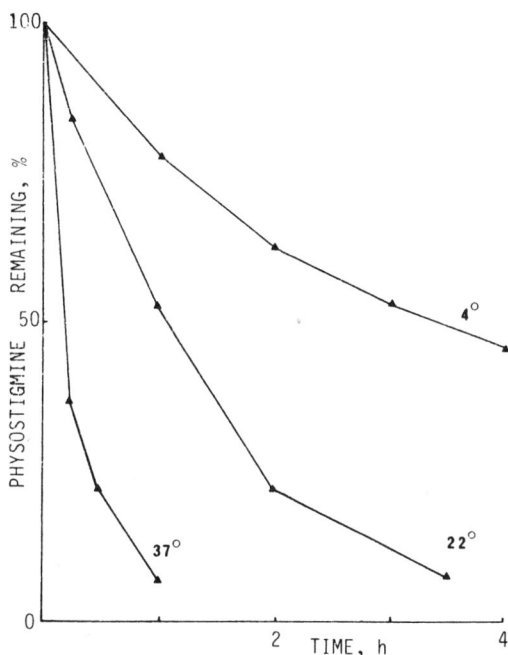

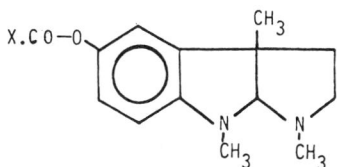

physostigmine   X=CH₃NH-

internal standard   X=(CH₃)₂N-

included. Three compounds were prepared for evaluation as an i.s.: the *N*-ethyl   and *N*-propyl homologues and *(above)*   the *N,N*-dimethyl analogue.   The *N*-ethyl homologue was not sufficiently resolved from physostigmine (it chromatographed between physostigmine and the propyl derivative).   The propyl homologue was rejected because it least resembled physostigmine in extractability in relation to pH [3]. This left the *N,N*-dimethyl analogue as the best choice of i.s.

A problem that we were aware of almost from the start was that physostigmine is unstable in plasma, causing difficulty in generating calibration curves, as shown in Fig. 2.   When incubated with plasma at 37°, physostigmine   (5 ng/ml)   disappearance followed apparent first-order kinetics with a half-life of 15 min.   Cooling in ice-water slowed the rate of loss but did not completely inhibit it.   At higher initial concentrations (e.g. 100 ng/ml) the kinetics of hydrolysis were almost zero-order – suggesting that the loss was   enzymatic,

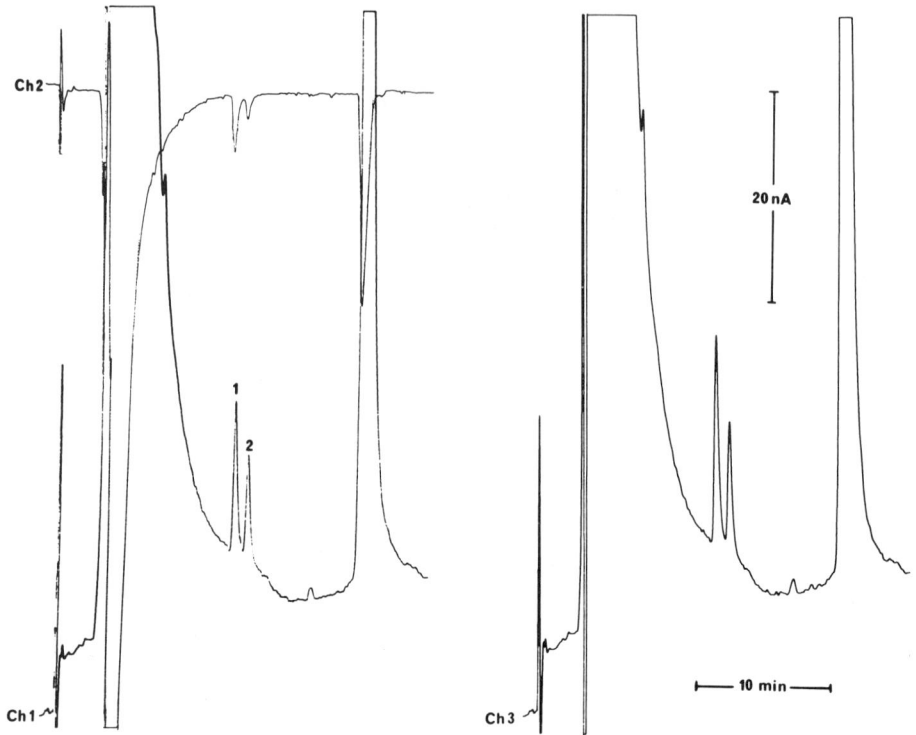

Fig. 3. Chromatogram of plasma spiked at 0.5 ng/ml. *Left:* oxidation (*upper.* +0.7 V) and reduction (*lower,* -0.2 V). *Right:* sum of oxidation and reduction signals.

due to cholinesterase. Neostigmine at 50 µg/ml completely inhibited the hydrolysis, and so was added to blood samples as soon as possible after they had been drawn. To avoid problems caused by neostigmine displacing physostigmine from red cells, whole blood rather than plasma was used for assay.

To 2 ml of blood containing neostigmine, 0.1 ml of i.s. in methanol was added, and 1 ml M NH$_4$OH and 5 ml of freshly distilled ether (or of benzene; advantageous when assaying urine samples, below). The tubes were shaken for 15 min, centrifuged and 4 ml of the organic layer transferred to a tapered tube and evaporated at 40° (air or N$_2$ stream). The residue was dissolved in 100 µl methanol and 50 µl injected into the chromatograph via a Kontron autosampler. The Coulochem detector [see R. Whelpton, #NC(C)-3 in Vol. 14, this series – *Ed.*] was operated with the first electrode at +0.7 V and the second at -0.2 V. The guard cell, positioned post-column before the analytical cell, was set at 0.4 V. Fig. 3 shows a representative run. The sensitivity of the assay was ~0.1 ng/ml using a 2 ml sample (C.V. 10%), but with a 4 ml sample as little as 25 pg in spiked plasma has been assayed with a C.V. of 20%.

SOLID–PHASE AS ALTERNATIVE TO LIQUID–LIQUID EXTRACTION

The renal clearance of physostigmine is ~50–100 ml/min; hence urine concentrations are much higher than those found in blood. However, ether extracts of urine were too dirty and benzene was used instead. To avoid the use of this toxic solvent and to simplify the assay, solid-phase extraction techniques were considered. The BondElut columns contained 100 mg of the chosen sorbent. A manifold to hold the columns was constructed by joining together standard Luer 3-way taps. A vacuum line was attached to the end tap. After the samples had been applied and washed under vacuum, the columns were removed from the manifold and eluted with methanol by centrifugation. The eluent was collected in polyethylene microcentrifuge tubes of capacity 1.5 ml, or 0.25 ml for small fractions, e.g. when examining the elution patterns of various types of silica (the tubes conveniently fit the Kontron autosampler, but must first be vortexed because the eluate is not homogeneous). Fig. 4 shows the collection assembly.

The columns were prepared by washing with methanol (2×1 ml), water (2×1 ml) and 0.1 M K_2HPO_4 (1 ml). The sample (1 ml) was mixed with i.s. solution (0.1 ml) and 1 ml applied to the column. The columns were washed with water (3×1 ml) and then eluted with methanol or further washed with 50% aqueous methanol (v/v; 2×0.1 ml) before elution. Fig. 5 shows the elution patterns obtained with 4 types of column. The sharpest elution was obtained when the sample was added as a solution in distilled water (Fig. 5, top). Washing with a small quantity of 50% methanol prior to elution resulted in an earlier but broader band with the nitrile columns, whereas with C-18 and C-8 columns the elution was a little later (Fig. 5, middle). When physostigmine was applied as a solution in urine, the elution bands were even broader (Fig. 5, bottom). The C-18 and C-8 columns retained urine pigments as a deep yellow band at the top of the columns, and although the 50% methanol wash removed some colour the first 100 µl fractions were so coloured that they were not injected into the chromatograph. Subsequent fractions showed marked tailing. The nitrile column retained very little coloured material, and physostigmine eluted in a reasonably shaped band with all the samples.

The i.s. eluted a little later than physostigmine; hence the physostigmine/i.s. ratio was different in each of the fractions. This prevented us reaching our goal of finding a system that would concentrate physostigmine and i.s. in discrete fractions of 100–200 µl. However, because of the higher concentrations in urine, it may not be necessary to concentrate the sample as distinct from remove physostigmine from the bulk of the biological material. The precision of this approach was tested by replicate assays of 0.5 ml urine samples using nitrile columns (CN BondElut) and eluting with 0.5 ml methanol. Intra-assay C.V.'s were satisfactory: 1.48% (6 obs.) for 100 ng/ml (column used 6 times); 0.64% (6) for 100 ng/ml with a second column; 1.29% (6) for 50 ng/ml; 1.92% (5) for 10 ng/ml.

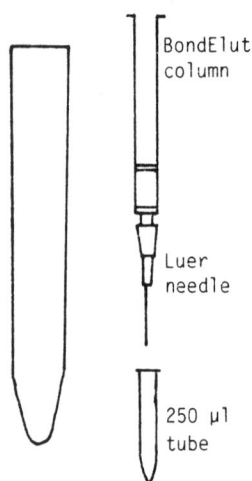

Fig. 4.
Elution
assembly
(see text).

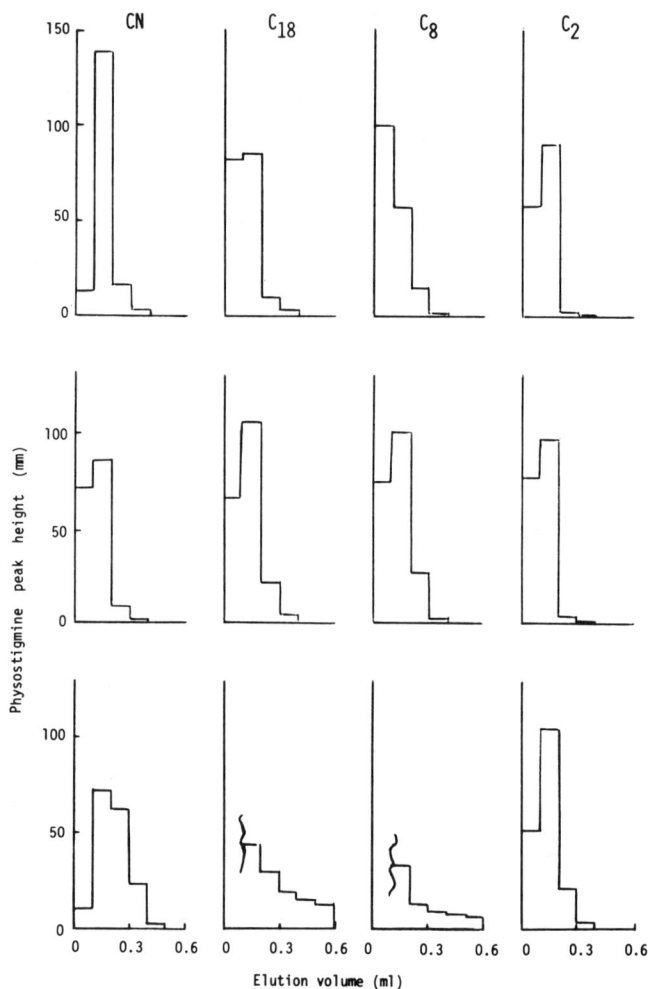

Fig. 5. Elution of physostigmine from BondElut columns of differ-ent types. *Top:* sample applied in 1 ml distilled water. **Middle:** *ditto* but washed with 50% methanol before elution. **Bottom:** *as for middle* but sample applied in 1 ml urine.

CONCLUDING COMMENTS

HPLC with EC detection offers a very sensitive method of assaying physostigmine in biological fluids. The method can be simplified by the use of solid-phase extraction columns, most suitably of nitrile type. Our remaining problem is loss by enzymic hydrolysis after taking blood samples. We are currently seeking an inhibitor that will inhibit the hydrolytic enzymes but have minimal effect on red cell partitioning and plasma-protein binding.

References

1. Groff, W.A., Ellin, R.I. & Skalsky, P.L. (1977) *J. Pharm. Sci.*
    66. 389-391.
2. Whelpton, R. (1983) *J. Chromatog. 272*, 216-220.
3. Whelpton, R. & Moore, T. (1985) *J. Chromatog. 341*, 361-371.

#B-7

HPLC-UV DETERMINATION OF SUBSTITUTED BENZAMIDES IN BIOLOGICAL FLUIDS FOR THEIR PHARMACOKINETIC STUDY

F. Bressolle, J. Bres and M. Snoussi

Groupe de Recherche en Pharmacocinétique
Faculté de Pharmacie
34060 Montpellier, France

Require- *Specific and sensitive assays for sulpiride, sultopride and*
ment   *a new substituted benzamide RIV 2093 (formulae: Fig. 1)*
        in plasma (also red blood cells, RBC) and urine.

End-step *RP-HPLC (at 50°) with 0.1 M ammonium acetate/methanol eluent;*
        (lower proportion of methanol for RIV 2093); detection at
        226 nm. In an earlier ('variant') method for sulpiride,
        with 197 nm detection, elution times were longer.

Sample   *Extraction by chloroform at pH 10, after an acid step if*
prepa-   *advantageous, or (RIV 2093) at 8.9. Internal standard*
ration   *(i.s.) added then or (RIV 2093) initially. Residue from*
        drying down the extract dissolved in mobile phase for HPLC.

Comments *In respect of linearity and other desired features the assays*
        perform well, and surpass previously reported methods (spec-
        trophotometry; TLC; HPLC). The methods are useful for drug
        monitoring as well as pharmacokinetic studies.

    The neuroleptic and antipsychotic benzamides are now widely
used as psychotherapeutic agents. They differ notably from the
other neuroleptics in having a much smaller volume of distribution
(1/kg): 0.6 for sulpiride [1], 1.43 for tiapride [2], 2.30 for a
new substituted benzamide, RIV 2093 (5-methylaminosulphonyl-N-[{1-
allyl-2-pyrrolidinyl}methyl]-2-methoxy-4-aminobenzamide), 2.2 to 3.4
for metoclopramide [3, 4] and 3.0 for sultopride [5, 6]. Sensitive
analytical techniques are required since plasma concentrations are low
(C_{max} 1000 – 300 ng/ml for sulpiride, 200 mg orally; 100 – 60 ng/ml for
metoclopramide, 20 mg orally) and, moreover, are unpredictable due to
wide variations in bioavailability as observed for metoclopramide
[3, 4] and sulpiride. Urinary data are informative since substituted benzamides are entirely (sulpiride [1], sultopride [5, 6]) or
largely excreted unchanged in urine.

Several methods, viz. colorimetry, UV spectrophotometry, spectro-fluorimetry, GC and quantitative TLC, have been proposed and reviewed [7, 8]. HPLC has been used for separation, identification and quanti-tative analysis of substituted benzamides [7] and appears to be a method of choice. Several HPLC methods have been developed for the analysis in body fluids of sulpiride [1, 8, 9], sultopride [6, 8], tiapride [2] and metoclopramide [3, 4]. These techniques have increa-sed specificity compared with the spectrofluorimetric assay, and allow the determination of any metabolites in urine (none detectable in plasma). Our own methodology [1, 8, 10] is now collated.

Reverse-phase HPLC methods with UV detection at 226 nm are presen-ted for the assay in plasma, RBC and urine of sulpiride, sultopride and RIV 2093. They have been used for many pharmacokinetic studies of these drugs. Our older HPLC method for sulpiride [1] is touched on.

MATERIALS

The test compounds and internal standards shown in Fig. 1 were obtained from Delagrange (Paris). Stock solutions of the drugs (0.1 g/l in purified water) were diluted 10- and 100-fold where appropriate (only 10-fold for sultopride). Chloroform was HPLC grade (E. Merck, Darmstadt). Methanol and, after ion-exchange treatment, water were double-distilled from glass. Sodium hydroxide, ammon-ium acetate, glycine and sodium chloride were analytical reagent grade (Merck). Buffers of pH 8.9 and 10 were obtained by mixing 0.1 M glycine (in 0.1 M NaCl) and 0.1 M NaOH, 88.5:11.5 and 51:49 by vol. respectively. Trichloroacetic acid was analytical reagent grade.

CHROMATOGRAPHY AND CALIBRATION CURVES

In the following, [] entries connote the superseded method for sulpiride. A Spectra-Physics chromatograph SP 8100 [8000] was used, with a Valco syringe-loading valve, an automatic sample injec-tion system (SP 8110) and a variable-wavelength detector (SF 770; Schoffel Insts., Cunow, France) operated at 226 [197] nm. A compu-ting integrator (SP 4100) was used to record the signal and determine peak areas. The flow rate was 1 ml/min. The chromatograph oven was kept at 50° [N/A], giving shortened, very reproducible retention times.

The column, 25 cm × 4.6 mm i.d., contained 10 µm Lichrosorb RP 8 [5 µm Hypersil-ODS]. Sample injection was by a 50 [10] µl loop. The mobile phase was 0.1 M ammonium acetate/methanol, 10:90 [70:30] or, for RIV 2093, 20:80 by vol. It was degassed with He and passed through a membrane filter (0.45 µm).

As the assay parameter, peak area ratios (analyte/i.s.) were plotted against analyte concentration, and standard curves obtained by least squares regression analysis. See later (Table 2) for the ranges studied, set up by spiking control material.

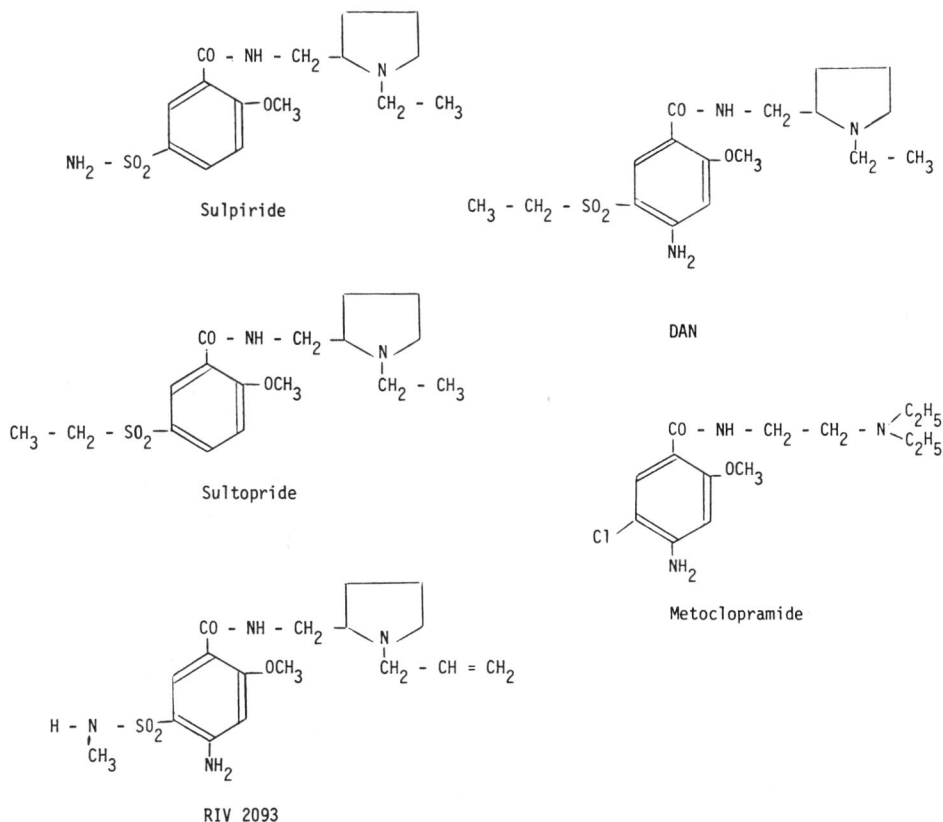

Fig. 1. Structures of drug and i.s. analytes. DAN = 5-ethylsul-phonyl-*N*-[(1-ethyl-2-pyrrolidinyl)methyl]-2-methoxy-4-aminobenz-amide. For RIV 2093, see text.

SAMPLE PREPARATION AND INTERNAL STANDARD (i.s.) ADDITION

Sample preparation hinged on an extraction step where the pH was set at 10 for sulpiride, taking into account the two pKa's of this drug: 9.05 for the tert-amine function and 10.0 for the sulphonamide function [11]. For sulpiride, sultopride (pKa 9.11), tiapride (9.05 and 12.66) and metoclopramide (9.36), pKa's were determined either spectrophotometrically or potentiometrically. For the determination of the two pKa's of RIV 2093 (8.60 and 11.7) we used solubility measurements.

Sulpiride assay [8].- Prior to extraction, 0.5 ml 2 M NaOH and 1 ml glycine buffer pH 10 were added to plasma (4 ml plasma) or urine (4 ml, or 0.5, 1 or 2 ml made up to 4 ml with dist. water). When necessary the pH was adjusted to 10 by adding 0.5 M

NaOH. After extraction with 20 ml chloroform and centrifugation, the tubes were kept at -20° for 1 h, and a 15 ml aliquot of organic phase removed. This procedure was repeated with a further 20 ml. To the combined organic phases (30 ml) an aliquot from a 10 mg/1 i.s. solution in methanol was added, viz. DAN, 0.2 ml or, if urine rather than plasma, 0.8 ml. [In the earlier method the i.s. was nicotinamide, 0.4 ml of a 1 mg/1 methanolic solution.] Each organic phase was evaporated to dryness at room temnperature and the residue dissolved with ultrasonication in the eluent (0.4 ml or, for urine, 1 ml). [The nicotinamide i.s. could not have been added to the starting sample because of inferior extractability compared with the drug.]

After RBC had been separated centrifugally from plasma, each being immediately put into -20° storage, portions (2, 3 or 4 g) of thawed RBC were weighed into tared extraction tubes. To each was added 2 ml water and 0.5 ml M H_2SO_4. After 5 min, 0.5 ml 2M NaOH was added; buffer addition and subsequent steps were as described above. The acid treatment of the RBC (which, after -20° storage, were already lysed) was conducive to a clean $CHCl_3$ extract; unlike trichloroacetic acid as used in sultopride assay (below), sulphuric acid did not cause degradation of the drug.

Sultopride assay [8].- To achieve clean extracts and so obviate chromatographic interferences, samples of plasma (2, 3 or 4 ml; water to 4 ml) or RBC (2, 3 or 4 g, + 2 ml water) were treated with 1.5 ml 20% (w/v) trichloroacetic acid; 5 min later, 1.5 ml 2M NaOH was added. If necessary the pH was adjusted to 10 by adding 0.5 M NaOH; likewise for urine samples (0.5-10 ml), where the initial step was merely addition of 0.2 ml 0.5 M NaOH. Assay continued as for sulpiride, except for i.s. addition, viz. 0.3 or (urine) 0.8 ml of sulpiride, 10 mg/1 in methanol, added to the $CHCl_3$ extract.

RIV 2093 assay [10].- To the starting sample (plasma, 1-4 ml; urine, 0.5-10 ml), aqueous metoclopramide was added as i.s., then 0.5 ml pH 8.9 buffer, and 0.1 M NaOH (0.2 ml, or more if pH not 8.9). Extraction and HPLC were performed as for the other drugs.

ASSAY PARAMETERS

HPLC patterns and retention times.- Patterns with different spike concentrations are shown in Figs. 2-4. With unspiked plasma, RBC or urine there were no interfering peaks in the regions of interest. The retention times (min) with the current method (HPLC at 50°) were 4.4 for sulpiride and 6.3 for DAN as i.s., markedly shorter for the drug than in the previous (ambient temperature) method where the values were 12 and, for nicotinamide as i.s., 6.8. In the sultopride assay the drug eluted at 5.4 and the i.s., sulpiride, at 4.4. For the RIV 2093 retention time, see Fig. 4.

Fig. 2. RP-HPLC patterns for sulpiride (1) and DAN as i.s., spiked into chloroform extracts of RBC. The stated two levels refer to the wt. of RBC.- See text, which also gives the HPLC conditions. The mm values connote position; chart speed 1 cm/min. AT denotes attenuation.

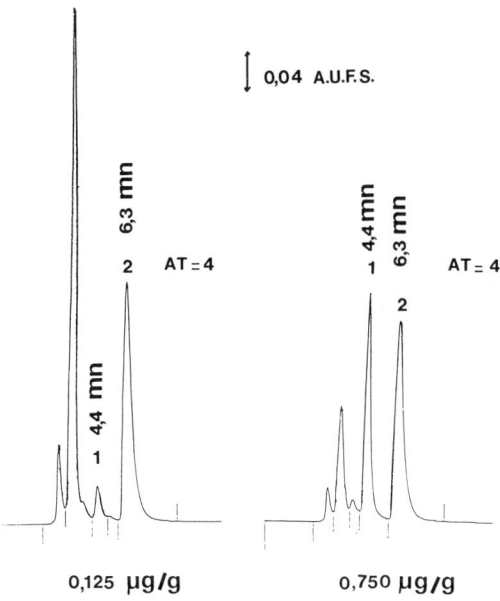

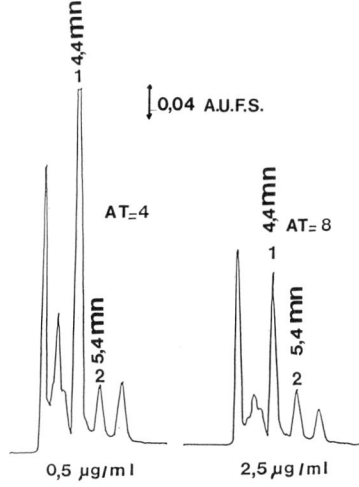

Fig. 3. RP-HPLC as in Fig. 2, for sultopride (2) and sulpiride as i.s. (1) spiked into 4 ml plasma (at high levels, in context of patients getting a 400 mg dose).

Fig. 4, *below.* RP-HPLC patterns for RIV 2093 (1) and metoclopramide as i.s. (2) spiked into 4 ml urine.

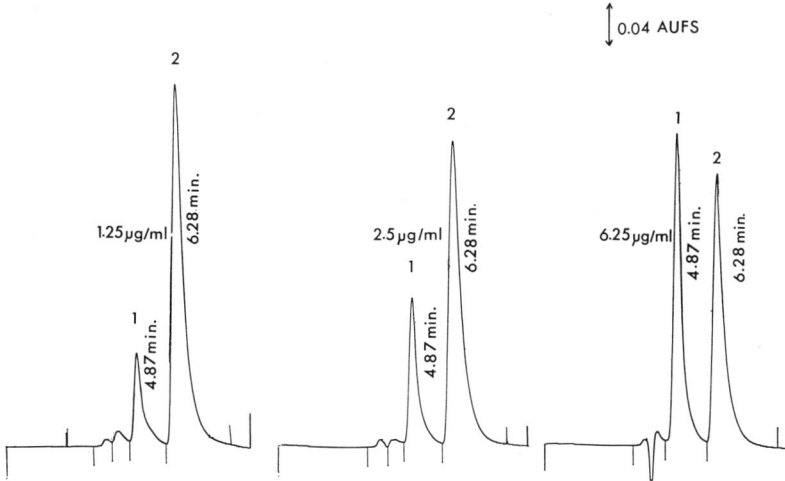

Table 1. Assay linearity for sulpiride (previous [1] & current [8] methods), sultopride and RIV 2093. The no. of calibration points is denoted]; Table 2 gives ranges. See text for amplification. **P** = plasma; **E** = erythrocytes (RBC); **U** = urine.

	Sulpiride [1]	Sulpiride [8]	Sultopride	RIV 2093
Linear regression analysis coefficient	**P:** 0.9998 10] $\pm 1.10^{-4}$ **U:** 0.999979 10] $\pm 1.3 \times 10^{-5}$	**P:** 0.9980 10]$\pm 4.7 \times 10^{-4}$ **E:** 0.99986 5] $\pm 1.5 \times 10^{-4}$ **U:** 0.9970 14] $\pm 2.10^{-3}$	**P:** 0.9983 10]$\pm 12.78 \times 10^{-4}$ **E:** 0.998016 10] $\pm 10.64 \times 10^{-4}$ **U:** 0.994496 14] $\pm 24.51 \times 10^{-4}$	**P:** 0.99993 12] $\pm 6.32 \times 10^{-5}$ **U:** 0.99980 12] $\pm 2.16 \times 10^{-4}$
Slope $ng^{-1} \cdot ml$	**P:** 146.4 $\pm 0.54 \times 10^{-4}$ **U:** 579 $\pm 1.9 \times 10^{-3}$	**P:** 0.821 $\pm 1.2 \times 10^{-2}$ **E:** 0.502 $\pm 6.10^{-3}$ **U:** 0.209 $\pm 3.10^{-3}$	**P:** 0.154 $\pm 2.10^{-2}$ **E:** 0.133 $\pm 1.10^{-3}$ **U:** 0.057 $\pm 1.10^{-3}$	**P:** 2.17 $\pm 1.68 \times 10^{-2}$ **U:** 0.0250 $\pm 8.74 \times 10^{-4}$
Intercept	**P:** 13.8 ± 0.0045 **U:** 12.7 ± 0.010	**P:** 0.0242 ± 0.010 **E:** 0.0154 ± 0.0147 **U:** 0.0492 ± 0.0373	**P:** -0.0025 ± 0.0032 **E:** -0.0058 ± 0.00922 **U:** -0.00986 ± 0.0198	**P:** -0.00425 ± 0.00751 **U:** 0.0165 ± 0.0144

Extraction efficiencies.- The drugs were spiked into control plasma or urine, and the i.s. was added after extraction. Peak area ratios of drugs to i.s. were compared with those for unextracted standards at concentrations equivalent to those for extracted standards. The efficiencies thus determined were 98% for sulpiride and sultopride, and 99% for RIV 2093.

Linearity.- Table 1 shows that for each drug, in comparison with i.s., the peak-area ratio varied linearly with concentration over the range studied (as given in Table 2; 0.02-1.5 µg/ml for the earlier sulpiride method [1]). The '$ng^{-1} \cdot ml$' slope values and the intercepts in Table 2 are based on the usual equation, the y-axis units being an arbitrary reflection of the amount of i.s. added.

Reproducibility.- The reproducibilities of the actual chromatographic methods were determined by injecting 10 aliquots from each of a number of worked-up samples from spiked urine. The concentrations

Table 2. Day-to-day reproducibility of the assay methods: coefficients of variation (C.V.'s), as %. No. of assays denoted n. RBC = red blood cells (erythrocytes).

µg/ml	Sulpiride[8]			Sultopride			RIV 2093	
	Plasma n = 10	RBC n = 5	Urine n = 14	Plasma n = 10	RBC n = 10	Urine n = 14	Plasma n = 12	Urine n = 12
0.050	4.14	3.02					1.86	
0.125	3.52	7.68					4.66	
0.250							1.62	
0.500				3.18	2.33		1.49	
0.750		0.592						
1.25	2.52			1.55	4.50		0.692	4.96
2.50	2.02	1.06		0.56	1.08			3.66
5.00	1.50	1.24		0.50	2.39			
6.25						1.98		2.49
10.00				1.31	0.57			
12.50			1.60			0.71		2.74
18.75			1.21					
25.00			1.53			2.28		3.66
50.00			1.43			1.01		

(µg/ml) and the observed C.V.'s were as follows.- Sulpiride (current method): 0.05, 2.10%; 1.25, 1.30%; 2.5, 1.00%; 5.0, 0.9%. Sultopride: 6.25, 0.23%; 25, 0.79%. RIV 2093: 6.25, 0.27%; 25, 0.45%. Table 2 shows the day-to-day variability for the complete assay of each drug, spiked into plasma, RBC or urine.

Within-run precision was assessed by performing 10 replicate assays on urine spiked with RV 2093: for 2.5 and 25 µg/ml the C.V.'s were respectively 0.68% and (unexpectedly higher) 1.85%.

Accuracy.- To check the accuracy of the assay for RV 2093, it was spiked into 5 aliquots (4 ml) of urine at each of 3 concentrations. The following sets of 5 values were obtained, and averaged to give observed concentration as % of theoretical (and relative error).-

5 µg/ml: 5.0   5.5   5.0   4.98   5.0   = 102.0% (+2%).
10 µg/ml: 10.2   10.15   10.13   10.08   10.13   = 101.25% (+1.25%).
17.5 µg/ml: 17.58   17.5   17.75   17.63   17.5   = 100.57% (+0.57%).
Evidently the method is of good accuracy.

Limit of detection.- Minimum detectable quantities (signal-to-noise ratio of 2:1) were 10 and 15 ng/ml extracted from 4 ml plasma (or RBC) for sulpiride and sultopride respectively, and 12 ng/ml extracted from 4 ml plasma for RIV 2093. In fact during all the pharmacokinetic studies of these drugs, 95% of the assayed samples were above 50 ng/ml (RBC and plasma; higher for urine).

Fig. 5. Levels of sulpiride
in plasma (**P**) and RBC (**E**)
following i.v. or oral administration to volunteers.

*From ref. [8], courtesy of
Elsevier (likewise for Fig. 6).*

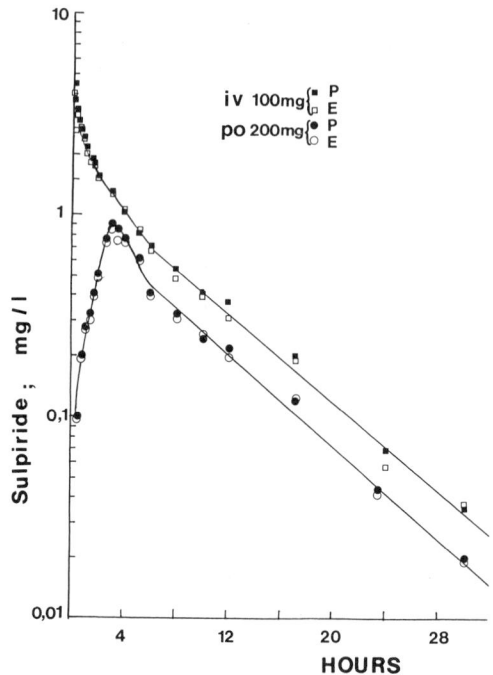

APPLICABILITY AND COMMENTS

The assay technique developed for sulpiride with improved HPLC
conditions in the later version [8], and likewise the technique for
sultopride, served well for the analysis of all samples collected
during pharmacokinetic investigations. Sulpiride given intravenously
(100 mg), intramuscularly (50 mg or more) [1] or orally (200 mg or
more) can be followed in plasma and RBC up to 30 h (Fig. 5) and in
urine up to 48 h. However, in some subjects the concentration is
very low throughout, due to very poor bioavailability (10-60%).

The distribution ratio of sulpiride between RBC and plasma is
close to 1.0. For sulpiride this ratio does not change with time
(Fig. 5), but for sultopride the ratio changes beyond 3 h. Half-lives
determined from either plasma or RBC concentrations were similar,
viz. 7 h for sulpiride and 5 h for sultopride [6].

The RIV 2093 method, which is selective, reliable and sensitive,
has been used to measure plasma and urine concentrations in pharmacokinetic studies on volunteers [10]. Plasma concentrations after
administration intravenously (50 mg) or orally (200 mg; bioavailability
~40%) can be followed up to 36 h (Fig. 6); the urinary recoveries
of unchanged drug were 57% and 23% respectively. During multiple
dosing (3 × 50 mg/day, orally) steady-state plasma levels of 130
to 80 ng/ml were reached on day 2 [10].

Fig. 6. RIV 1093 plasma
levels following i.v. and
oral administrations to a
healthy volunteer.   The
'extended least-squares
method' (MSDOS PHARM program)
was used to calculate the
exponential parameters.
From ref. [10].

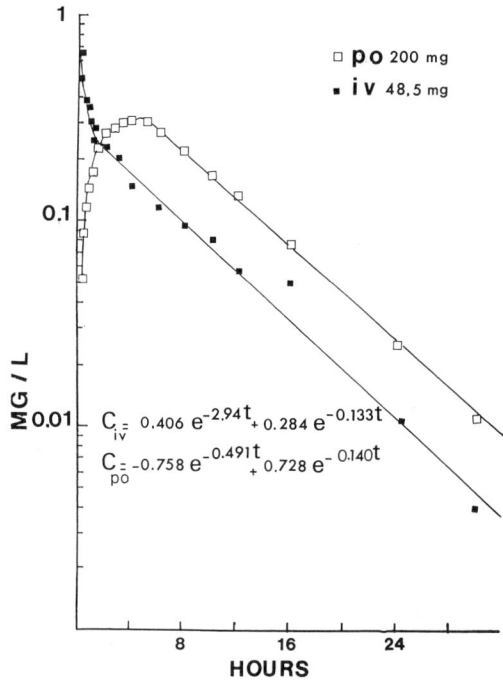

$$C_{iv} = 0.406\ e^{-2.94t} + 0.284\ e^{-0.133t}$$
$$C_{po} = -0.758\ e^{-0.491t} + 0.728\ e^{-0.140t}$$

References

1. Bressolle, F., Bres, J., Blanchin, M.D. & Gomeni, R. (1984)
    J. Pharm. Sci. 73, 1128-1136.
2. Rey, E.,   d'Athis, P., Richard, M.O., de Lauture, D. & Olive, G.
    (1980) *Int. J. Clin. Pharmacol. Ther. Toxicol. 20*, 62-67.
3. Huizing, G., Brouwers, J.R. & Westhuis, P. (1980) in *The Serum
    Concentration of Drugs, Clinical Relevance, Therapy and Practice*
    (Merkus, F.W., ed.), Excerpta Medica, Amsterdam, pp. 125-133.
4. Block, W., Pingoud, A., Khan, M. & Kjellerup, P. (1981)
    Arzneim.-Forsch./Drug Res. 31, 1041-1045.
5. Bres, J., Gaillot, A.F., Monsoncles, D., Penuchet, J.C. &
    Vidal, G. (1981) *Progress in Clinical Pharmacy, III* (Turakka, H.
    & Van der Kleijn, E., eds.), Elsevier/North Holland Biomedical
    Press, Amsterdam, 61-70.
6. Bres, J. & Bressolle, F. (1985) *Therapie   40*, 433-439.
7. Verbiese-Genard, N., Hanocq, M., Van Damme, M. & Molle, L. (1979)
    Int. J. Pharm. 2,   155-166.
8. Bressolle, F. & Bres, J. (1985) *J. Chromatog. 341*,   391-399.
9. Verbiese-Genard, N., Hanocq, M. & Molle, L. (1980) *J. Pharm.
    Belg. 35*, 1-40.
10. Bressolle, F., Bres, J. & Snoussi, M. (1985) *J. Chromatog. 343*,
    443-448.
11. Van Damme, M., Hanocq, M., Topart, J. & Molle, L. (1976)
    Analusis 4, 299-307.

#NC(B)

NOTES and COMMENTS relating to

CNS-ACTIVE DRUGS AND THEIR METABOLITES

Comments relating to particular contributions

#B-1, B-2, B-4, B-6 & B-7, and #NC(B)-1 & -3, p. 215

Forum presentation by R. Schmid on assaying CNS-active drugs - p. 217

#NC(B)-1

APPLICABILITY OF DISPOSABLE EXTRACTION COLUMNS TO CNS-DRUG ANALYSIS

J.P. Desager

Université Catholique de Louvain
Laboratoire de Pharmacothérapie
53, Avenue E. Mounier, 1200 Bruxelles, Belgium

Require-ment	*Assay of adinazolam and demethyladinazolam in plasma and urine at levels of 2-250 ng/ml (see* Comments *for other drugs).*
End-step	*HPLC with C-18 column and methanol/pH 7 buffer eluent; detection at 226 nm.*
Sample preparation	*Extraction (of unbound drug) by CN-type column. Eluate (ethyl acetate, pH 9.3) dried down, and residue redissolved.*
Comments	*Binding to plasma proteins (especially strong after freezing) resists 6 M HCl hydrolysis or acetonitrile deproteinization. Similar methodology for amitriptyline/nortriptyline and alprazolam/4-OH-alprazolam but with NP-HPLC.*

Our analytical experience covers a wide range of CNS-active drugs, e.g. amitriptyline, maprotiline, nomifensine, chlorpromazine, triazolam and alprazolam. Most of the assays were performed by GC or HPLC after liquid-liquid extraction, often necessitating large volumes of solvent and one or two drying-down steps; the assays were therefore time-consuming and rather expensive. The relatively new technique of solid-phase extraction, at first distrusted by analysts especially if concerned with biomedical samples, has now achieved world-wide application. It is economical, through reduction of solvent consumption and handling time, and meets present-day quality assurance criteria. Design of solid-phase extraction procedures exploits selective interactions that depend on the analyte, the bonded silica and the sample matrix.

Relevant features of the analyte.- Through its characteristic functional groups, the analyte can undergo interactions of 4 types: Van der Waals and hydrogen bonding - both low-energy (<10 kcal/mol),

and ionic and covalent bonding - both of higher energy (~100 kcal/mol).
If the energy of these interactions increases, the selectivity increases too.

Relevant features of the bonded silica.- The best way to develop
selective interactions is to modify chemically the surface of a
support such as the widely used silica. A porous silica matrix provides
a large surface area, but only one-third of this is available for
interactions. After chemical modification there remain many silanols,
which must be pre-solvated to stabilize the surface; trapping of
the analyte occurs only through the solvated surface.

Relevant features of the sample matrix.- The matrix will affect
the specific interactions, to an extent depending on the relative
content of endogenous components. In large amount they may swamp the
active sites on the solvated surface.

General guidelines for a robust method can be drawn from these
and other considerations. Analyte stability may need to be safeguarded
by adjusting the pH and preventing oxidation. Pre-solvation of the
silica surface must be thorough, and dominating components of the
sample matrix must be compatible with the surface. Eluent pH and
ionic strength must be conducive to surface stability. The analyte
should not co-migrate with the solvent in which it is applied or with
the wash solvent, and should have a high affinity for the support
(equilibrium constant K >1000); but it should elute with <5 bed-vols.
of the eluting solvent (here K <0.001). With good retention of
the analyte on the column, there may be higher recovery than with
solvent extraction, in a form suitable for GC or HPLC analysis.

As initial strategy clearly shown by Stewart et al. [1] to
be advantageous, solid phases of different types should be screened.
The choice for many HPLC applications is C-18 silica; it retains many
compounds, but for this very reason it may be the least desirable for
selectively separating off the compound of interest from endogenous
components. With any potential analyte we routinely ascertain
retention with different solid phases and a range of pH. Kits with
different phases are now available to optimize extraction, and some
tips are given by manufacturers of extraction columns. This screening
is a step in selecting which phase gives minimal background interferences from the samples. More than 20 different phases are now available,
and new ones are in prospect, mainly those exhibiting strong (pseudo-
covalent) binding of analyte. The latter types exhibit high affinity
for some sulphur compounds and are promising for drugs such as chlorpromazine which is very difficult to assay in biological samples.

The use of supposedly equivalent columns from different manufacturers may give comparable results only if two parameters are varied:
solvent strength, and sample pH.

APPLICATIONS TO DRUGS IN PLASMA

Throughout we used CN-BondElut columns (Analytichem Internat[1]., Harbor City, CA), and using the 10-port VacElut manifold. The HPLC pump and autosampler with a loop (302, 231) were from Gilson (Middleton, WI), and the detector from Pye Unicam (LC3; Cambridge, U.K.). Selection of columns and eluents followed guidelines that we have published elsewhere [2], with protection by an in-line filter (0.5 μm; Rheodyne, Cotati, CA) and a pre-column (Brownlee, Santa Clara, CA).

Amitriptyline and nortriptyline.- In our GC method as practised for many years [3], the expected peaks for these drugs were lacking on occasion, for no apparent reason. This led us to try solid-phase extraction. The best results were obtained by adding 100 μl of 2 M NaOH (and desipramine as internal standard (i.s.) to 1 ml plasma and applying it to a CN-BondElut column pre-conditioned with methanol/water. After a 2 ml water wash, the drugs were eluted with 2 ml of acetonitrile. Solvent was blown off and the residue dissolved in 250 μl of mobile phase. Fig. 1 shows a typical chromatogram for a spiked plasma sample.

Alprazolam and 4-hydoxyalprazolam.- This anxiolytic drug is one of a new class of compounds, the triazolobenzodiazepines. The published assay method for the parent drug and main metabolite in plasma [4] is time-consuming. Again, with sample preparation as above, we had good results with CN-BondElut columns (with triazolam, which is in the same chemical class, as internal standard). HPLC runs were short and clean (Fig. 2).

Adinazolam and _N_-desmethyladinazolam.- For this new drug, also a triazolobenzodiazepine (Fig. 3), the method of Peng [5] gave us poor assay results: accurate determination in plasma was precluded by many interfering peaks, arising mainly from the toluene extractant (even if glass-distilled; Burdick & Jackson Inc., MI). With the above procedure for processing the samples, we could detect only traces of drug and metabolite. This finding was unexpected, and hardly tallied with the increasing doses regularly and repeatedly taken by the volunteers (Fig. 4).

Good recoveries of spiked-in drug were obtainable with fresh plasma, but not if the spiked samples had been frozen. Evidently the analytes were washed off, not reaching the active sites on the columns. We assumed that a strong link between analytes and matrix constituents was formed upon freezing, and tried unsuccessfully to disrupt the bond with common deproteinizing agents - HCl (1 M or 6 M), acetonitrile and phosphate buffers.

Going back to Peng's method [5], we tried ethyl acetate/K_2HPO_4 (0.1 M) for extracting the plasma; the residue from drying down was dissolved in K_2HPO_4 solution for application to the CN column. Thereby, with repeated washings, a working method (below) was attained.

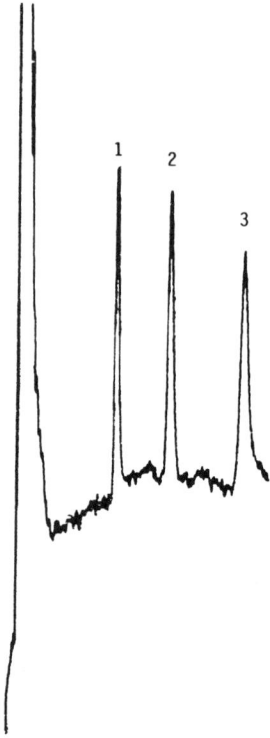

Fig. 1 *(left)*. Typical chromatogram of nortryptyline (**1**, 250 ng/ml; peak at 7.42 min), desipramine (**2**, 500 ng/ml, as i.s.; at 11.05 min) and amitriptyline (**3**, 500 ng/ml; at 16.05 min) from a spiked human plasma, extracted as in text. Column: Zorbax-SIL 5 μm, 250 × i.d. 4.6 mm. Mobile phase: acetonitrile /water/methanol/ammonia (1000:80:80:6 by vol.), 1.5 ml/min. Loop: 200 μl. Detection at 220 nm.

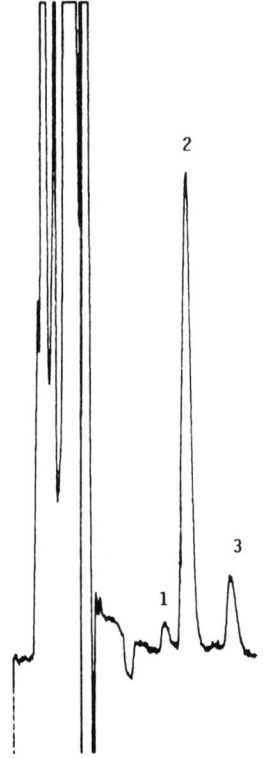

Fig. 2 *(right)*. Typical chromatogram of 4-hydroxy-alprazolam (**1**, 0.7 ng/ml; at 5.05 min), triazolam (**2**, 200 ng/ml, as i.s.; at 5.87 min) and alprazolam (**3**, 18.7 ng/ml; at 7.39 min) from a patient's plasma, extracted as in text. Column and loop as above; acetonitrile/water (6:0.35).

Fig. 3. Triazolobenzodiazepine structures.

I : R$_1$ = CH$_2$N(CH$_3$)$_2$, R$_2$ = H   ADINAZOLAM

II : R$_1$ = CH$_2$NHCH$_3$, R$_2$ = H   N- DEMETHYL METABOLITE

III : R$_1$ = CH$_2$CH$_3$, R$_2$ = CH$_2$N(CH$_3$)$_2$ INTERNAL STANDARD

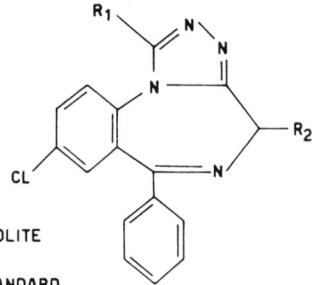

Method adopted for adinazolam and its metabolite

To 1.5 ml plasma (thawed) were added 2 ml 0.1 M K$_2$HPO$_4$, 200 μl i.s. (Fig. 3; 10 μg/ml) and 5 ml ethyl acetate. After manual shaking for 1 min, the tubes were centrifuged at 2000 rpm for 10 min. The organic layer was transferred to a tube containing a few 2 mm glass beads and reduced to dryness (N$_2$ stream; N-EVAP). The residue was taken up in 1 ml 0.1 M K$_2$HPO$_4$, vortexed and applied to the extraction

Fig. 4. Chromatograms for *N*-desmethyladinazolam (**1**, 50 ng/ml), the i.s. as in Fig. 3 (**2**, 2 µg/ml) and adinazolam (**3**, 50 ng/ml) from a spiked human plasma, extracted onto a CN column. *Left:* frozen specimen. *Middle:* freshly prepared sample (see text). *Right:* initial extraction into ethyl acetate - the method adopted (see text).

Column: Supelco LC-18 3 µm, 75 × i.d. 4.6 mm. Mobile phase: methanol/0.05 M pH 7 phosphate buffer (65:35 by vol.), 1 ml/min. Loop: 500 µl. Detection at 226 nm.

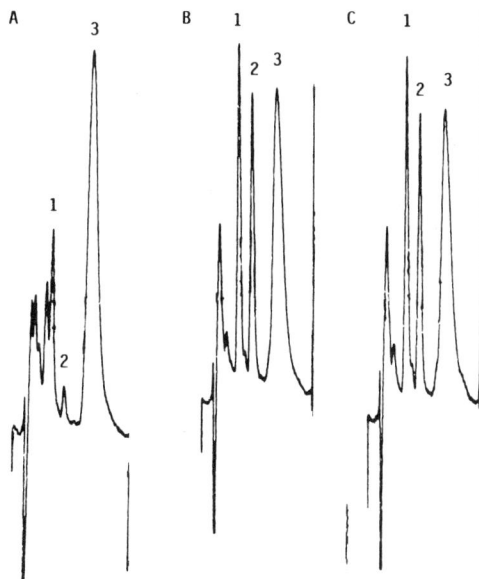

column (Analytichem, CN-BondElut; conditioned with 1 ml methanol and 1 ml water). The column was washed 5 times with 1 ml water. The drugs were eluted with 0.9 ml of the mobile phase, and 0.4 ml injected by auto-injector (Gilson 231 with Rheodyne valve), allowing a second injection if necessary. For urine, solvent extraction was omitted; 1 ml was applied directly to the CN extraction column.

HPLC was performed as in the legend to Fig. 4, using a Gilson 302 pump, a Brownlee RP18-5 µm (OS-GU 3 cm) pre-column which was changed after 200 injections, a Rheodyne 7302 0.5 µm filter, and a Pye LC3 detector with a Shimazdu CR 1A integrator. For the peaks shown in Fig. 4 the retention times were as follows, with the adopted method as in the *right* chromatogram (and with the less satisfactory conditions used in the above-mentioned pilot work), expressed in min: **1**, 3.5 (*left*, 3.49; *middle*, 3.49); **2**, 4.8 (*left*, 4.74; *middle*, 4.77); **3**, 7.19 (*left*, 7.03; *middle*, 7.12).

The sensitivity of the method was 1 ng/ml plasma for adinazolam and 10 ng/ml for the metabolite. The C.V.'s did not exceed 5%. A calibration sample containing 50 ng/ml of each drug was used daily.

DISCUSSION AND CONCLUSIONS

The problems encountered in the determination of adinazolam plasma concentrations illustrate well the fact that solid-phase extraction does not always suffice as the sole pre-chromatographic step. A mixed method was needed in the present instance because, on the one hand, a tight bond to endogenous material results from freezing, whilst on the other hand solvent extraction alone, as performed with toluene in initial work, gave too many interferences. With our successive extractions - ethyl acetate, then solid-phase - reproducibility is good (C.V. <5%), and only a few columns have proved ineffective (3 per thousand). With the auto-sampler, >90 samples could be prepared and injected within 24 h.

A wide variety of compounds may be efficiently extracted from biological matrices with bonded sorbents. For a given compound of interest, a range of extraction protocols may be developed, and there is essentially no one 'correct' protocol for any isolation. As the number of functional groups in a molecule increases, the range of bonded sorbents appropriate to the separation increases too. However, to ensure that a particular method is valid, it is important to consider the possible secondary interactions associated with complex molecules. The bonded sorbent merely facilitates the ease, efficiency and selectivity of the protocol.

A trend can be foreseen towards the use, in place of the disposable extraction columns, of a pre-column onto which, by-passing the HPLC column, plasma or urine is injected directly, followed by its switching to the analytical solvent and column. Two pumps and 2 or 3 injection valves are needed; but there is the advantage that the preconcentration column could be used repeatedly [cf. the pre-concentrator described by H.M. Ruijten, art. B-1 in Vol. 14.-*Ed.*]. The future will also see the development of more selective solid-phase materials, mainly of the 'covalent' type.

References

1. Stewart, J.T., Reeves, T.S. & Honigberg, I.L.(1984) *Anal. Lett.* *17 (B16)*, 1811-1826.
2. Desager, J.P. & Sclavons, M. (1982) *Chromatographia 15*, 451-452.
3. Desager, J.P. & Vanderbist, M. (1978) in *Blood Drugs and Other Analytical Challenges* [Vol. 7, this series] (Reid, E., ed.), Horwood, Chichester, pp. 325-326.
4. Bombardt, P.A., Brewer, J.E. & Adams, W.J. (1983) *Abstracts, 185th National ACS Mtg.* (Seattle, WA, March 1983), American Chemical Society, Washington, DC, p. 183.
5. Peng, G.W. (1984) *J. Pharm. Sci. 73*, 1173-1174.

#NC(B)-2

A Note on

ISOMERISM OF THE RING-SULPHOXIDES OF THIORIDAZINE
AND OF SOME OTHER PHENOTHIAZINE DRUGS

A.S. Papadopoulos and J.L. Crammer

Institute of Psychiatry
Department of Psychiatry
Denmark Hill, London SE5 8AF, U.K.

The ring-sulphoxide of thioridazine (Tz; Fig. 1), a phenothiazine used extensively in psychiatry, is found in blood samples in two isomeric forms (Fig. 1) [1]. These isomeric ring-sulphoxides (diastereoisomeric racemates; see below) can be prepared from Tz by oxidation with H_2O_2 and resolved by TLC [2]. Sulphoridazine (Sz; Fig. 1), having a sulphone rather than a sulphide side-chain and itself clinically active [3], likewise gives rise to two ring-sulphoxide isomers; we have identified these by mass spectrometry (MS), various microchemical tests and the ability of trifluoroacetic anhydride (TFAA) to isomerize asymmetric sulphoxides [4]. We have also examined other phenothiazine drugs similarly oxidized with H_2O_2 for resulting isomeric sulphoxides resolvable by TLC. When phenothiazine metabolites have to be determined quantitatively, it may be important to recognize the presence of isomers and measure them individually.

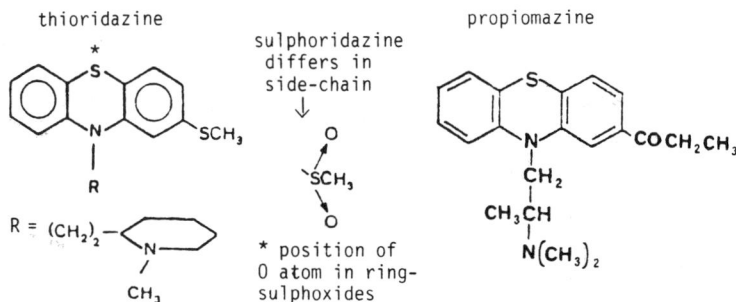

Fig. 1. Chemical structures of the phenothiazines now considered.

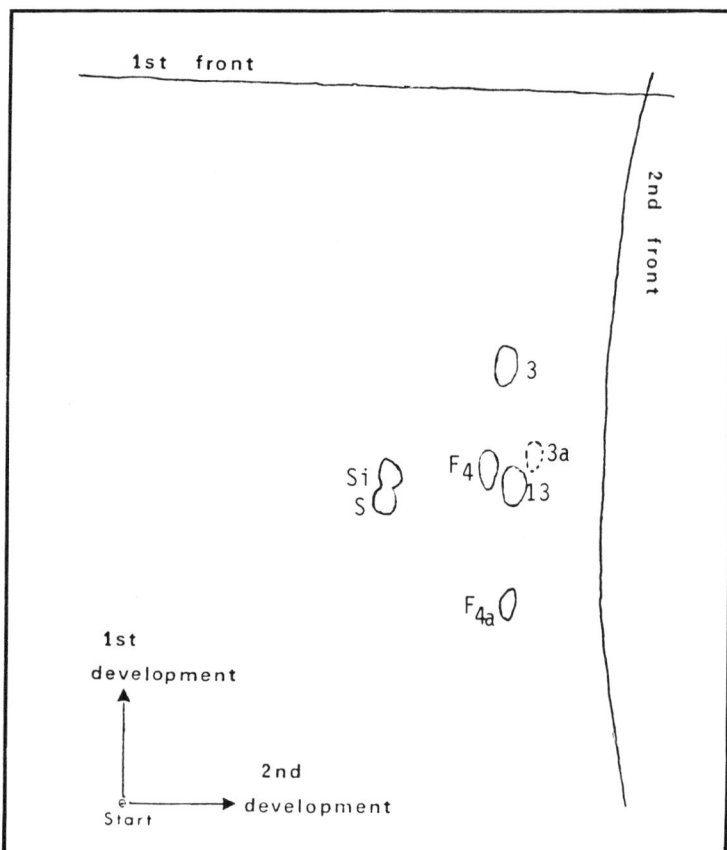

Fig. 2. Urine from a patient receiving Sz (50-100 mg/day): 2-D TLC pattern for solvent-extracted material (details in [5], including spray reagents). Plates: silica gel (Anderman 5553); solvents: see text. Identifications: 3, Sz; 3a, nor-Sz; 5, Sz ring sulphoxide: 5i, isomer of 5; F_4, 7-hydroxy-Sz; F_{4a}, 7-hydroxy-nor-Sz; 13, piperidone derivative of Sz sulphoxide.

EXTRACTION AND SEPARATION

Urine (10 ml) from Sz-treated patients was made alkaline with 5 ml M NaOH and extracted with redistilled chloroform (3 × 15 ml). The pooled extracts were evaporated to dryness (N_2, 65°), and the residue dissolved in methanol (~0.1 ml) and resolved by 2-D TLC (Fig. 2).

IDENTIFICATIONS

Our authentic Sz-ring sulphoxide appeared by TLC to be homogeneous. Metabolite 5 in Fig. 2 was identical in R_F and colour after

spraying [5].   From these and other tests (below) it was identified
as the Sz-ring sulphoxide of our reference preparation. Metabolite 5i
did not correspond to any of our standards, and was shown as follows
to be an isomer of this sulphoxide.

Metabolites 5 and 5i were further purified by TLC with, as
developing solvent, chloroform/ethanol/ammonia of s.g. 0.88 (80:20:1
by vol.) and examined as follows.-
(i) Each showed the same GC retention time (3% OV-17 on Gas Chrom Q,
80-120 mesh, N_2 carrier at 40 ml/min; 264°) as the Sz-ring sulphoxide
standard.
(ii) Each could be reduced (with 1.2 g zinc powder and 2 ml 0.1 M
HCl) back to Sz, as identified by R_F, MS spectrum and GC retention time.
(iii) Each was shown by EI-MS (VG ZAB IF instrument) to match the
sulphoxide standard.   The following peaks of m/z >90 and >2% above
base peak intensity were observed, expressed as m/z (& % relative intensity at 70 eV): 97 (5), 98 (100), 99 (8), 112 (2), 126 (3), 196 (2),
197 (4), 198 (5), 211 (2), 230 (5), 277 (6), 303 (2), 401 (3), 402 (4).
M^+ at 18 eV only: 418 (0.5).

When Sz (0.9 μmol in ~0.3 ml methanol) was oxidized with H_2O_2
(0.3 μmol in 30 μl water) for 1-2 h at room temperature, two products
were formed which matched metabolites 5 and 5i respectively by TLC
and the Sz-ring sulphoxide standard by MS; each could be reduced to Sz.
Moreover, treatment of the standard (0.08 μmol in ~100 μl acetonitrile) with TFAA (7 μmol in 0.3 ml acetonitrile) for 1 h in sealed
microvials produced a substance resembling metabolite 5i by TLC.

RING SULPHOXIDES OF OTHER PHENOTHIAZINES

Oxidation with H_2O_2 as described for Sz was performed with propiomazine (Fig. 1), mesoridazine, chlorpromazine, promethazine, thioproperazine, thioethylperazine, ridazine, mepazine, trifluoropera-
zine and methdilazine.   After 2-D TLC (acetone/ammonia, 96:4; ethyl
acetate/acetic acid/water, 5:2:2), the formed ring-sulphoxides were
eluted from the silica layer and examined in two TLC systems, viz.
acetone/ammonia as above, and chloroform/ethanol/ammonia (80:20:1).
Only propiomazine gave rise to what appeared to be two isomeric ring-
sulphoxides.

DISCUSSION

Bourquin et al. [6] reported that the ring sulphoxide of a 2-bromo-
phenothiazine, with the same N^{10} side-chain as Tz and Sz, formed two
separable sulphoxides which were diastereoisomeric racemates.   They
identified the prime centre of asymmetry as the carbon atom next to
the piperidyl nitrogen of the N^{10} side-chain.   They also observed
(personal communication) that Tz-ring sulphoxide formed two separable
diastereoisomeric racemates.   This evidently applies also to the
two isomeric sulphoxides of Sz.

Isomeric sulphoxides appear to be formed only by phenothiazines which have both an asymmetric centre in their N^{10} side-chain and a substituent at position 2 of the phenothiazine nucleus; propiomazine (Fig. 1) is an example besides Tz and Sz. Further, judging from our results (not given above) with the sulphoxide of mesoridazine, the nature of the substituent at position 2 appears to determine whether or not any formed isomers can be easily separated by TLC.

Acknowledgements

We are grateful to Mr. D.M. Carter (School of Pharmacy, Univ. of London) and Dr. D.A. Cowan (Chelsea College) for mass spectrometry. Dr. R. Whelpton gave valuable criticism and advice during the progress of the work. Thanks are due also to certain U.K. companies for gifts of various substances: Sandoz Products Ltd., May & Baker, Wyeth Labs., Lundbeck, Smith Kline & French Research, and Westwood Pharmaceuticals.

References

1. Poklis, A., Wells, C.E. & Juenge, E.C. (1982) *J. Anal. Toxicol.* *6*, 250-252.
2. Juenge, E.C., Wells, C.E., Green, D.E., Forrest, I.S. & Schoolery, J.N. (1983) *J. Pharm. Sci. 72*, 617-621.
3. Axelsson, R. (1977) *Curr. Ther. Res. 21*, 587-605.
4. Jones, N.D. (1979) *Comprehensive Organic Chemistry*, Vol. 3, Pergamon, Oxford, p. 129.
5. Papadopoulos, A.S., Crammer, J.L. & Cowan, D.A. (1985) *Xenobiotica 15*, 303-316.
6. Bourquin, J.P., Schwarb, G., Gamboni, G., Fisher, R., Ruebsch, L., Guldimann, S., Theus, V., Schenker, E. & Renz, J. (1959) *Helv. Chim. Acta 42*, 259-281.

#NC(B)-3

A Note on

RELEVANCE OF METABOLISM TO METHODS FOR DETERMINING NOMIFENSINE IN BIOLOGICAL SAMPLES

M. Uihlein, W. Heptner and I. Hornke

Hoechst Aktiengesellschaft
Postfach 800320, D-6230 Frankfurt am Main 80, W. Germany

In man, complete information on the fate of a drug is hard to obtain, since only blood - the distributing compartment - and the excretion compartments are available for analysis. Thus, in some cases, this limited information may easily result in misleading deductions.

This applies to nomifensine, which is rapidly distributed and has an extremely high volume of distribution. The main metabolite, nomifensine-*N*-glucuronide, is immediately formed after absorption of the drug. Like all glucuronides, its distribution is confined to the blood plus, at most, the extracellular volume. This leads to nomifensine being only a minor component in the blood compared to its glucuronide, although it is the main and most relevant agent in the body as a whole. Therefore, in spite of the low analyte concentrations, every effort should be made to determine it specifically and sensitively.

Nomifensine-*N*-glucuronide, however, is extremely unstable at any non-physiological pH, and during storage even at optimum pH and under optimal conditions. As it is rapidly cleaved to the parent compound, a wide variety of blood values and pharmacokinetic data has been obtained for nomifensine in comparable studies due to the different histories of the samples collected.

As a consequence, if reliable information is to be provided, only the sum of nomifensine and the glucuronide concentrations obtained after complete hydrolysis of the glucuronide should be determined.

SENIOR EDITOR'S REINFORCEMENT *of the foregoing Forum Abstract*

Some points relevant to analysis have been noted in a publication by the Hoechst authors [1], which cites earlier publications on aspects such as metabolism and assay methodology before the instability

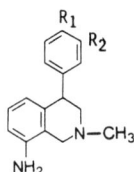

	R_1	R_2
nomifensine	H	H
metabolite M1	OH	H
M2	OH	OCH_3
M3	OCH_3	OH

at neutral pH was fully appreciated: the ratio of glucuronide to parent drug in freshly obtained urine was truly ~15% if the pH were 7.0 (<2% if pH 6.0). If the glucuronide were to be measured, besides keeping the pH alkaline during isolation the subjects were dosed with NaHCO₃ besides the drug. Within 24 h of administering radiolabelled drug the urine contained 90% of the dose, mainly (90%) unstable conjugates of which one-third comprised the *N*-glucuronides of metabolites M1, M2 and M3 (above); a small proportion of *O*-glucuronides was found besides. With precautions against the instability, the proportion of parent drug in humans given 100 mg nomifensine maleate orally was only 1.5%. In practice "the determination of free nomifensine appears to be inappropriate".

Reported GC methods typically entail HFB derivatization, with measurement by ECD or AFID (NPD). RIA has also been described. However, HPLC and TLC are the only techniques that allow simultaneous assay of M1, M2 and M3 as well as the parent drug. Initial hydrolysis of *N*-glucuronides is suitably performed at room temperature with HCl or, with fewer HPLC interferences, H₃PO₄. After washing with diethyl ether, which further reduced interferences, ether extraction is performed at pH 10-11, and the residue from drying down is applied in the mobile phase ('TEAP' buffer, pH 2.5, containing acetonitrile and methanol, each ~10%) to a C-18 column; detection was at 200 nm. (An NP-HPLC approach was previously reported.) The sensitivity as stated for urine was 10 ng/ml, with ±33% C.V. (±5% at 1 µg/ml).

The TLC method, allowing assay in urine down to 0.2 µg/ml, entailed extraction of the analytes at pH 10 with ethyl acetate, and plate development with ammoniacal ethyl acetate/ethanol. Finally the plates, after 2 h at ~75°, showed fluorescent spots for nomifensine and M1, and coloured spots for M2 and M3. The spots were measured with a TLC scanner.

Total nomifensine in plasma or urine could be conveniently determined by RIA, according well with HPLC and similar in sensitivity; dextran-coated charcoal was used to separate free and bound tracer. The metabolites and *O*-glucuronides showed <1% cross-reactivity.

Reference

1. Heptner, W., Hornke, I. & Uihlein, M. (1984) *J. Clin. Psychiat.* *45*, 21-25.

#NC(B)-4

A Note on

HPLC DETERMINATION OF DICLOFENSINE AND METABOLITES
IN PLASMA*

J.A.F. de Silva[†] **and N. Strojny**

Department of Pharmacokinetics, Biopharmaceutics
    and Drug Metabolism
Hoffman-La Roche Inc.
Nutley, NJ 07110, U.S.A.

Requirement   *A sensitive assay for total (free and conjugated) diclofensine and demethylated metabolites; also a simplified assay for the free parent drug only.*

End-step   *Conversion of the analytes to isoquinolinium derivatives, then RP-HPLC with fluorescence detection.*

Sample preparation   *Deproteinization by heating at pH 5.4; enzymic fission of glucuronide (if applicable); solvent extraction at alkaline pH, and drying down for the derivatization steps which are preceded, if applicable, by alkylation (using 2-iodopropane) of the O- and N-desmethyl metabolites.*

Comments   *Sensitivity limit ~60 ng/ml or better, for parent drug and a major metabolite; 300 ng/ml for two other metabolites. With the simplified procedure for free parent drug (with pre-concentration of the HPLC load sample), 0.4 ng/ml plasma could be measured. Method development entailed establishing pre-HPLC and HPLC conditions that gave good recoveries and clean chromagrams.*

AMPLIFICATION OF SOME POINTS

In common with another antidepressant, nomifensine, diclofensine has an isoquinoline moiety (demethylation loci: 2 and/or 7):-

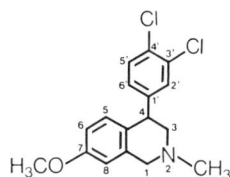

H₃CO—...—N—CH₃ (structure)

* Editors' précis of a lengthy text; see [1] for a full version.

[†] Addressee for correspondence, at 419 Harding Dr., S. Orange, NJ 07079.

Treatment of the plasma (0.1 ml, containing, as i.s., the *N*-ethyl analogue of the drug; 60 ng): kept 3-5 min, with occasional mixing, at 90° after adding pH 5.4 phosphate buffer, as also used to wash the centrifugal pellet obtained. Supernatant shaken over-night at 37° with Glusulase® for fission of the glucuronide of the 2-*O*-desmethyl metabolite (unless only the free drug is to be deter-mined). Analyte(s) extracted at alkaline pH into diethyl ether con-taining 5% (v/v) ethanol, as also added if centrifugation led to an emulsion. Extraction repeated; then drying-down at 40° (N$_2$).

Fluorophore generation, to give detection sensitivity unattain-able by UV detection.- A two-step procedure [2] was tried: it entailed an oxidative dehydrogenation reaction in aqueous mercuric acetate at 100° to form moderately fluorescent dihydroisoquinol-ines, then photochemical dehydrogenation to give the highly fluores-cent isoquinolinium derivatives by insertion of a second double bond. However, the metabolites were not thereby convertible to highly fluorescent products, such as were achievable as follows.- An initial alkylation was performed with 2-iodopropane (better than other reagents in respect of yield and HPLC retention times): to the analytes in acetone, KOH pellets pre-washed in acetone were added, besides the reagent, and the mixture was kept at 70-75° for 30 min. The mixture was then diluted with aqueous ethanol/ acetic acid, as an aid to clean oxidation reactions with good recoveries, and extracted twice with acid-washed ether; the residues from drying-down were exposed to a vacuum before redissolving in 0.05 M H$_2$SO$_4$. After reaction with mercuric acetate in a boiling water bath, the photochemical reaction (conditions critical) was performed to give the fluorescent products. (Whilst the described alkylation was important for sensitive detection of the metabolites, in respect of the parent drug it adversely affected detection.)

HPLC (with 'WISP' auto-injection) was performed with a radial-compression column of 5 μm Nova-Pac (C-18). The samples were loaded in admixture with the mobile phase, viz. 0.25 M 'TEAP', pH 2.5/0.25 M acetic acid/methanol/acetonitrile/tetrahydrofuran (1.5:3.5:1.25:3.75:0.25 by vol.); the tetrahydrofuran content is adjustable to optimize resolution and analysis time (final metabolite peak can be eluted within 11 min). Detection: 254/>389 nm.

Validation, and pharmacokinetic studies: reported elsewhere [1], along with fuller rationale and experimental details than in the foregoing outline.

References

1. Strojny, N. & de Silva, J.A.F. (1985) *J. Chromatog.* *341*, 313-331.
2. de Silva, J.A.F., Strojny, N. & Munno, N. (1973) *J. Pharm. Sci.* *62*, 1066-1074.

Comments on material in #B

Comments on #**B-1**, S.H. Curry - OVER-VIEW
        & #**B-2**, M. Danhof - BENZODIAZEPINES

J. Chamberlain, commenting to S.H. Curry on his implication that use of the NPD in GC has waned: where a GC method is used in our own laboratories, we invariably use a NPD; the scant attention paid to NPD's during the Forum probably reflects their reliability such as we have found over the last 10 years. **M. Danhof, answering a query** on whether any peripheral tissue might be useful as a receptor source for the RRA of benzodiazepines: brain is preferred since it is the tissue of action and is particularly easy to handle for receptor preparation. **P. Ashton, responding to S.H. Curry** who had invited thoughts on up-and-coming HPLC systems or detectors for assaying benzodiazepines: HPLC with negative ion CI-MS might be advantageous [cf. art. by H. Brandenberger & R. Ryhage in Vol. 7, this series - *Ed.*].

Comments on #**B-4**, K.K. Midha - PHENOTHIAZINES
         #**B-6**, R. Whelpton - PHYSOSTIGMINE
        & #**B-7**, J. Bres - BENZAMIDES

Comment by R.H. Whelpton to K.K. Midha.- Because of difficulties with *N*-oxides due to their lability, in any assay where they might be formed it is vital to have authentic specimens available - a point which might be noted by fine-chemical manufacturers. **Whelpton, replying to query by D. Dell:** in physostigmine one would guess the ring-methyls to be responsible for the electroactivity. **S.H. Curry, remark to J. Bres:** an interesting feature of sulpiride, easing the assay problems, is that it is a CNS-active drug with no metabolites.

Comments on #**NC(B)-1**, J.P. Desager - CARTRIDGES IN CNS DRUG ASSAYS
        & #**NC(B)-3**, M. Uihlein - NOMIFENSINE

M.D. Osselton, to J.P. Desager.- You described loss of drug due to protein binding, not reversed by acid digestion. Have you tried prior sample treatment with proteolytic enzymes? This should release bound drugs and the column should retain the unwanted material.[⊗] **Reply.-** I didn't try this; our experience of this approach for liberating cholesterol from tissue was disappointing. **Answer by M. Uhlein to D. Dell:** there was no way to stabilize our *N*-conjugate.

[⊗] M.D. Osselton's art. in Vol. 10, this series, describes his approach.- *Ed.*

SOME CITATIONS *contributed by Senior Editor*
See end of #NC(D) also (method comparisons)

GC assay of 1,4-benzodiazepines as benzophenones has been reviewed [1]. An NP-HPLC method has been described for **alprazolam** in serum, initially extracted with toluene at alkaline pH; after drying down and dissolving the residue in acetone/acetonitrile, HPLC is performed with acetonitrile/water (94:6 by vol.) with detection at 214 nm [2]. Consideration is given to breakdown products.

Assay by **GC-ECD of midazolam** and, after silylation, of its 1-hydroxy metabolite in plasma and urine has been described [3], with a packed column. **RP-HPLC** with 215 nm detection has been performed after ether extraction with Na_3PO_4 present, for study of **midazolam** pharmacokinetics [4].

Conventional and capillary **GC-ECD of flurazepam** and metabolites in plasma can achieve ng/ml sensitivity levels [5]. Radiolabel along with 240 nm absorption was followed in the RP-HPLC of **toloxatone** (an antidepressant) and metabolites, extracted from urine at acid pH with or without enzymic hydrolysis [6]. For *cis*-**thiothixene** (an antipsychotic) in plasma, the *trans*-isomer was used as i.s. [7]: extraction was at alkaline pH with hexane (+ isoamyl alcohol, 1.5%) and HPLC was performed with a cyanopropyl column, enabling 0.5 ng/ml to be measured with detection at 229 nm.

Monitoring of **clonazepam** in plasma can be performed on a dried-down solvent extract by RP-HPLC (C-8) with detection at 306 nm [8]. Assay of urinary **nitrazepam by HPLC,** with metabolites, has been described from a forensic laboratory [9]. After solid-phase extraction and C-18 separation, the analytes were detected at 254 nm. Rat brain and other tissues were analyzed by RRA for **triazolobenzophenones** formed as active metabolites of 1-(2-*o*-chlorobenzoyl-4-chlorophenyl)-5-gly-cylaminomethyl-3-dimethylcarbamoyl-1*H*-1,2-triazole.HCl.2H$_2$O (a triazoyl benzodiazepine) [10]. Metabolite investigation entailed use of TLC, RP-HPLC and RRA (in succession for determining tissue levels, on ethanol extracts of frozen tissues), and GC-MS (SCOT capillary column) to identify the metabolites.

By **GC-ECD, zomepirac** [11] and 2-amino-*N*-(1,1-dimethylhexyl)acet-amide [12] have been assayed in plasma with good sensitivity. For assay of **naloxone,** benzene-extracted at alkaline pH from serum, RP-HPLC was performed at pH 4.8, with detection at 220 nm. The detection limit was 3 ng/ml [13]. **Baclofen** is amenable to GC-ECD [14].

References

1. Gasparic, J. & Zimak, J. (1983) *J. Pharm. Biomed. Anal. 1*, 259-279.
2. Adams, W.J., Bombardt, R.A. & Brewer, J.E. (1984) *Anal. Chem. 56*, 1590-1594.

3. Heizmann, P. & von Alten, R. (1981) *J. High Res. Chrom. C. Comm.* 4, 266–269.
4. Vree, T.B., Baars, A.M., Booji, L.H.D. & Driessen, J.J. (1981) *Arzneim.-Forsch./Drug Res.* 31, 2215–2219.
5. Coassolo, Ph., Aubert, C. & Cano, J.P. (1984) *J. High Resolu. Chromatog. Chromatog. Comm.* 7, 258–264.
6. Vajta, S., LeMoing, J.P. & Rovei, V. (1984) *J. Chromatog. 311*, 329–337.
7. Narasimhachari, N., Dorey, R.C., Landa, B.L. & Friedel, R.O. (1984) *J. Chromatog. 311*, 424–429.
8. Heazelwood, R.L. & Lemass, R.W.J. (1984) *J. Chromatog. 336*, 229–233.
9. Kozu, T. (1984) *J. Chromatog. 310*, 213–218.
10. Fujimoto, M., Hashimoto, S., Takahashi, S., Hirose, K., Hatakeyama, H. & Okabayashi, T. (1984) *Biochem. Pharmacol. 33*, 1645–1651.
11. Ng, K-T. & Kalbron, J.J. (1983) *J. Chromatog. 276*, 311–318.
12. Parsons, D.N. (1983) *J. Chromatog. 276*, 197–201.
13. Terry, M.D., Hisayasu, G.H., Kern, J.W. & Cohen, J.L. (1984) *J. Chromatog. 311*, 213–217.
14. Kochak, G. & Honc, F. (1984) *J. Chromatog. 310*, 319–326.

Some approaches practised for CNS-active drugs

- *by R. Schmid (Psychiatric University Hospital of Vienna): the following is based on a Forum Abstract*

Having tried different bonded solid-phase materials for extraction of tricyclic antidepressants from plasma, we favour cyanopropyl silica; this approach to selective and quantitative isolation prior to GC or HPLC is very fast and efficient. With capillary GC we can measure underivatized tricyclics down to pg levels, with NPD (AFID). A deactivation procedure must be applied during analysis because tricyclics are readily adsorbed onto active column sites.   If we also need values for hydroxy metabolites, which cannot easily be analyzed by GC, we perform RP-HPLC with short small-bore columns, using oxidative EC detection for good sensitivity and specificity. Thereby, with imipramine and desmethylimipramine as internal standards, we can rapidly separate clomipramine, desmethylclomipramine and the hydroxy metabolite corresponding to each.

Question by P.G. Ashton at the Forum: how is the final extract treated after the CN-BondElut extraction prior to GC? **R. Schmid's reply:** the final extract is usually in 600 µl of ethanol, and its volume is reduced prior to GC injection unless the drug level is high.

Section #C

SEPARATION TECHNOLOGY APPLICABLE TO VARIOUS DRUGS AND
TO ENANTIOMERS

#C-1

NOVEL CAPILLARY GAS-CHROMATOGRAPHIC PHASES APPLICABLE TO DRUGS

B. Caddy and W.M.L. Chow

Forensic Science Unit
University of Strathclyde
204 George Street, Glasgow G1 1XW, U.K.

The incorporation of various barbiturate moieties into a poly-siloxane liquid phase as a means of introducing selectivity forms the main theme of this article, in which the emphasis is on qualitative rather than quantitative analysis. Such liquid phases have also been assessed for their ability to resolve drugs of misuse and abuse.

There have been enormous advances in making capillary columns for GC, largely due to the discovery of ways to deactivate glass (quartz) surfaces and of methods to render these surfaces compatible with a variety of liquid phases [1]. The development of immobilized phases [2], whereby the liquids are covalently bonded to the walls of the columns, offers many advantages over simple coated capillaries, including the ability to decontaminate such columns by solvent washing. This property can be particularly useful when dealing with samples of biological origin. Finally, the introduction of the external polyimide coatings [3] onto quartz columns, thereby making them flexible, has led to an explosion in the use of these highly resolving systems.

Notwithstanding such advances, developments have been almost exclusively confined to the use of well deactivated non-polar columns. Such systems usually demonstrate, even for capillary columns, a lack of selectivity for polar compounds of related structure, e.g. the barbiturate group. Many capillary systems have been described which even in the non-deactivated form can resolve certain barbiturate mixtures [4]. However, no single column seems to possess an adequate resolving power or selectivity for all these compounds. In fact, in the analysis of these drugs it is common practice to use a combination of two capillary columns, one containing a non-polar and the other a polar phase [5]. Resolving power can be increased by various physical modifications including increasing the film thickness and column length. Such changes do not always solve the problem and usually lead to longer analysis times or a higher operating temperature, both of which can prove unsatisfactory. An alternative is to prepare liquid phases having greater sensitivity.

Early workers are stated [6] to have improved the performance of packed columns by column priming, viz. injection of the analyte in large amounts onto the column prior to loading for analysis. Whilst such a procedure is not to be recommended, clearly it effectively saturates any active support sites; but in doing so these workers also changed the nature of the 'liquid' phase. Accepting this as a starting point for our researches and the chromatographer's axiom that like compounds separate like, we embarked upon a series of investigations into the incorporation of the barbiturate nucleus into the immobilized liquid phase of capillary columns.

Our choice in considering which polymer would best serve as the base for these investigations was the polymethylsiloxane phase SE54, which is thermally stable and, moreover, possesses some vinyl groups which could allow incorporation of a suitable barbiturate moiety, **B** [see opposite for this and other abbreviations - *Ed.*]. SE54 is also effective in separating some underivatized **B**'s, as shown with a standard mixture of 13 common **B**'s in Fig. 1; hence an SE54 column could serve as a reference point for judging all other columns.

Next a decision had to be made as to which monomer should be incorporated into the polymethylsiloxane and how incorporation of the **B** could best be achieved. In order to achieve a certain compatibility between the silicone polymer and the **B**, it was decided to employ a vinyl silicone derivative whose structure is given in Fig. 2a. It was synthesized and incorporated into the polymer during the column coating procedure by means of a free-radical reaction initiated by dicumyl peroxide [7]. The effect of incorporating this monomer was shown to depend on its concentration and the time of curing; but generally the higher the concentration the higher the polarity. However, 10% incorporation of the monomer gave results much inferior to the standard SE54: tailing was considerable, bralloB did not elute, and cycloB and phenoB were not resolved. One reason for this poor performance may have been the acidic hydrogens in the molecule. To test this hypothesis, a column incorporating a methylated **B** monomer (Fig. 2b) was investigated. Such columns were slightly acidic in nature but demonstrated greater selectivity and better performance. The selectivity, as expected, improved with higher levels of incorporation of monomer.

FURTHER INVESTIGATION OF COLUMNS WITH MONOMER INCORPORATED

The problem of column 'activities' (adsorptive losses) still existed. It was thought that one reason for this was the presence of small amounts of residual peroxide and/or breakdown products. This

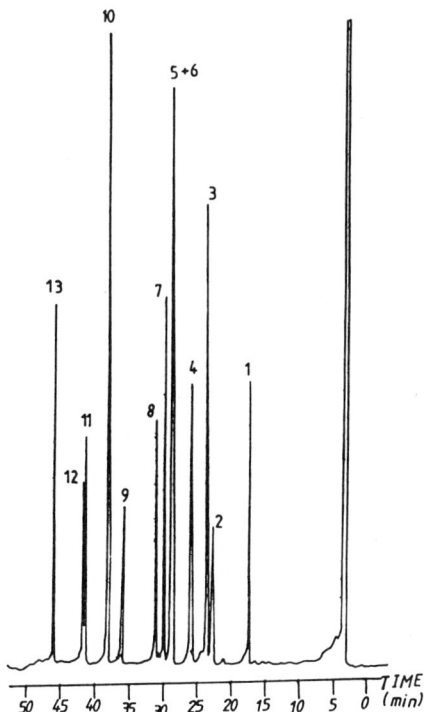

Fig. 1. Use of SE54 reference column to chromatograph a test mixture: 120° for first 2 min, programmed at 2°/min up to 220°, and held at 220° for 32 min. Column 20 m × 290 μm i.d., DPTMDS-persilylated. Detector: FID.
Peaks:
1 = B;   2 = alloB;   3 = aproB;
4 = butal*B*;   5 = amyloB;
6 = nealB;   7 = pentoB;
8 = vinB;   9 = bralloB;
10 = methylphenylB;   11 = phenoB;
12 = cycloB;   13 = heptaB.

Abbreviations used above and elsewhere in the article: **B** = barbital *or in certain contexts* barbiturate *(Editor's abbreviation; see Fig. 3 for* di$_0$AB, di$_1$AB etc.*)*; butal*B* = butalbital (allylbarbital). *Authors' own abbreviations:* CE = coating efficiency, TZ = separation efficiency (Trennzahl value); in designations for persilylating agents (deactivators; % values are w/w) such as DPTMDS: TMDS (DMDS) = tri- (di-)methylsilazane, DP (TP) = di- (tri-)phenyl, DV = divinyl, F_3/F_4 (trade name) is a mixed siloxane deactivating agent. DCUP = dicumyl peroxide. PEG 20M = polyethylene glycol, M_r~20,000. Throughout, 'octanol' is octan-1-ol.

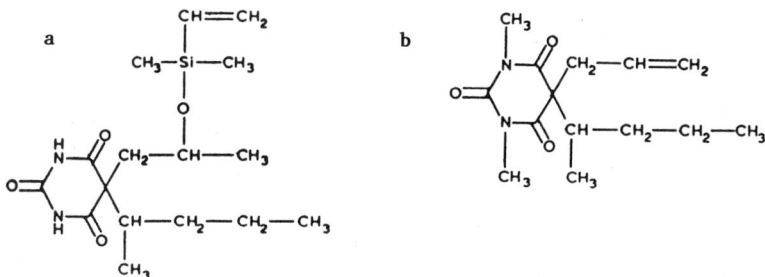

Figs. 2a *(left)* **and 2b** *(right).* Compounds incorporated into the SE54 liquid phase: **a**, 5-(2-vinyldimethylsiloxypropyl)-5-(1-methylbutyl)barbituric acid; **b**, 1,3-dimethyl-5-allyl-5-(1-methylbutyl)-barbituric acid.

Fig. 3. As for Fig. 2: *N,N'*-di-allylamylobarbital (di$_o$AB), and higher homologues. *NOTE: chains only 3-C for* di$_o$AB.

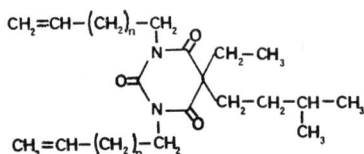

Value of n	Editor's abbreviation
0	di$_o$AB
1	di$_1$AB
2	di$_2$AB
3	di$_3$AB

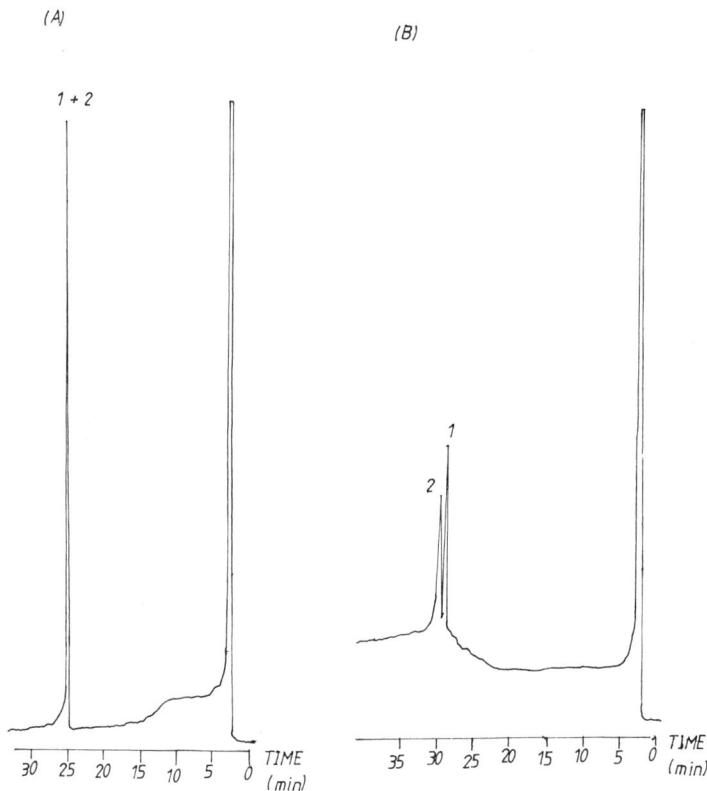

(A) (B)

1 + 2

2

1

TIME (min)

TIME (min)

30 25 20 15 10 5 0   35 30 25 20 15 10 5 0

Fig. 4. Use of treated SE54 columns (23 m × 230 μm i.d.; DPTMDS-persilylated) for a mixture of amyloB (peak 1) and nealB (peak 2); 4°/min temp. rise but otherwise as for Fig. 1 except that upper limit in A was 150°. Incorporated: A, 1% (w/w) DCUP; B, 30% di$_o$AB and 3% DCUP.

was minimized by using less reagent and carefully washing the immobilized phase with solvent. However, while some selectivity had been introduced, these columns were still unable to resolve butaB, butoB and butalB. One reason for this failure may have been the point of attachment of the monomer within the SE54 3-D matrix, via position 5 of the B

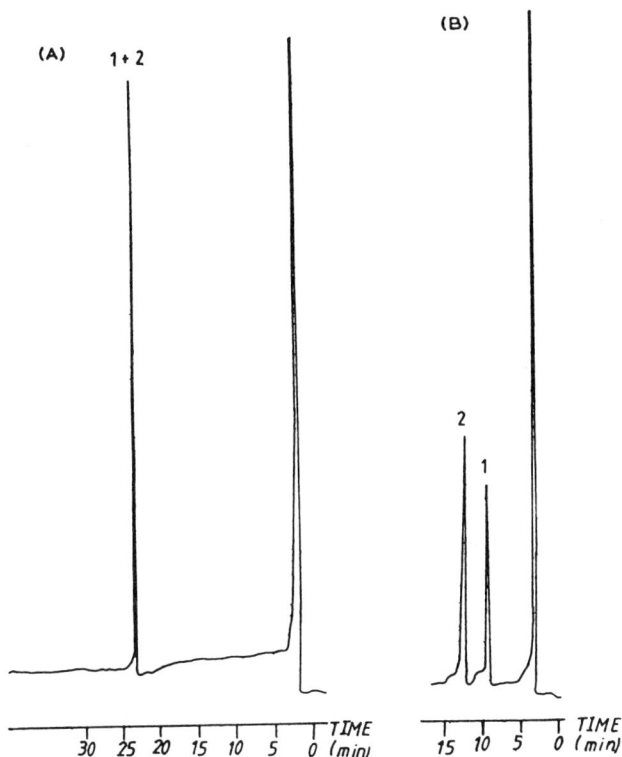

Fig. 5. A & B as for Fig. 4 A & B respectively, but with hexo**B** and bralloB (unresolved under optimal conditions in A, resolved in B). A: 120° for 1 min, then up to 180° (4°/min) and kept there 10 min. B: 210° for 4 min, then up to 240° (4°/min) and kept there 10 min.

which may have caused steric hindrance to the chromatographed species. This may have been important since most **B**'s differ from each other by the substitution pattern at position 5. Greater selectivity might therefore be obtained by attaching the monomer through some other position in the **B** nucleus. For this reason the N,N'-diallyl derivative of amylo**B** (di₀AB, Fig. 3) was synthesized and incorporated at different concentrations into the SE54 matrix. Evidence for its incorporation into the matrix came from the longer retention of amylo**B** and neal**B** with a need for a higher temperature on the new phase. There was some improvement in selectivity, manifest by their near-baseline resolution although with some tailing (Fig. 4). One surprise was that amylo**B** eluted before neal**B**, implying that the latter has greater selectivity towards the incorporated monomer. This might be due to incomplete incorporation of di₀AB into the SE54, resulting in the presence of at least one intact **N**-allyl group. Buto**B** was separable from buta**B** but not completely from butal**B**. Furthermore, resolution of bralloB and hexo**B** was possible on the new-phase column but not on the standard SE54 column (Fig. 5).

Table 1. Evaluation of SE54-based columns (Pyrex, 0.23 mm i.d.). The values for the 3 components of the Grob mixtures represent observed peak heights as % of that expected if no adsorption had occurred (as determined from peak heights of hydrocarbons and methyl esters). Abbreviations are given in conjunction with Fig. 3.

TZ	Length	di₀AB incorporated in stat. phase, %	Octanol	2,6-dimethyl-phenol	2,6-dimethyl-aniline
25.9	22 m	none	60	68	82
24.9	13 m	2	75	69	94
19.0	15 m	4	62	79	90
15.5	15 m	10	84	100	52
13.5	23 m	20	83	97	51
9.0	23 m	30	72	100	57
8.3	21 m	50	87	–	–

As indicated by running Grob test mixtures [8], columns with N,N'-diallylamylo**B** incorporated into the SE54 are acidic, whereas the reference SE54 columns are slightly basic. Furthermore, the elution sequence is changed: 1-octanol elutes after undecane (Grob I) on the new column, and 2,6-dimethylphenol, 2,6-dimethylaniline and 2-ethylhexanoic acid elute after dodecane (Grob II). This increase in retention of the polar components of the Grob mixtures is to be expected in view of the increased phase polarity, and is supporting evidence for incorporation of the monomer into the SE54 matrix. What remained to be achieved was a means of reducing tailing and an assessment of the effect of varying the concentration of monomer.

With a view to resolving **B** pairs that are difficult to separate, SE54 columns with 2, 4, 10, 20, 30, 50 and 100% (w/w) incorporation of the monomer were prepared and their performance compared with that of a reference SE54 column. Polarity, acidity and activity were tested with Grob mixtures I and II, and selectivity with a standard **B** mixture. A column with 2% monomer hardly differed from the reference column, except that peak tailing was worse. Evidently 2% incorporation was too little to significantly affect separation of the **B**'s.

Column polarity began to increase with incorporations from 4% to 50%, as evidenced by increased retention of the polar components of a Grob mixture. With 20% it was similar to that with 30% but higher than with 10%. Generally the Grob mixture elution patterns were different for different % incorporations, suggesting that each column should be regarded as of particular polarity.

As shown in Table 1, acidity increased with % incorporation; activity was low towards octanol, its peak height being generally 60-80% of that expected.

Table 2. Resolution (R) of pairs of barbital (**B**) derivatives on SE54 columns (Pyrex, 0.23 mm i.d.) differing in % incorporation of the barbiturate monomer. The R nos. were calculated thus:

$$R = \frac{2\Delta t}{1.7(W_{h1} + W_{h2})}$$

where Δ_t = distance between the two peak maxima, W_{h1} (W_{h2}) = peak width at half-height of component 1 (2).

Length	di$_o$AB incorporated in stat. phase, %	amyloB and nealB	butoB and butalB (i.e. butalbital)	hexoB and bralloB
15 m	4	0.8	–	4.1
15 m	10	1.0	0.8	4.6
23 m	20	1.0	1.0	–
23 m	30	1.1	1.1	5.7
21 m	50	1.5	1.2	11.1

Attempts to prepare columns with 100% incorporation of monomer were at first unsuccessful because the coatings separated into visible droplets (see later). The higher the % incorporation of the monomer, the higher was the selectivity towards separation of the **B** mixture, especially for difficult pairs not separable on the reference column. Table 2 summarizes the results. With 4% monomer, complete baseline separation of bralloB and hexoB was achieved (Fig. 6). With 50%, complete baseline separation of amyloB and nealB and ~80% separation of butoB and butalB were achieved.

With a mixture of 13 common **B**'s as in Fig. 1, increasing % incorporation gave stronger retention of certain components selectively (viz. those with peak designations 2, 6, 9 & 11 in legend to Fig. 1). Two components (5 & 6) that were unresolved by the reference column were resolved with 10% incorporation, but a different pair (6 & 7) was merged. Performance was best with 4% incorporation [not illustrated]: all 13 components showed some resolution in one run (temperature program as in legend to Fig. 7).

To extend the assessment of the column that had performed best (4% monomer), it was tested with 22 common barbiturates which are encountered in toxicological cases and which included some pairs that are difficult to separate. All showed some resolution except bralloB and cyclopentoB which eluted together (peak 14/15; Fig. 7). Fig. 8 shows the same test on the reference SE54 column, which failed to resolve the peak pairs 6 & 7, 8 & 9, 13 & 14 and 20 & 21. The column with 4% incorporation retained some components more strongly as compared with the reference column, viz. alloB (peak 3), butalbital (butalB peak 7), nealB (9), bralloB (14), cyclopentoB (15), ibomal (16), phenoB (18) and 5-ethyl-5-p-tolylB (20).

In **Figs. 6-8**, *overleaf*: SE54 columns (+ monomer in **6** & **7**), 15 m × 230 µm; 120° for 2 min, then 8°/min rise, to 230° (**6**) or 240° and kept there for 5 min (**7** & **8**).

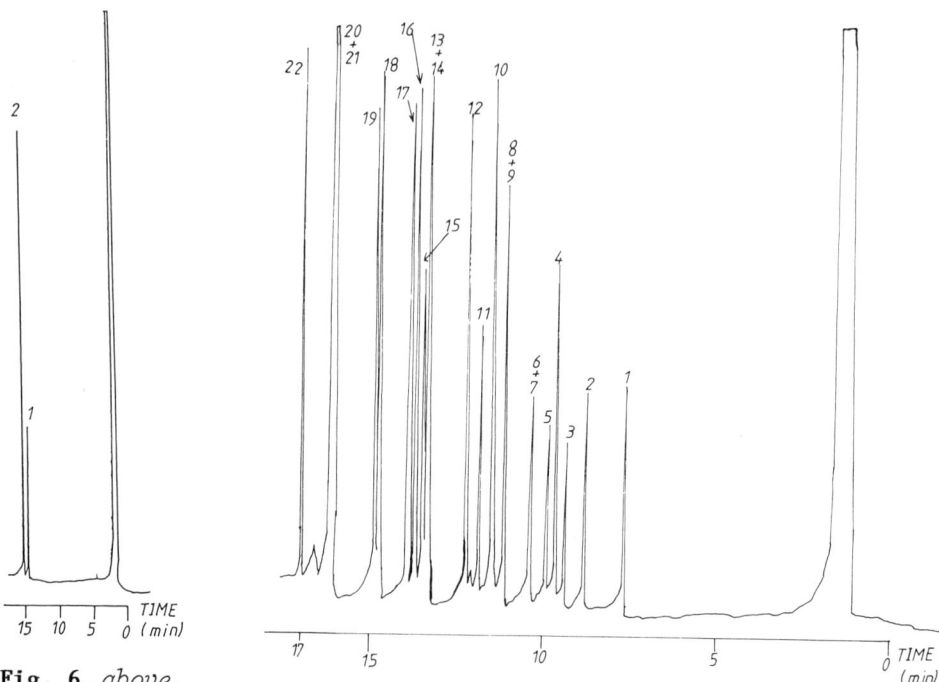

Fig. 6, *above.*
HexaB (1) and
bralloB (2)
separation, with
4% di₀AB as also
in the run of:
Fig. 7, *top right,*
with a 22-compon-
ent mixture as
also in:
Fig. 8, *right.*
Reference column.
*Besides peaks
named in text:*
1 = **B**; 2 = proB;
4 = aproB; 5 =
ethyl-crotylB;
6 = butoB;
8 = amyloB;
10 = pentoB;
11 = vinoB;
12 = quinalB;
13 = hexoB; 17 =
methyl-pentylB;
19 = cycloB;
21 = heptaB;
22 = reposal.
See also foot of page 227.

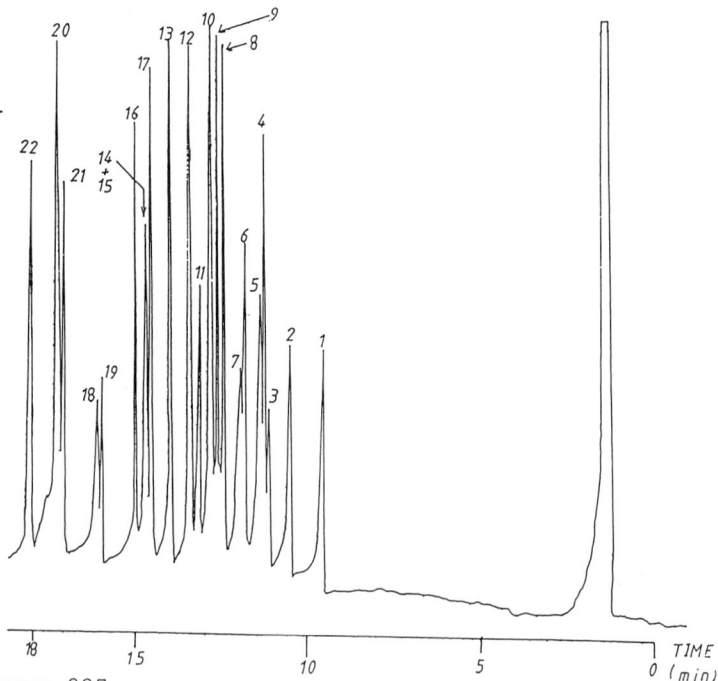

Table 3. Separation efficiencies (TZ) with different treatments of the columns (Pyrex, 0.23 mm i.d.). TZ is the average for two comparisons of methyl esters: decanoate and undecanoate, and undecanoate and dodecanoate. Abbreviations: see below Fig. 1. The Grob test mixture was run with the column at 40° initially (except column 2: 100°), rising by 8°/min.

Column, no. & length	di$_o$AB incorporated in stat. phase	DCUP, v/w	HF roughening	Deactivation: agent & temp.; t connotes TMDS, thus DPt = DPTMDS etc.	TZ
1, 22 m	none	0.4%	–	DPt, 400°	25.9
2, 23 m	30%	3%	–	DPt, 400°	9.0
3, 17 m	30%	3%	–	F$_3$/F$_4$, 400°	1.3
4, 10 m	30%	3%	+	DPt, 400°	7.5
5, 14 m	30%	3%	–	TPt, 400°	1.2
6, 14 m	30%	1.5%	–	1:3 v/v DVt/DPt, 350°	22.4
7, 15 m	30%	1.5%	–	1:1 v/v DVt/DPt, 350°	22.7
8, 15 m	30%	1.5%	–	DVt, 350°	29.1
9, 14 m	30%	3%	–	PEG 20M, 280°	14.4
10, 12 m	30%	3%	+	PEG 20M, 280°	7.0
11, 15 m	100%	6%	–	DVt, 350°	9.4

OPTIMIZATION OF PERFORMANCE WITH THE PREFERRED MONOMER TYPE

Although SE54 columns incorporating various percentages of di$_o$aB coated onto a leached, DPTMDS-persilylated surface were both selective and efficient, with upwards of 20% incorporation the efficiency fell drastically as evidenced by the 2,6-dimethylaniline results in Table 1. In order to fully utilize the unique selectivities of SE54 columns with a high di$_o$AB content, two approaches were tried.

In the first, the surface area of the inner walls of the columns was increased by controlled treatment with HF, prior to the leaching [9]. The second approach consisted in chemical modification of the surface using different deactivating agents capable of generating surfaces more compatible with the stationary phase [10].

SE54 with 30% (w/w) of di$_o$AB incorporated was employed to assess the effects of different surface pre-treatments (Table 3). Very low efficiency was obtained using DPTMDS as persilylating agent (TZ = 9.0; Table 3; CE = 33%: Table 4). Clearly improvements were necessary if the high efficiency of the standard SE54 column (TZ = 25.9: Table 3; CE = 88%: Table 4) was to be matched.

Roughening by HF increased the surface area of the inner walls of the column by forming silica whiskers [9]. Whisker walls are highly active and have to be deactivated. The total surface energy of the deactivated whisker walls was increased, enabling them to 'hold'

Table 4. Column characteristics (Nos. as in Table 3). All except No. 1 had 30% di.AB incorporated in the stationary phase. For the abbreviations DPt etc. see column heading in Table 3. Values for k' and HETP refer to hexadecane at 140°. n.d. = not determined.

Column no.	DCUP, %, & HF roughening		Deactivation agent	k'	HETP, mm	Coating eff'y, CE	k' decr. after solvent rinse
1	0.4%;	–	DPt	7.8	0.22	88%	2.6%
2	3%;	–	DPt	20.0	0.63	33%	0%
6	1.5%;	–	1:3 DVt/DPt	7.3	0.29	67%	11%
7	1.5%;	–	1:1 DVt/DPt	6.2	0.28	69%	7.8%
8	1.5%;	–	DVt	6.5	0.25	77%	5.2%
9	3%;	–	PEG 20M	8.6	0.38	53%	n.d.
10	3%;	+	PEG 20M	13.0	0.65	32%	n.d.

stationary phases of high surface tension. Surprisingly, the efficiencies of the HF-treated columns (nos. 1, 4 & 10, Table 3) were lower than for the corresponding columns without HF treatment. Maybe this was due to the difficulty of creating uniform whiskers throughout the inner surface of the column, precluding uniform coating with the stationary phase and resulting in inefficient columns.

The wettability towards the newly generated stationary phase was worse if the surface had been persilylated with F_3/F_4 or TPDMDS rather than DPTMDS, as evidenced by a drastic decrease in TZ values (Table 3). However, the efficiency improved for the column deactivated with PEG 20M as compared with the DPTMDS-persilylated column, and the TZ value increased by a factor of ~1.6 (Table 3). Furthermore, the PEG 20M-deactivated surface affected the overall polarity, leading to a more polar column. Selectivity in **B** separation was better for the PEG 20M-deactivated column than for the DPTMDS-persilylated column, the only limitation of the former being thermal stability (280° limit). The TZ value, although improved, was still low when compared with the standard SE54 column (Table 3).

Very efficient columns were obtained from 30% incorporation of di.AB when persilylation was performed with DVTMDS, 1:1 DVTMDS/DPTMDS or 1:3 DVTMDS/DPTMDS (Table 3). The TZ values increased ~2.5-3-fold (Table 3) and were comparable to that of the standard SE54 column; CE values were also high (Table 4). These columns showed similar polarity to the DPTMDS column, were slightly basic in character, and showed little tailing. The columns also showed very weak, but clearly observable, activity (adsorptiveness); but they can be used up to at least 300°. The selectivity in separating **B**'s improved markedly and, with DVTMDS-persilylation, 21 out of 22 **B**'s, including the difficultly separable pairs, were resolved with an analysis time of <21 min (Fig. 9).

Table 5. Characteristics of the new stationary phases (cf. Fig. 3). As in Table 4, k' and HETP refer to hexadecane.

SE54 stationary phase	Octanol retention value, mm	TZ	k'	HETP, mm	CE	k' decr. after solvent rinse
+ 30% di₁AB	18.5	27.3	5.75	0.23	85.2	3.5
+ 30% di₂AB	16.0	27.4	4.89	0.24	80.4	3.9
+ 30% di₃AB	14.0	27.4	5.65	0.22	89.2	4.0

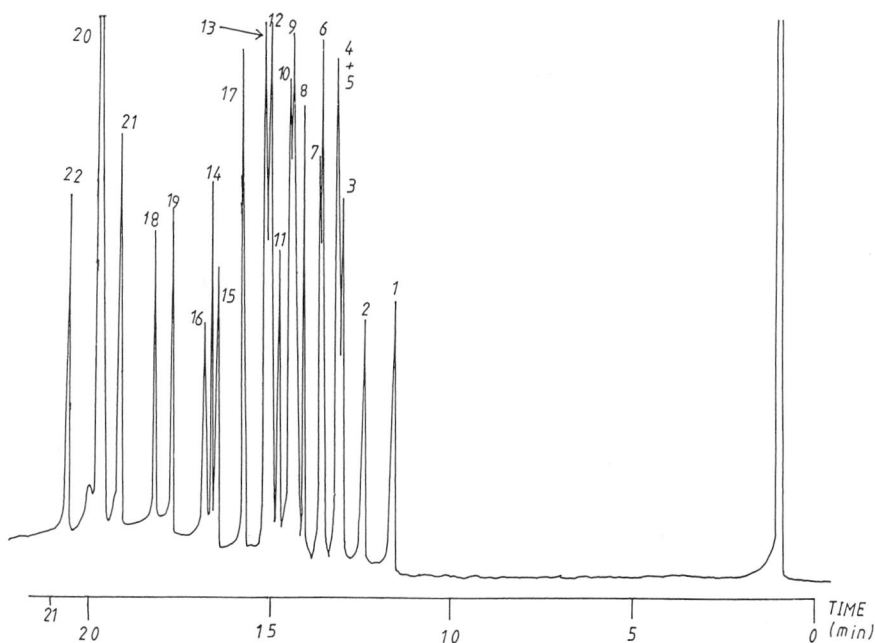

Fig. 9. As for Fig. 7, but 30% monomer; deactivation by DVTMDS.

A further series of columns was prepared containing amyloB in which each *N*-substituent was lengthened successively by single methylene units as indicated in Fig. 3 (di₁AB, di₂AB, di₃AB). From the elution sequence of undecane and dodecane and from the decreasing retention value of l-octanol (Table 5), it was apparent that there was a progressive decrease in polarity with lengthening of the incorporated monomer. This is what might be expected from the stepwise introduction of non-polar methylene groups. Columns incorporating di₁AB or di₂AB are slightly basic in character, whereas di₃AB confers slight acidity. All three phases showed very good tailing behaviour and are very efficient as evidenced from their high TZ values (Table 5), They also showed very high CE values and can be routinely used up to at least 300°. All phases were immobilized and extracted with dichloro-

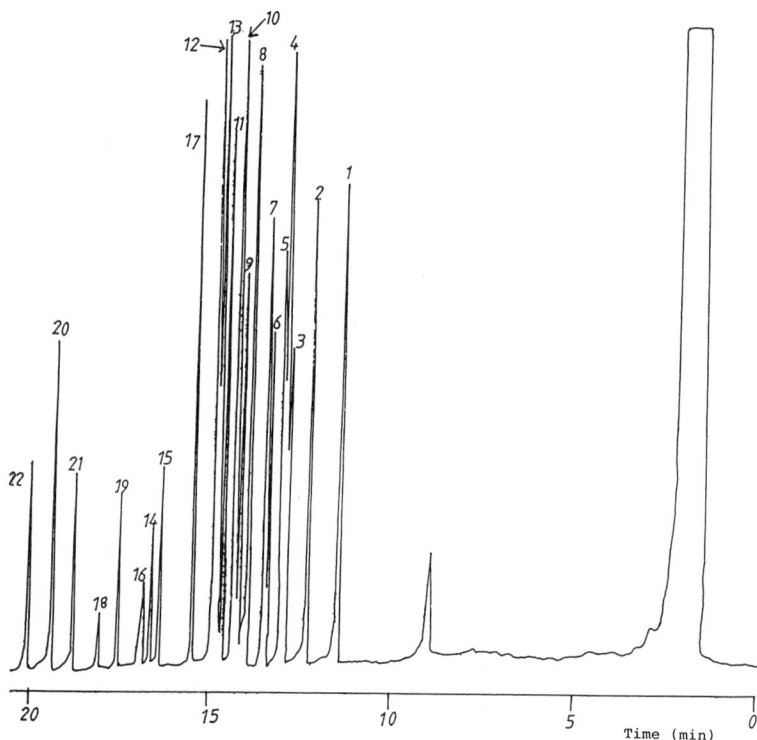

Fig. 10. As for Figs. 7 & 9, but with 30% of di$_1$**AB** incorporated.

methane, the resulting decrease in k' values being only ~3.5-4%. For the mixture of 22 underivatized **B**'s, Fig. 10 shows the pattern for an SE54 column incorporating the monomer di$_1$**AB**.

To illustrate the versatility of these columns, some other drug groups were examined. The similarity of the 7-membered benzodiazepine ring to the **B** nucleus in terms of polarity suggested that they might chromatograph well on the new columns. Partial resolution of 6 common benzodiazepines requires 25 min on a standard SE54 column, whereas a better result can be obtained in 15 min on a column which has di$_3$**AB** incorporated (Fig. 11). The separation of some drugs of abuse is shown for columns incorporating di$_2$**AB** or di$_1$**AB** (Figs. 12 & 13).

CONCLUDING REMARKS

It is hoped that our remarks will stimulate others to approach their difficult resolution problems by selectively modifying the structures of stationary phases. As we have shown, such a process is now viable for immobilized capillary column systems.

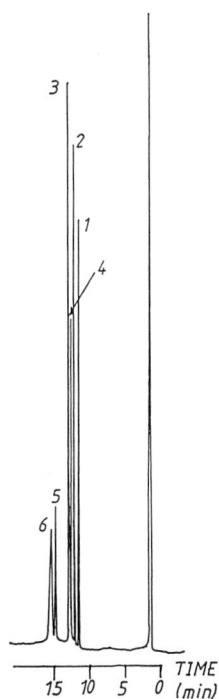

Fig. 11. Separation of 6 commonly abused benzodiazepines on a column with di$_3$A**B** incorporated: 130° for 2 min; 16°/min rise to 300° and kept there for 5 min.
1 = oxazepam
2 = diazepam
3 = desmethyl-diazepam
4 = librium⊗
5 = nitrazapam
6 = clonazepam

⊗ chlordiazepoxide

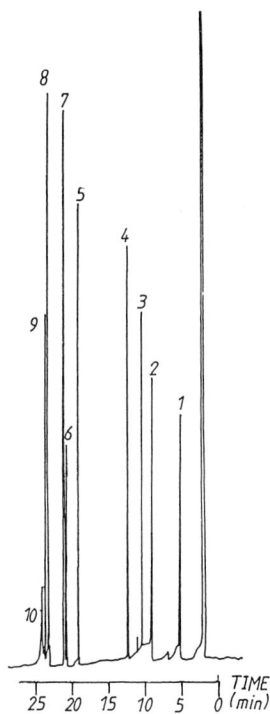

Fig. 12. Separation of several important drugs of abuse in a human urine drug screen on a column with di$_2$A**B** incorporated: 100° for 2 min; 8°/min rise to 280° and kept there for 5 min.
1 = amphetamine
2 = ephedrine
3 = phendimetrazine
4 = benzocaine
5 = procaine
6 = methaqualone
7 = cocaine
8 = codeine
9 = ethylmorphine
10 = morphine

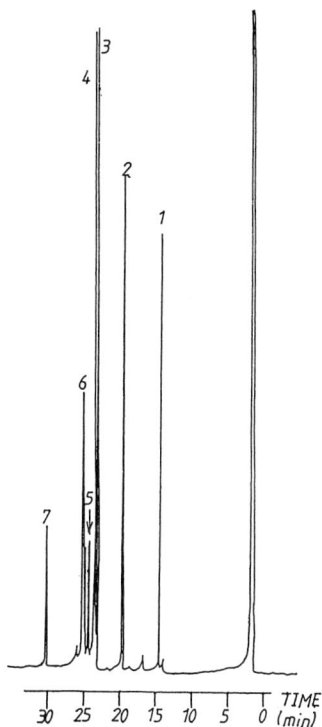

Fig. 13. Separation of some common narcotic analgesics on a column incorporating di$_1$A**B**.
1 = pethidine
2 = methadone
3 = dipipanone
4 = codeine
5 = morphine
6 = heroin
7 = dextromoramide

(LSD 25 tartrate applied to this column gave a sharp LSD 25 peak at 22 min.)

References

1. Blomberg, L.G. (1984) *J. High Resolu. Chromatog. Chromatog. Comm. 7*, 232–244.
2. Grob, K., Grob, G. & Grob, jr., K. (1981) *J. Chromatog. 211*, 243–246.
3. Lee, M.L., Kong, R.C., Woolley, C.L. & Bradshaw, J.S. (1984) *J. Chromatog. Sci. 22*, 136–142.
4. Gough, T.A. & Baker, P.B. (1983) *J. Chromatog. Sci. 21*, 145–153.
5. Alm, S., Jonson, S., Karlsson, H. & Sundholm, E.G. (1983) *J. Chromatog. 254*, 179–186.
6. McMartin, C. & Street, H.V. (1966) *J. Chromatog. 23*, 232–241.
7. Bamberg, L.G., Buijtem, J., Markides, K. & Wannman, T. (1982) *J. Chromatog. 239*, 51–60.
8. Grob, K., Grob, G. & Grob K., Jr. (1981) *J. Chromatog. 219*, 13–20.
9. Onuska, F.I., Comba, M.E., Bistricki, T. & Wilkinson, R.J. (1977) *J. Chromatog. 142*, 117–125.
10. Grob, K. & Grob, G. (1980) *J. High Resolu. Chromatog. Chromatog. Comm. 3*, 197–198.

#C-2

LIQUID-SOLID SAMPLE PREPARATION

R.D. McDowall*, J.C. Pearce, G.S. Murkitt and R.M. Lee

Department of Drug Analysis
Smith Kline & French Research Ltd.
The Frythe, Welwyn, Herts. AL6 9AR, U.K.

Sample preparation is frequently an essential step in the deter-mination of drugs in biological fluids. Until recently the need for selective extraction of analytes has usually been met by liquid-liquid extraction. However, due to recent developments in bonded-silica chemistry an alternative is feasible for many drugs and meta-bolites. They can be trapped on a solid phase (e.g. C-18 or CN silica), freed from contaminants by washing, then eluted and analyzed chromatographically. Liquid-solid extraction is rapid and offers good precision and accuracy. It is the basis of two automated sample processors which are commercially available and can notably aid produc-tivity. The capabilities of one of these ('AASP') are outlined.

The instrumental analysis step in assaying biological materials for drugs is usually preceded by some form of sample preparation, designed to largely remove potentially interfering endogenous com-pounds while concentrating the analyte to facilitate its detection. The assay specificity partly comes from the instrumental analysis but may partly come from the preliminary clean-up. This can be performed in various ways, but only liquid-liquid and liquid-solid methods will be considered here.[†]

---

* to whom any correspondence should be addressed

[†] *Senior Editor's note.*-There has been condensation of the less advan-ced material in the authors' MS., especially on sample-preparation modes - as surveyed earlier in this series, e.g. by J.A.F. de Silva (Vol. 10), R.P. Maickel (Vol. 14) [cf. Reid, E. (1976) *Analyst 101*, 1-18]. Ion-pair extraction is exemplified in Vols. 12 (M.J. Stewart) & 14 (K. Ensing & R.A. de Zeeuw). Contributors who used solid-phase aids (including cartridges), especially pre-HPLC, include P.R.J. Ceelen et al. (this vol.; use of AASP), A.P. Woodbridge (Vol. 10), R.C. Williams (Vol. 14; Du Pont PREP automated processor). Some diagrams in the present authors' MS. do not appear here.

LIQUID–LIQUID EXTRACTION

Sample preparation commonly entails direct extraction of the biological material with a water-immiscible solvent, the choice governing the recoveries of drug and metabolites and the selectivity that is achieved if there is minimal extraction of endogenous substances. Difficulty in extracting highly polar molecules may be overcome by use of a suitable ion-pairing agent [1]. The major disadvantage of liquid-liquid extraction is emulsion formation; this causes loss of analyte by occlusion within the emulsion, and lower recoveries ensue. Emulsion formation may be minimizable by less rigorous mixing, or by use of large volumes of extracting solvent, whose later removal may entail delay and risk.

Liquid-liquid extraction can be used in assaying large numbers of samples and operated batch-wise; but the transfer steps involved make the process labour-intensive and tedious. Extraction may be incomplete (75% for oxmetidine [2]), quite apart from the losses in the extraction procedure.

LIQUID–SOLID EXTRACTION

An alternative to liquid-liquid extraction is to treat the biological sample with an adsorbent which, with appropriate relative affinity, will retain the analyte and allow its elution with a suitable solvent. Adsorbents such as charcoal, celite, florisil and alumina have been used for many years with varying degrees of success. This approach, whilst avoiding emulsion formation, may still require the eluting solvent to be removed before analysis.

Impetus to the liquid-solid approach has come from advances in bonded-silica chemistry, primarily for HPLC column packings. Now there are commercially available cartridges, generally silica-based and optimized for sample preparation (Bond Elut, Analytichem International; Sep-Pak, Waters Associates), as illustrated in Fig. 1. They consist of polypropylene or polyethylene containers packed with sorbent. Available bonded groups include C-2 to C-18, diol, amine, cyano, phenyl and ion-exchange. The biological sample is applied to the top, and liquid flow is usually achieved by applying negative pressure to the bottom, possibly using a manifold that allows 8 or 10 cartridges to be processed simultaneously. The analytes eluted by a suitable solvent are collected in tubes positioned directly beneath each cartridge. Any endogenous substances that had been adsorbed may remain behind when the analyte is eluted.

AUTOMATED LIQUID–SOLID EXTRACTION PROCEDURES

One first-generation automated sample processor (PREP; Du Pont) was described by R.C. Williams in Vol. 14, this series. The other

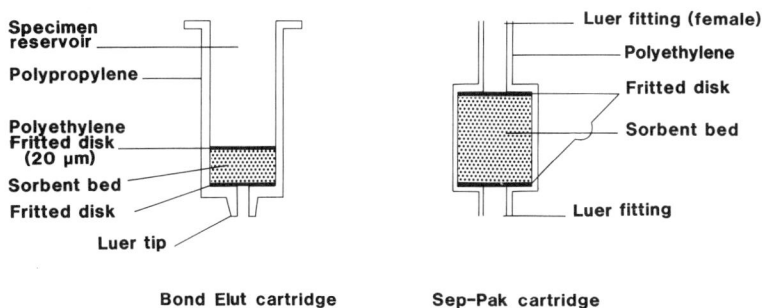

Bond Elut cartridge   Sep-Pak cartridge

Fig. 1. Diagrammatic representation of cartridge types.

as now considered is the Advanced Automated Sample Processor (AASP, Varian Assoc.; microprocessor-controlled). It is designed to integrate extraction on bonded-phase columns with automated on-line injection of the eluate into an HPLC system. Samples are prepared at the bench using a cassette of 10 miniature columns[*]. These are similar in design to Bond Elut columns but fit into a modified Vac-Elut manifold in which positive pressure (nitrogen or air) is applied to drive the sample through the sorbent bed; then the columns may be washed to remove undesirable compounds. The cassettes, retaining the analyte(s) of interest, are then loaded into the Auto-Injector, up to 10 (i.e. 100 samples) at any one time.

The auto-injector consists of two hoppers: an in-feed containing the loaded cassettes and a waste that receives used cassettes pending disposal. Connecting the two hoppers is the cassette-feeding mechanism which takes the next cassette and encapsulates each column in turn into a high-pressure sealing chamber. Elution is effected by switching the solvent flow from the HPLC pump through this chamber and onto the analytical column. The fluid pathway is determined by a pneumatically activated Valco 10-port injection valve controlled by the AASP microprocessor (Fig. 2). This valve can also be re-set after a predetermined time period. Thus, the analytes of interest are selectively eluted off the extraction cartridges leaving unwanted endogenous compounds behind and so obviating much lengthening of the chromatography and hence reduced sample throughput.

The AASP's operational modes are 'Manual' for processing individual cartridges, 'Remote' for automatic analysis controlled from an external device, and 'Auto' for automatic analysis controlled by the AASP itself. Besides the off-line column washes, a purge facility is available. Prior to injection the cartridge can be flushed with up to 9 (25 µl) aliquots of a suitable solvent from a separate reservoir (Fig. 2), the eluent in this instance being sent to waste.

---

[*] The same bonded-phase packing that are available for the Bond Elut cartridges are available for use with the AASP also.

COMPRESSION

ELUTION

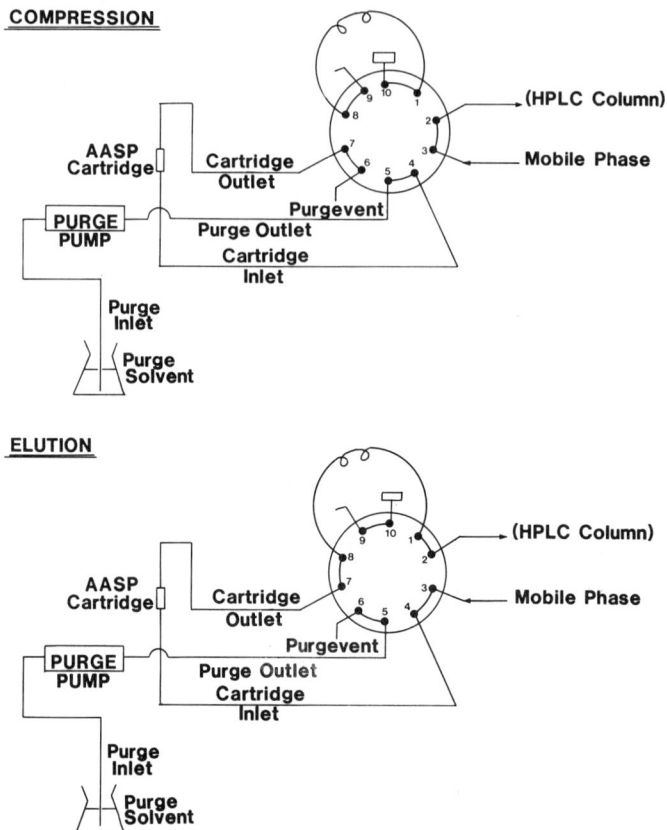

Fig. 2. AASP fluid pathways during compression and elution cycles.

ADVANTAGES OF LIQUID–SOLID EXTRACTION METHODS

LSE methods show the following advantages. Firstly, there is minimal introduction of impurities into the assay. Secondly, the housing of the packings in high-purity polypropylene or polyethylene vessels means that leaching of plasticizers is virtually eliminated. There is also total elimination of emulsion formation that is a notable disadvantage of liquid–liquid extraction. Since a high proportion of the analyte in the sample reaches the column, a reduced amount of biological sample may suffice. Moreover, the columns are disposable and are removable from the laboratory merely as biohazard waste. The solvents used in the final elution are water-soluble and constitute a reduced safety hazard. However, the major advantage of the newer methods of sample preparation is speed, enabling more samples to be processed. These methods are especially suitable for molecules that are volatile or labile, as all operations are done at room temperature, with no solvent evaporation steps.

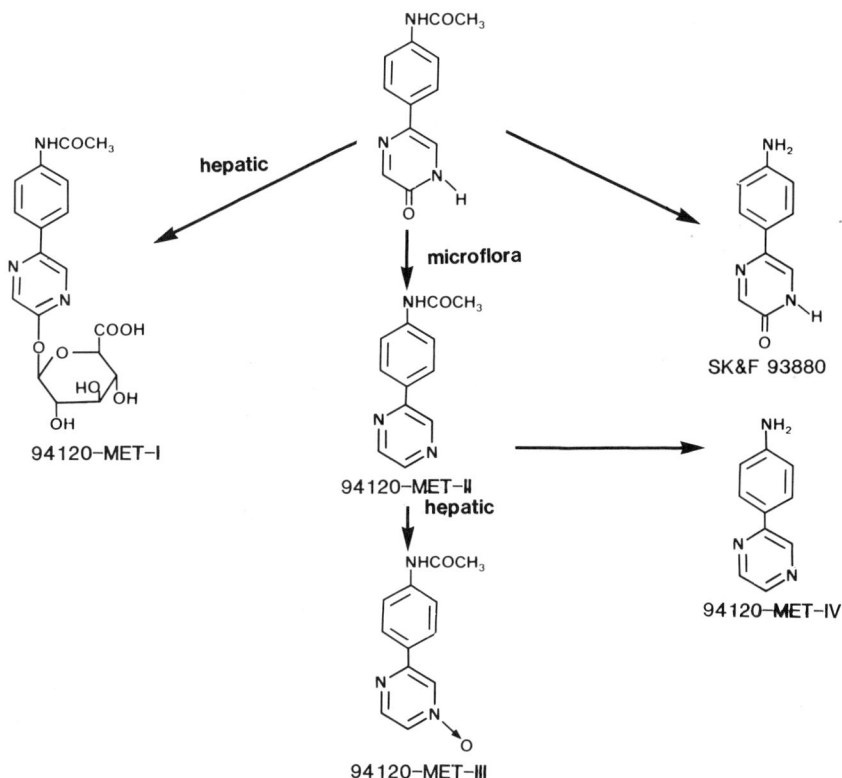

Fig. 3. Metabolic pathways of SK&F 94120 (SK&F 93880 = postulate)

DISADVANTAGES OF LIQUID-SOLID METHODS

We have found that plasma which has been frozen and thawed often contains precipitated fibrin that impedes flow through the columns so that uninterrupted analysis calls for its removal, effected by routinely centrifuging every plasma sample. When preparing samples manually the operator's concentration should be undivided lest he should add the wrong solution at the wrong time and elute the analytes instead of washing the column.

AN ILLUSTRATIVE APPLICATION OF LIQUID-SOLID EXTRACTION

SK&F 94120, 5-(4-acetamidophenyl)pyrazin-2(1H)-one (parent compound in Fig. 3), is a novel positive inotropic agent, potent and orally active, with vasodilator activity considered useful for treating congestive heart failure [3]. In developing an assay for SK&F 94120 in plasma we decided to use liquid-solid rather than liquid-liquid extraction. Initially we used C-18 Bond Elut cartridges. However, the availability of the AASP focused our attention on this instrument as conducive to sample throughput, reproducibility and sensitivity.

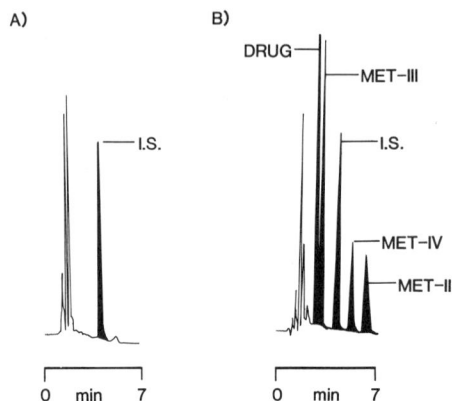

Fig. 4. Typical chromatograms of extracts of rat plasma: **A)** control, **B)** spiked with SK&F 94120 and 3 metabolites; spiking with internal standard in both cases. HPLC on 300 × 3.9 mm i.d. μ-Bondapack column at 35°, with acetonitrile/10 mM ammonium acetate (1:4 by vol.) containing 0.03% (v/v) orthophosphoric acid; 2 ml/min. Detection at 280 nm (Hg lamp & filter).

The compound is metabolized (Fig. 3; P.M. Osborne et al., unpublished observations) mainly to a glucuronide (94120-Met-I), a pyrazine (94120-Met-II) produced by gut microflora, and two further metabolites of this compound: the amine and the N-oxide (94120-Met-IV and -III respectively). SK&F 93880 (Fig. 3) is a postulated metabolite that has not as yet been identified in animal species.

As mentioned above, plasma samples thawed at room temperature were centrifuged at 2000 **g** for 10 min to remove fibrous material. An aliquot (100 μl) was then transferred to a 1.5 ml polypropylene centrifuge tube, to which were added, followed by vortex mixing, 100 μl water and 500 μl of internal standard solution. The latter contained 500 ng SK&F 94857, the N-propionyl homologue of SK&F 94120. The medium for spiked-in compounds was plasma.

The AASP C-18 cassette was activated by passing 1 ml methanol and then 1 ml water through each column. Then 300 μl of each sample was loaded, and air applied until the reservoir was empty. Then 1 ml water was applied, to remove residual plasma from the cartridge bed as well as any highly polar material adsorbed onto the column. The cassette was transferred from the manifold to the AASP for HPLC.

Fig. 4 shows typical chromatograms, for analytes eluted from the AASP extraction cartridges after spiking into control plasma. No endogenous compounds with retention times corresponding to either SK&F 94120 or the internal standard have been encountered in pre-dose or control samples from cynomolgus monkeys, rats, mice and dogs.

Metabolites II, III and IV can also be quantified by this procedure. A major metabolite of SK&F 94120 in rat, dog and monkey has been tentatively identified as a glucuronide conjugate (on the pyrazine oxygen). The applicability of this assay to measure this conjugate intact is under investigation.

Recovery.- SK&F 94120 and 94857 were recovered quantitatively over the range 0.5-10.0 µg/ml plasma, as shown by comparing peak areas for standards taken through the extraction procedure and for standards injected directly onto the HPLC column.

Precision and bias.- Replicate plasma samples containing known concentrations of SK&F 94120 were assayed over two separate days (n observations). For the above range, the following summarized results show excellent precision (expressed as C.V.) and bias (% error; *italicized entries*):-
- 0.5 µg/ml (n = 12): 3%, *-1%*
- 1.0 µg/ml (n = 6): <1%, *<-1%*
- 2.5 µg/ml (n = 6): 2%, *<-1%*
- 5.0 µg/ml (n = 6): 2%, *+1%*
- 7.5 µg/ml (n = 6): 2%, *<+1%*
- 10.0 µg/ml (n = 12): 2%, *<-1%*.

*Comparison with Bond Elut method.-*Employment of the AASP resulted in a 50% saving in sample preparation time, by virtue of the reduction in liquid sample handling, and also in a markedly improved precision: C.V. 2% for 0.1, 1 or 5 µg/ml dog plasma whereas Bond Elut (manual) gave 14%, 11% and 19% respectively.

However, the particular Bond Elut results with which the AASP results were compared were not typical. Although 80% of the drug is bound to the sorbent after plasma has been passed through the cartridge, elution with 250 µl of mobile phase recovers only 50% of the original amount of drug in the plasma. In contrast, most Bond Elut methods in the literature give >90% overall recoveries with good precision and accuracy (within 10%).

CONCLUDING COMMENTS

The major advantages of liquid-solid extraction sample preparation are those of speed and versatility over the more conventional method of liquid-liquid extraction. Although the technique is still in its infancy it is growing rapidly. This growth will be helped by two factors.- (i) Information and understanding of the mechanisms of isolation will be forthcoming, enabling more applications to be devised. (ii) The technique is relatively easy to automate (cf. art. by Pearce et al., #NC(C)-7, below,   describing the use of a Zymark robot to automate the off-line sample preparation stage of the AASP). This will, we hope, provide the impetus for manufacturers to develop fully automated systems based on liquid-solid extraction technology. The authors look forward to the day when the biological sample will be placed in an instrument for automated liquid-solid extraction and quantitative HPLC analysis. The role of the analyst will then be to set up and monitor the performance of the system and evaluate the data generated.

Acknowledgements

The authors are grateful to Mr. J.W. Kitteringham and to Dr. T. Walsgrove, Dept. of Synthetic and Isotope Chemistry, SK&F, The Frythe, for synthesis of authentic reference compounds.

References

1. Schill, G. (1978) *Separation Methods for Drugs and Related Organic Compounds*, Apotekarsocieteten, Stockholm, 182 pp.
2. Lee, R.M. & McDowall, R.D. (1983) *J. Chromatog. 275*, 377-385.
3. Coates, W.J., Eden, R.J., Emmett, J.C., Gristwood, R.W., Owen, D.A.A., Slater, R.A., Taylor, E.M. & Warrington, B.H. (1985) *Br. J. Pharmacol. 84*, 22P.

#C-3

APPLICABILITY OF HPLC CHIRAL STATIONARY PHASES TO PHARMACOKINETIC AND DISPOSITION STUDIES ON ENANTIOMERIC DRUGS

Irving W. Wainer*

Division of Drug Chemistry
U.S. Food and Drug Administration
200 C Street, Washington, DC 20204, U.S.A.

The scope of this article is evident from the section headings.
• *Resolution of enantiomeric drugs on HPLC chiral stationary phases (CSP's).* # *Resolution of enantiomers as diastereoisomers.* # *Resolution of enantiomers on CSP's.*
• *Commercially available CSP's.* # *Type I CSP's.* # *Type II CSP's.* # *Type III CSP's.* # *Type IV CSP's.*
• *Type I CSP's in pharmacological studies.* # *An overview.* # *Studies of the stereoselectivity of propranolol disposition and clearance.* # *Stereochemical aspects of the metabolism of ibuprofen.* # *Glutethimide metabolism in glutethimide-intoxicated patients.* # *Pharmacological studies of the stereoselective metabolism of polycyclic aromatic hydrocarbons.*
• *Pharmacokinetic applications using other CSP's.* # *An overview.* # *Determination of (R)- and (S)-disopyramide in human plasma.*
• *A look toward the future.*

The development of chiral stationary phases (CSP's) for use with HPLC provides the capabilities for the rapid and facile resolution of enantiomeric drugs. The separations are carried out on the enantiomers themselves rather than on diastereoisomeric derivatives, often without derivatization. The application of these CSP's to investigation of the pharmacokinetics and metabolism of the stereoisomers of optically active drugs is an important area of study, since the enantiomers often have different potencies, pharmacological actions, plasma-disposition kinetics and metabolic fates, and in some cases enantiomer interconversion occurs *in vivo*.

* Present address: St. Jude Children's Research Hospital, P.O. Box 318, Memphis, TN 38101.

Often a drug exhibits more than one of these properties. The
l-isomer of the β-adrenergic blocking agent propranolol is ~100 times
as potent as the *d*-isomer [1] and has a longer plasma half-life [2].
For the anticoagulant warfarin (**1**, Fig. 1) the (*R*)-(+)-enantiomer has
a 75% longer half-life than the (*S*)-(-)-isomer, whereas the (*S*)-(-)-
enantiomer is 3 times as active as the (*R*)-(+)-enantiomer [3]. The
metabolism of warfarin is also highly stereoselective and the enantiomers yield different metabolites [4]. The (*R*)-(+)-enantiomer is
reduced to the (*R*,*S*)-warfarin alcohol (**1a**, Fig. 1), whereas the
(*S*)-(-)-isomer is ring-hydroxylated to produce 7-hydroxy-(*S*)-warfarin
(**1b**, Fig. 1).

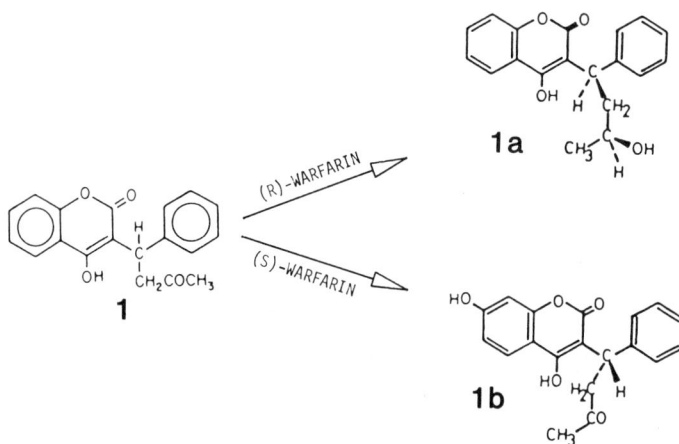

Fig. 1. Metabolism of warfarin enantiomers (**1**). See text for **1a**, **1b**.

The enantiomers of barbiturates and related compounds also have
different activities and/or metabolic pathways. The (*S*)-(+)-enantiomer
of hexabarbital, for example, has a greater hypnotic activity than the
(*R*)-(-)-isomer [5] and a higher brain/blood ratio, suggesting a stereoselective carrier mechanism [6]. Similar differences have been observed
in other enantiomeric barbiturates [7, 8]. Differences in metabolism
and disposition have also been detected for the enantiomers of phensuximide [9], mephenytoin [10] and glutethimide [11].

Another class of compounds which displays metabolic differences
between the enantiomers is the group of α-methylarylacetic acid anti-
inflammatory agents. For this series of optically active compounds,
the pharmacologically inactive (*R*)-(-)-isomers of ibuprofen, naproxen
and benoxaprofen have been shown to be converted *in vivo* into the
active (*S*)-(+)-enantiomers [12-14].

The development of safe and efficacious drugs requires a knowledge
of the pharmacological fate of both enantiomers of an optically active
molecule. The magnitude of this task is reflected by the fact that in

the U.S.A. in 1982, among frequently prescribed drugs 12 of the first 20
and 114 of the first 200 were optically active molecules [15].

RESOLUTION OF OPTICALLY ACTIVE DRUGS ON HPLC CSP's

Resolution of enantiomers as diastereoisomers

There are a number of approaches to the separation and analysis
of enantiomeric drug substances from body fluids. One of the most common
is the synthesis of diastererisomers by using an optically active
derivatizing agent.   There are, however, a number of significant
problems. One concerns the stereochemical purity of the derivatizing
agent, which should contain only one of the two possible enantiomers.
If it contains even a small amount of the other isomer, false determinations will result. An example is the work done in this laboratory
on the pharmacokinetics of the enantiomers of propranolol [16], where
(-)-*N*-trifluoroacetyl-1-prolyl chloride (TPC) was used as the derivatizing agent. The commercial TPC was found to be contaminated with
4-15% of the (+)-enantiomer and racemized rapidly during storage in
reagent form.

An additional complication is that enantiomers can have quite
different rates of reaction and/or equilibrium constants when they
react with another chiral molecule. As a result, the generation
of two diastereoisomeric products may occur in proportions different
from the starting enantiomeric composition.

Resolution of enantiomers on CSP's

Problems with diastereoisomer formation can be avoided by resolving the drug isomers as enantiomers using CSP's. The CSP and the
enantiomeric solutes form temporary diastereoisomeric complexes, which
differ in stability and hence are separable chromatographically. The
mode of action of CSP's needs to be considered in adopting this approach.
The initial theory of the mechanism of chiral resolution in a chromatographic system was developed by Dalgliesh [17] to explain the resolution of aromatic amino acids by paper (cellulose) chromatography.
The proposed model consisted of a '3-point' attachment between the
solute and CSP achieved through attractive interactions, which included hydrogen bonding and adsorption of the aromatic moiety. The
'3-point' interaction model has been widely used as the basis not only
for understanding the mechanism of chiral resolution but also for
designing new CSP's [18, 19]. However, chiral recognition models
based on only two interactions [20, 21] or just one [22-24] have
been proposed. Lochmuller & Souter [25] have even suggested that
an environmental chirality where there are no attachments could
distinguish between enantiomers.

In this article, where the term 'CSP' connotes HPLC, GC-CSP's
as used by Frank ([26] & #NC(C)-4, this vol.)   are not considered, nor

actual techniques for HPLC with CSP's as reviewed elsewhere [27-31].
The emphasis is on application of commercially available CSP's to
pharmacological problems.

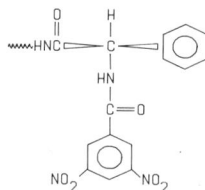

COMMERCIAL AVAILABLE CSP's

The first commercial CSP for HPLC was introduced by Pirkle
in 1981 [32].   As depicted above (in covalent form), it consists
of (R)-N-(3,5-dinitrobenzoyl)phenylglycine [denoted (R)-DNB-Øgly in
the listing below] attached, through an ionic bond, to an aminosilica
support.   By 1985 the number on the market had attained 19. Here
the chiral discriminating agents are listed with numbers assigned
(and CSP supplier stated*); they are based on four general mechanisms
(I-IV) for the formation of the solute-CSP complexes.-

        I. π-Complex and hydrogen bonding interactions:
1, (R)-DNB-Øgly, covalent binding to silica support (B, R); **2**, (R)-
DNB-Øgly, ionic binding (B, R); **3**, (S)-DNB-Øgly, covalent binding
(R); **4**, (S)-DNB-leucine, covalent (B, R);   **5**, (S)-DNB-leucine, ionic
binding (R); **6**, (R)-α-methylbenzyl urea (S).

        II. Inclusion complexes:
7-9, cellulose ester, with manufacturer's designations 'OA', 'OB',
'OK' (D); **10**, cellulose ether, 'OE' (D); **11**, cellulose carbamate,
'OC' (D); **12** & **13**, chiral polymethacrylate, 'OT' & 'OP' (D);   **14** &
15, β- and γ-cyclodextrin (A).

        III. Diastereoisomeric metal complexes:
16 & **17**, ligand exchange, 'WH' and 'WM' (D).

        IV. Protein complexes:
18, bovine serum albumin (AN); **19**, α_1-acid glycoprotein (L).

Type I CSP's

The mechanism of chiral resolution for Type I CSP's depends on
specific polar interactions with the solute.   These include   π-π
interactions between an aromatic moiety on the CSP (the 3,5-dinitro-
benzoyl group on CSP's 1-5, for example) and one on the solute, hydrogen
bonding interactions, amide dipole-dipole interactions and steric
interactions [18, 19, 27].

---

* *Abbreviations for suppliers* (U.S.A. except for L):   A, Advanced
Separation Technologies Inc., Whippany, NJ 07981; AN, Anspec. Co.,
Inc., Ann Arbor, MI 48107; B, Baker Chemical Co., Phillipsburg, NJ
08865; D, Daicel Chemical Ind., Ltd., New York, NY 10166-0130; L, LKB,
Bromma, Sweden; R, Regis Chemical Co., Morton Grove, IL 60053; S,
Supelco Inc., Bellefonta, PA 16823.

Type I CSP's can be used for a variety of compounds; however, the chiral analytes often have to be derivatized before chromatography. This is especially true for cationic drugs such as amines and for anionic drugs such as carboxylic acids [27]. Without derivatization the analyte often lacks the necessary interaction sites.

Another drawback of Type I columns is the fact that they function most satisfactorily with non-aqueous mobile phases. This precludes the direct injection of biological fluids and hinders the development of fully automated procedures.

Type II CSP's

The naturally occurring chiral polymer cellulose was one of the earliest liquid-chromatographic CSP's [17]. Since then a number of other polymers have been developed, chiefly based on derivatives of cellulose (CSP's 7-11) [33, 34] and on β- and γ-cyclodextrin (CSP's 14, 15) [30]. The latter are macrocyclic polymers formed by the action of *Bacillus macerous* amylase on starch [30]. A synthetic chiral polymer, (+)-poly(triphenylmethyl methacrylate), has also been used [35].

The mechanism proposed for these CSP's involves the entry of the enantiomers into chiral cavities present in the polymer. The difference in fit between the enantiomers, which affects the stability of the solute-CSP complexes, yields the observed resolution. This type of chromatographic chiral resolution has been termed 'inclusion chromatography' [36].

Type II CSP's can resolve a large variety of enantiomeric molecules and can be used with both aqueous and non-aqueous mobile phases. However, there are some limitations. The low column efficiencies lead to broad peaks that hinder their application to bioanalytical problems. In addition, although the separation of some underivatized cationic and anionic molecules has been reported for the cyclodextrin columns [30], some form of derivatization seems necessary for the cellulose CSP's [37]. (In art. #C-4, later in this vol., K.G. Feitsma & R.A. de Zeeuw discuss some attempted chiral separations with Type II CSP's.-*Ed.*)

Type III CSP's

Chiral ligand-exchange chromatography has been the subject of some recent reviews [29, 38, 39]. Separation depends on the formation of diastereoisomeric ternary complexes involving a transition metal (M), a single enantiomer of a chiral molecule (R_1, the selector-ligand) and the racemic chiral analyte (R_S and S_S, the selectand-ligands). The diastereoisomeric mixed chelate complexes formed in this system are represented thus: R_1-M-R_S and R_1-M-S_S. When these differ in stability, the less stable one is eluted first to achieve the desired separation.

The most common transition metal ion used in these separations is copper (II), and the selector-ligands are usually amino acids and, as for the chiral analytes, are limited to molecules that can form coordination complexes with transition metal ions. Ligand-exchange chromatography can be performed by using an achiral support (e.g. C-18) and adding all three components to the mobile phase. A more effective approach is to bind the selector-ligand to a silica support (CSP's 16 & 17), leaving just the metal ion and the analyte in the mobile phase; this gives better reproducibility as well as efficiency.

The Type III CSP's are most effective when amino acids and derivatives are the selectand-ligands. Their applicability to other classes of compounds is limited, although resolution has been achieved with carboxylic acids, amino alcohols (as Schiff bases), barbiturates, hydantoins and succinimides [29].

Type IV CSP's

One basis for the pharmacological differences between enantiomeric drugs is the stereoselective binding of the molecules to plasma proteins. Thus, Walle et al. [40] have demonstrated a difference in the binding of (+)- and (-)-propranolol to both human α_1-acid glycoprotein (AGP) and human serum albumin (HSA). Other serum albumins, including BSA, have also displayed enantioselective binding [41, 42].

These properties have been used to develop the Type IV CSP's, in which AGP or BSA is bound to a silica support. The AGP-CSP was developed by Hermansson [43], and the BSA-CSP by Allemark et al. [31, 44]. These CSP's appear to be very widely applicable; e.g. the AGP-ASP was used to resolve >40 commonly used enantiomeric cationic drugs without derivatization [45].

Because Type IV CSP's are effective for diverse underivatized analytes and are compatible with aqueous mobile phases, they are powerful analytical tools for pharmacological studies. However, they occasionally show low efficiency, which limits some applications.

TYPE I CSP's IN PHARMACOLOGICAL STUDIES

An overview

Although the ability to resolve enantiomeric drugs on CSP's has rapidly expanded, the transfer of this technology to pharmacological studies is only beginning, and has mostly been with the Type I CSP's due, in part, to these being the first on the market [32] and to the excellent quality control of the product. However, the key reason is the wide applicability of these phases.

The 28 drugs in the following list that have been resolved on these CSP's (Pirkle-type) were run with or without derivatization.-

Amphetamines, all run with a 'DNB' CSP, **1** in preceding list:
as amide derivative: amphetamine [refs. 46, 47]; *as carbamate:* amphetamine [48], methamphetamine [48], benzphetamine [48], methoxy-phenamine [48], p-hydroxyamphetamine [48].

Ephedrines, run with CSP **2** (1st entry) or **1** (other entries):
as oxazolidine: ephedrine [49]; *as carbamate:* ephedrine [48], pseudoephedrine [48]; *as oxazolidone:* norephedrine [50]; *as carbamate:* norephedrine [48], norpseudoephedrine [48].

β–Blocker, run with CSP **1:**
as oxazolidone: propranolol [51]; *as amide:* propranolol [32].

α–Methylaryl acetic acid anti–inflammatories, run with CSP **1:**
as amide: ibuprofen [52], naproxen [52], fenoprofen [52], benoxa-profen [52].

Tropic acid/amide, run with CSP **1:**
as amide: tropic acid [53]; *underivatized:* tropic amide [53].

Barbiturates, run with CSP **5** (2nd entry) or **4** (other entries):
underivatized: hexobarbital [54], mephobarbital [54], butabarbital [54], secobarbital [54].

Succinimides, run with CSP **2, 4** and **5** respectively:
underivatized: ethosuximide [54], methsuximide [54], phensuximide [54].

Hydantoin, run with CSP **4:**
underivatized: mephenytoin [54].

Benzodiazepinones, run with CSP **1,** alternatively **4** for 2nd entry:
underivatized: lorazepam [55], oxazepam [55].

Miscellaneous, run with CSP **5, 1** and **2** respectively:
underivatized: glutethimide [54], etodolac (an analgesic and anti-inflammatory agent) [56], oxygenated derivatives of polycyclic aromatic hydrocarbons (PAH's) [57, 58] – *not drugs; >100 run.*

The most useful derivatives for cationic amines such as amphet-amine and its analogues are naphthoyl amides [46] or carbamates [48], both formed by rapid and facile reactions in good yields; the added naphthyl chromophore aids HPLC detection of trace amounts. Already the naphthoylamide method has been used in determining the enantiomeric purity of amphetamine preparations [47].

Formation of oxazolidine or oxazolidone derivatives as cited above for ephedrines involves the use of an aromatic aldehyde and of phosgene respectively. The listed carbamate method is currently being applied to a pharmacokinetic study of norephedrine in rabbits, using a Type II CSP (a cellulose carbamate, CSP 11). Of the options listed for propranolol, an amino-alcohol, the oxazolidone approach has been applied in pharmacokinetic studies [51, 59], and should be applicable to other β-blockers.

Strongly anionic drugs such as carboxylic acids also need to be derivatized before running them on Type I CSP's. Besides the listed anti-inflammatories, which (similarly for tropic acid) may be resolved as their 2-naphthalenemethylamides, etodolac has been resolved after conversion into a methyl ester [56]. For ibuprofen there has been an application to equine blood [60].

As is evident from the list, Type I CSP's are applicable without derivatization to various drugs, mainly cyclic amides and imides including barbiturates, succinimides, benzodiazepinones, hydantoins and glutethimide [54, 55]. The application to oxygenated PAH's by Yang and co-workers, including stereoselective metabolism by rat liver microsomes, concerns benzo[a]pyrenes [57] and 7,12-dimethyl-benz[a]anthracene [58, 61].

Studies of the stereospecificity of propranolol disposition and clearance

For propranolol, marketed and administered as a racemic mixture, pharmacological studies have demonstrated stereochemical differences in potency [1] and plasma half-life [2]. For rapidly and accurately determining propranolol enantiomers in biological samples, Wainer et al. [51] used a Type I CSP after extraction and derivatization, as exemplified in Fig. 2. With a fluorescence detector, as little as 0.5 ng/ml of each enantiomer can be identified and quantitated. Fig. 3 shows a whole-blood time-concentration curve obtained in a human subject given 80 mg.

The analytical procedure can be adapted for large clinical studies and screenings. Thus, it was used in studying the effect of cimetidine on the oral clearance and metabolism of propranolol enantiomers [59]. Cimetidine decreased the oral clearance of d-propanolol more than that of l-propanolol (40.3 vs. 36.5%) and stereoselectively inhibited propranolol metabolism.

Stereochemical aspects of the metabolism of ibuprofen

Ibuprofen is widely used as a non-steroidal agent to relieve acute and chronic rheumatoid arthritis, and is also available as a non-prescription analgesic. It is notable that the (R)-(-)-enantiomer (therapeutically inactive) is converted in vivo into the active (S)-(+)-enantiomer; the reverse transformation does not occur [12]. In the initial pharmacokinetic and metabolic studies the enantiomers were derivatized to form diastereoisomeric amides and then separated by GC [12]. This method has inherent problems of a nature discussed in general terms above, including possible inaccuracies due to enantiomeric contamination of the derivatizing agent. To obviate these problems, Wainer & Doyle [52] developed an HPLC method for enantiomer resolution using a Type I CSP. The acids were converted to their benzyl- or 1-naphthalenemethylamides and resolved on the covalent form of the (R)-N-3,5-dinitrobenzoyl)phenylglycine CSP.

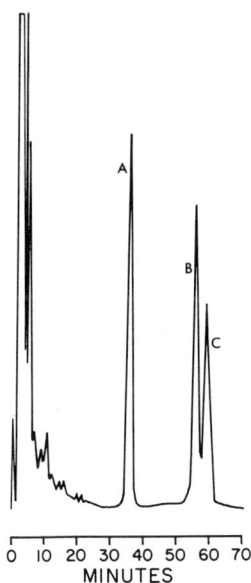

Fig. 2. Chromatogram of whole-blood extract from a subject 2.5 h after an 80 mg oral dose of *dl*-propranolol. A, *d*-meto-prolol (internal standard); B & C, *l*- and *d*-propranolol.

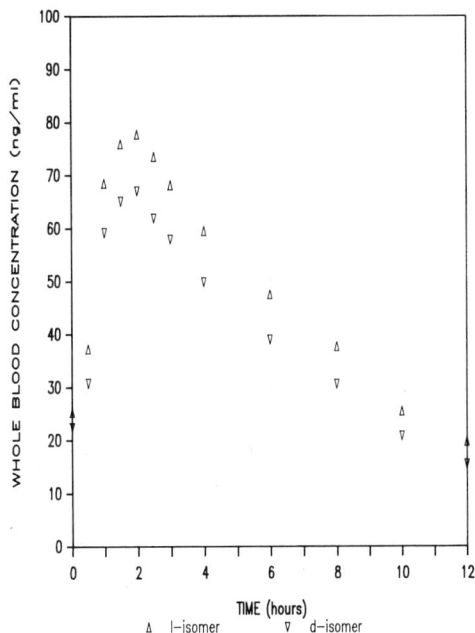

Fig. 3. Time-concentration curves for blood levels of propranolol administered as for Fig. 2. *Both Figs.:* initial ether extraction at pH 10, then phosgene; HPLC, 20°: hexane/2-propanol/acetonitrile.

Crowther et al. [60] analyzed urine from adult mares given 2 g of racemic ibuprofen orally. The analysis involved acidification of the urine, extraction with hexane/dichloromethane/diethyl ether (1:1:1 by vol.), concentration, and initial TLC separation on a silica gel plate. The ibuprofen extracted from the scraped-off area that contained it was derivatized and analyzed by HPLC with a Type I CSP. Thereby it was demonstrated that in horses, as in man [62], urine taken during 2 h after the dose contained predominantly the (S)-(+) drug enantiomer.

A variant of the Type I CSP approach is to couple the column to a mass spectrometer (CSP-LC/MS), allowing both detection of the chiral analyte at low concentrations and structural identifications. Resolution and identification by use of this system have been performed with the benzylamide of ibuprofen, as shown in Fig. 4 for equine urine (see above) and authentic racemate, and also with the 1-naphthalene-methylamides of fenoprofen and benoxaprofen and the 1-naphthoylamide of amphetamine [60]. For the positive-ion CI-MS, the reagent gas was the eluate (2% fed in), viz. hexane with a small admixture of 2-pro-panol. The MS detection obviated endogenous interferences.

A

296

M/Z

TI

B

296

M/Z

TI

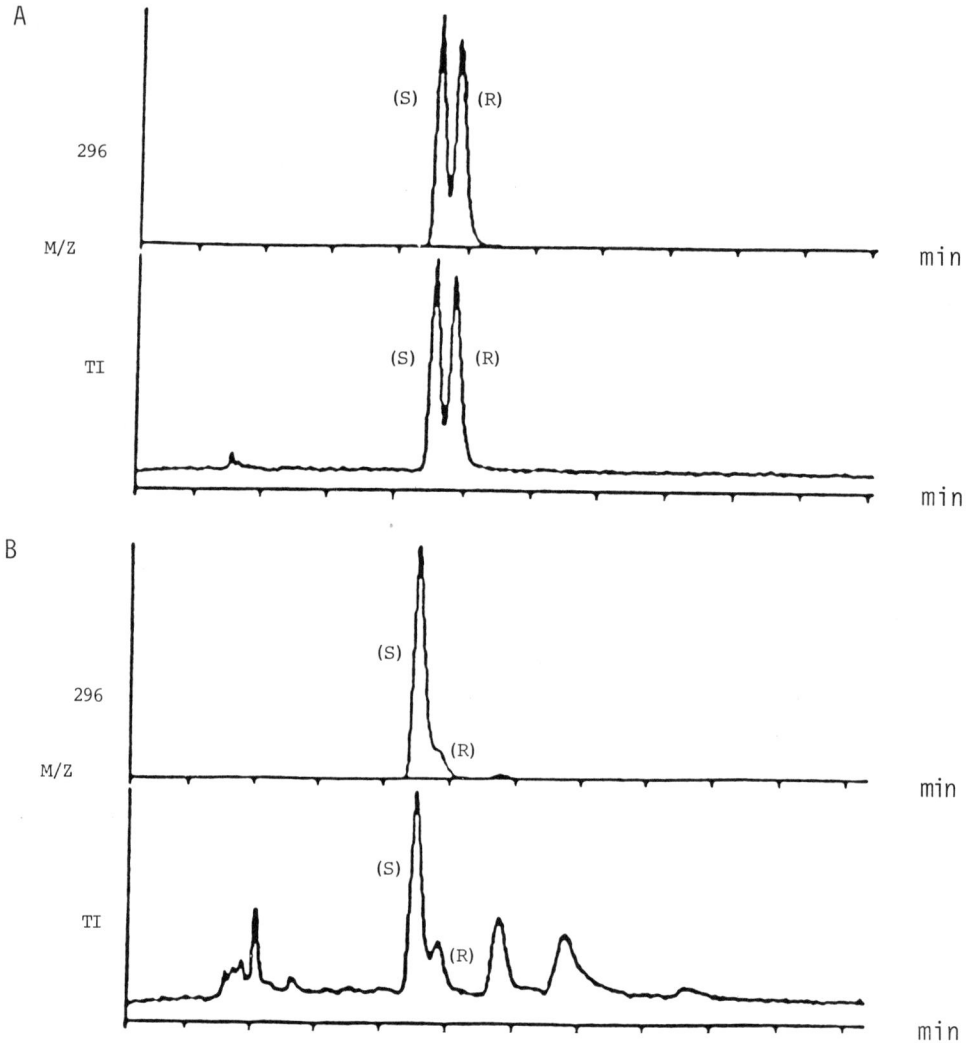

Fig. 4. CSP-LC/MS, with monitoring of m/z 296 and of total ion current (TI), of: A, authentic (R,S)-ibuprofen benzylamide mixture; B, the benzylamide prepared from TLC-isolated material from an extract of equine urine collected 2 h following ibuprofen administration. *From ref. [60]©, courtesy of AmericanChemical Society.*

Glutethimide metabolism in glutethimide-intoxicated patients

Glutethimide, a non-barbiturate sedative, has caused numerous toxic reactions in humans; its metabolism plays an important role in its morbidity and mortality. 4-Hydroxyglutethimide, a metabolite which possesses marked sedative hypnotic activity, is known to accumulate in the plasma of drug-intoxicated humans [63]; it was shown in initial metabolic studies to arise from a stereoselective metabolic process in which the (R)-enantiomer of the drug is converted to this metabolite to a greater extent than the (S)-enantiomer [64]. Hydroxylation of the ethyl moiety of the molecule is also stereospecific [64]. The metabolite (1-hydroxyethyl)glutethimide is derived primarily from (S)-glutethimide, whereas iso-(1-hydroxyethyl)glutethimide comes almost exclusively from (R)-glutethimide.

The method of Yang et al. [54] for resolving glutethimide on a Type I CSP has now been adapted for blood and urine (I.W. Wainer & M.C. Alembik). The enantiomers of both glutethimide and 4-hydroxyglutethi-mide can be resolved at levels as low as 1.25 µg/ml by this gradient-elution procedure, which is now being used to screen samples from glutethimide-intoxicated patients.

Pharmacological studies of the stereoselective metabolism of PAH's

Stereoselective oxygenation of PAH's by microsomal enzymes gives optically active intermediates [62], often with enantiomer differences in mutagenicity and carcinogenicity [63]. Yang & Fu [e.g. 61], in microsomal studies with PAH's as mentioned above, isolated the meta-bolites and, without derivatization, determined enantiomeric composi-tions using CSP 2 ('DNB' moiety, ionic form). Having shown that the major enantiomers of *trans*-dihydrodiols from 7-bromobenz[a]anthra-cene were stereochemically R,R, they investigated the *trans*-5,6-dihydrodiols formed in the metabolism of 7,12-dimethylbenz[a]anthra-cene by microsomes from untreated, 3-methylcholanthrene-treated and phenobarbital-treated rats: the R,R/S,S enantiomeric ratios were respectively 11:89, 6:94 and 5:95 [61]. The 12-methyl group in this PAH thus seems to play an important role in determining the stereo-selective metabolism at the K-region 5,6-double bond, and the stereo-selectivity seems to depend on the type of substrate metabolized rather than on the precise nature of the metabolizing enzyme system.

PHARMACOKINETIC APPLICATIONS USING CSP's OTHER THAN TYPE I

An overview

In contrast to Type I CSP's, Type II–IV CSP's are just beginning to be applied to pharmacological studies, partly because they have only recently become commercially available. Their use is likely to increase rapidly in the next few years. The recently introduced AGP phase due to Hermansson [43] is particularly promising; it has already shown broad applicability to cationic drugs [45]. An initial study with this CSP is now considered.

Determination of (R)- and (S)-disopyramide in human plasma

Although the (R)- and (S)-enantiomers of disopyramide are equi-potent as antiarrhythmic agents [65], the (S)-isomer is 3-4 times as

Fig. 5. Separation of (R)-
disopyramide (peak 1) and
(S)-disopyramide (peak 2)
isolated from human plasma.
A: Blank plasma, with the
retention times indicated
by *arrows*. B: Blank plasma
spiked with racemic disopyramide (1.5 µg/ml).
C: plasma sample from a
patient obtained 1 h after
administering racemic disopyramide. Not marked: mono-
despropylpyramide, a metabolite whose (S)-isomer
would have coincided with
(R)-disopyramide; hence use
of a RP-2 pre-column, with
some band-broadening as
a penalty. Mobile phase:
pH 6.2 phosphate buffer
with 4.3% v/v 2-propanol and
1.95 mM **N,N**-dimethyloctyl-
amine. **Main separation on**
an AGP CSP; 254 nm detector.
From [68], by permission.

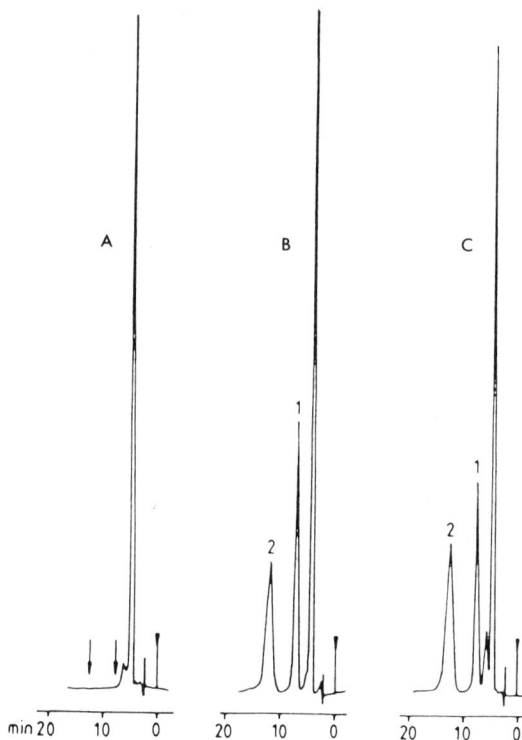

potent as an anticholinergic agent [66]. Differences in the plasma
disposition of the two isomers have also been observed in dogs [67].

A study by Hermansson & Eriksson [68] of these stereochemical
differences in humans was based on the direct resolution and quantitation of (R)- and (S)-disopyramide on an AGP CSP (Type IV). The
column was coupled in series with an RP-2 column serving as a pre-
column. The method was able to detect each enantiomer at concentrations <15 ng/ml, and results for the racemic drug in plasma were
reproducible over the range 3.0 to 1 µg/ml. Fig. 5 shows chromatograms
from spiked plasma and from a patient 1 h after drug administration.
The free plasma concentration of (S)-disopyramide exceeded by ~100%
(peak area basis) that of the (R)-isomer. This is relevant to the
possible advantage of administering only the (R)-isomer to minimize
unwanted anticholinergic effects.

A look toward the future

The rapid development of CSP's for HPLC has now made possible
the determination of the enantiomeric composition of most drug substances. Hence routine determination of the pharmacokinetics and
metabolism of each isomer is in sight. Soon the CSP's now available and

those due to be marketed will be regarded as standard HPLC items comparable to today's RP- and NP-columns; they will be found in every analytical and pharmacological laboratory. CSP's are all the more likely to come into their own when integrated with automated systems and [cf. 68] coupled-column technology. With such advances, large-scale screening will be practicable and will be accompanied by pharmacological investigations of the stereochemical aspects of efficacy and toxicity. It is possible that unknown properties of many common pharmaceuticals will be discovered and that the development of new drug substances will be immeasurably aided.

Acknowledgements

I acknowledge the help of Dr. T.D. Doyle and my co-workers at the Food and Drug Administration in preparing the manuscript and especially Ms. Alice Marcotte for her invaluable editorial assistance.

References

1. Barrett, A.M. & Cullum, V.A. (1968) *Br. J. Pharmacol. 34*, 43-55.
2. Kawashima, K., Levy, A. & Spector, S. (1976) *J. Pharmacol. Exp. Ther. 196*, 517-523.
3. O'Reilly, R.A. (1974) *Clin. Pharmacol. Ther. 16*, 348-354.
4. Lewis, R.J., Trager, W.F., Chan, K.K., Breckenridge, A., Orme, M., Rowland, M. & Schary, W. (1974) *J. Clin. Invest. 53*, 1607-1617.
5. Wahlstrom, G. (1966) *Life Sci. 5*, 1781-1790.
6. Rummel, W., Bradenburger, U. & Buch, H. (1967) *Med. Pharmacol. Exp. 16*, 496-504.
7. Wahlstrom, G. (1968) *Acta Pharmacol. Toxicol. 26*, 81-91.
8. Buch, H., Buzello, W., Nueroh, O. & Rummel, W. (1968) *Biochem. Pharmacol. 17*, 2391-2398.
9. Dudley, K.H., Bius, D.L. & Grace, M.E. (1972) *J. Pharmacol. Exp. Ther. 180*, 167-179.
10. Kupfer, A. & Bircher, J. (1979) *J. Pharmacol. Exp. Ther. 209*, 190-195.
11. Kennedy, K.A. & Fisher, L.J. (1979) *Drug Metab. Dispos. 7*, 319-324.
12. Kaiser, D.G., Vangiessen, G.J., Resicher, R.J. & Wechter, W.J. (1976) *J. Pharm. Sci. 65*, 269-273.
13. Goto, J., Goto, N. & Nambara, T. (1982) *J. Chromatog. 239*, 559-564.
14. Bopp, R.J., Nash, J.F., Ridolfo, A.S. & Shepard, E.R. (1979) *Drug Metab. Dispos. 7*, 356-359.
15. Anon (1983) *Pharmacy Times, April*, p. 25.
16. Silber, B. & Riegelman, S. (1980) *J. Pharmacol. Exp. Ther. 215*, 643-648.
17. Dalgliesh, C.E. (1952) *J. Chem. Soc. 137*, 3940-3942.
18. Pirkle, W.H., Hyun, M.H. & Bank, B. (1984) *J. Chromatog. 316*, 585-604.

19. Pirkle, W.H., Hyun, M.H., Tsipouras, A., Hamper, B.C. &
    Bank, B. (1984) *J. Pharm. Biomed. Anal. 2*, 173-181.
20. Lochmuller, C.H. & Ryall, R.R. (1978) *J. Chromatog. 150*,   511-
    514.
21. Dobashi, A. & Hara, S. (1983) *J. Chromatog. 267*, 11-17.
22. Lochmuller, C.H., Harris, J.M. & Souter, R.W. (1972) *J.
    Chromatog. 71*, 405-413.
23. Wainer, I.W. & Alembik, M.C. (1986) paper submitted to *J.
    Chromatog.*
24. Wainer, I.W., Doyle, T.D., Fry, F.S., Jr. & Hamidzadeh, Z. (1986)
    J. Chromatog. 355, 149-156.
25. Lochmuller, C.H. & Souter, R.W. (1973) *J. Chromatog. 113*, 283-
    303.
26. Frank, H., Thiel, D. & Langer, K. (1984) *J. Chromatog. 309*,
    261-267.
27. Wainer, I.W. & Doyle, T.D. (1984) *LC Liq. Chromatog. HPLC Mag.
    2*, 88-98.
28. Pirkle, W.H. & Finn, J.M. (1983)   *Asymmetric Synthesis*, Vol. 1
    (Morrison, J.D., ed.), Academic Press, New York, pp. 87-123.
29. Lindner, W. & Pettersson, K. (1985) in *Liquid Chromatography
    in Pharmaceutical Development: An Introduction* (Wainer, I.W.,
    ed.), Aster Publ. Corp., Springfield, OR, pp. 63-131.
30. Armstrong, D.W. (1984) *J. Liq. Chromatog. 7*, 353-376.
31. Allenmark, S. (1985) *LC Liq. Chromatog. HPLC Mag. 3*, 348-353.
32. Pirkle, W.H., Finn, J.M., Schreiner, J.L. & Hamper, B.C. (1981)
    J. Am. Chem. Soc. 103, 3964-3966.
33. Okamoto, Y., Kawashima, K. & Hatada, K. (1984) *J. Am. Chem. Soc.
    106*, 5357-5359.
34. Ichida, A., Shibata, T., Okamoto, I., Yuki, Y., Namikoshi, H. &
    Toga, Y. (1985) *Chromatographia 19*, 280-284.
35. Okamoto, Y., Honda, S., Okamoto, I. & Yuki, H. (1981) *J. Am.
    Chem. Soc. 103*, 6971-6973.
36. Hesse, G. & Hagel, R. (1973) *Chromatographia 6*, 277-280.
37. *Enclosure* (1985) with Chiralpak and Chiralcel columns, Daicel
    Inc., 611 W. 6th St., Suite 2152, Los Angeles, CA 90017-3191.
38. Davankov, V., Kurganov, A. & Bochkov, A. (1983) *Adv. Chromatog.
    22*, 71-93.
39. Lindner, W. (1982) in *Chemical Derivatization in Analytical
    Chemistry*, Vol.2 (Lawrence, J.F. & Frei, R.W., eds.), Plenum,
    New York, pp. 145-190 (Chap. 4).
40. Walle, A., Walle, T., Bal, S.A. & Olanoff, L.S. (1983) *Clin.
    Pharmacol. Ther. 34*, 718-723.
41. Alebic-Kolbac, T., Rendic, S., Fuks, Z., Sunjic, V. & Kajez, F.
    (1979) *Acta Pharm. Jugosl. 29*, 53-70.
42. Allenmark, S. (1982) *Chem. Scr. 20*, 5-10.
43. Hermansson, J. (1983) *J. Chromatog. 269*, 71-80.
44. Allenmark, S., Bomgren, B. & Boren, H. (1983) *J. Chromatog. 264*,
    63-68.
45. Schill, G., Wainer, I.W. & Barkan. S.A. (1986) *J. Liq.
    Chromatog.*, in press.

46. Wainer, I.W. & Doyle, T.D. (1983) *J. Chromatog. 259*, 465-472.

47. Wainer, I.W., Doyle, T.D. & Adams, H.M. (1984) *J. Pharm. Sci. 73*, 1162-1164.

48. Doyle, T.D., Adams, W.M., Fry, F.S., Jr. & Wainer, I.W. (1986) *J. Liq. Chromatog.*, in press.

49. Wainer, I.W., Doyle, T.D., Hamidzadeh, Z. & Aldridge, M. (1983) *J. Chromatog. 261*, 123-126.

50. Wainer, I.W., Doyle, T.D., Hamidzadeh, Z. & Aldridge, M. (1983) *J. Chromatog. 268*, 107-111.

51. Wainer, I.W., Doyle, T.D., Donn, K.H. & Powell, J.R. (1984) *J. Chromatog. 306*, 405-411.

52. Wainer, I.W. & Doyle, T.D. (1984) *J. Chromatog. 284*, 117-124.

53. Wainer, I.W., Doyle, T.D. & Breder, C.D. (1984) *J. Liq. Chromatog. 7*, 731-741.

54. Yang, Z-Y., Barkan, S.A., Brunner, C., Weber, J.D., Doyle, T.D. & Wainer, I.W. (1985) *J. Chromatog. 324*, 444-449.

55. Pirkle, W.H. & Tsipouras, A. (1984) *J. Chromatog. 291*, 291-298.

56. Demerson, C.A., Humber, L.G., Abraham, N.A., Schilling, G., Martel, R.R. & Pace-Asciak, C. (1983) *J. Med. Chem. 26*, 1778-1780.

57. Yang, S.K., Weems, H.B. & Mushtaq, M. (1984) *J. Chromatog. 316*, 569-584.

58. Yang, S.K. & Weems, H.B. (1984) *Anal. Chem. 56*, 2658-2662.

59. Donn, K.H., Powell, J.R. & Wainer, I.W. (1985) *Clin. Pharmacol. Ther. 37*, 191.

60. Crowther, J.B., Covey, T.R., Dewey, E.H. & Henion, J.D. (1984) *Anal. Chem. 56*, 2921-2926.

61. Yang, S.K. & Fu, P.P. (1984) *Biochem. J. 223*, 775-782.

62. Brooks, C.J.W. & Gilbert, M.T. (1974) *J. Chromatog. 99*, 541-551.

63. Hansen, A.R., Kennedy, K.A., Ambre, J.T. & Fisher, L.J. (1975) *N. Engl. J. Med. 292*, 250-252.

64. Kennedy, K.A. & Fisher, L.J. (1974) *Drug Metab. Dispos. 7*, 319-324.

65. Burke, T.R., Jr., Nelson, W.L., Mangion, M., Hite, G.J., Mokler, C.M. & Ruenitz, P.C. (1980) *J. Med. Chem. 23*, 1044-1048.

66. Giacomini, K.M., Cox, B.M. & Blaschke, T.F. (1980) *Life Sci. 27*, 1191-1197.

67. Giacomini, K.M., Giacomini, J.C., Swezey, S.E., Harrison, D.C., Nelson, W.L., Burke, T.R. Jr., & Blaschke, T.F. (1980) *J. Cardiovasc. Pharmacol. 2*, 825-832.

68. Hermansson, J. & Eriksson, M. (1984) *J. Chromatog. 336*, 321-328.

#C-4

ATTEMPTS TO OBTAIN SEPARATIONS OF CHIRAL ANTICHOLINERGIC DRUGS

Karla G. Feitsma, Ben F.H. Drenth, Kor H. Kooi,
Jan Bosman and Rokus A. de Zeeuw

Department of Analytical Chemistry and Toxicology
State University, A. Deusinglaan 2
9713 AW Groningen, The Netherlands

Where a drug has enantiomeric forms, each should be measurable in the same sample, as now investigated with oxyphenonium and some quaternary atropine analogues. Resolution was attempted with a chiral-HPLC system, containing d-camphorsulphonic acid as a mobile phase component or (cf. W.H. Pirkle's work) with chiral stationary phases. Neither approach was successful, due to the relatively long distance between the chiral centre and the quaternized nitrogen.

We therefore tried to resolve the optical antipodes of the acid parts of the cholinergics (easily obtained by hydrolysis). An HPLC system having β-cyclodextrin as the chiral stationary phase was chosen. Using aqueous mobile phases, cyclohexylphenylglycollic acid (the acid moiety in oxyphenonium), cyclohexylphenylacetic acid and mandelic acid (e.g. in homatropine) were resolved. However, tropic acid could not be separated into enantiomers with this system. Consideration is given to the influence of temperature and sample concentration on selectivity and resolution and to difficulties in quantitative analysis.

Stereoselectivity has always been an interesting phenomenon in the field of pharmacology. Due to advances in analytical and organic chemistry we now have the ability to obtain a better insight into this area. Stereochemical principles can contribute to our under-standing of the pharmacological actions of drugs, and may strengthen the basis for preparing drugs that have a profile of activities specifically directed to the desired therapeutic effect. Many commonly used drugs have one or more asymmetric centres, but generally only the racemic mixtures are available. However, the desired acti-vity is often limited to one enantiomer. The co-administration of

therapeutically less active or inactive enantiomers may influence
the profile of action as compared to that of the therapeutically
active enantiomer alone.   Moreover, it is undesirable to dose with
xenobiotics that are not only virtually inactive but can even cause
toxic reactions.

As early as 1904 a study was published concerning the action of
the optical isomers of atropine [1]. For a number of anticholinergics
different parasymphaticolytic activities for l- and d-forms were reported by Ellenbroek et al. [2] and Barlow et al. [3]. Preliminary
results recently published [4] show different excretion rates for
l- and d-oxyphenonium, a potent anticholinergic compound that has
been on the market for 35 years.

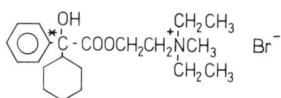

$$\text{C-COOCH}_2\text{CH}_2\overset{+}{\text{N}}\text{CH}_3 \quad \text{Br}^-$$

oxyphenonium bromide

For evaluation of the events in living systems after administration of such drugs, assays are required that allow the determination
of the two enantiomers separately in the same sample. This article
concerns attempts to fulfil this aim for certain anticholinergics,
in particular oxyphenonium, by chiral HPLC especially.

EXPERIMENTAL

Chemicals.- Acetonitrile, methanol, H_3PO_4 (85% w/v), $K_2HPO_4.3H_2O$
and KH_2PO_4 were of analytical grade (E. Merck, Darmstadt).   Tropic
acid was the synthetic grade (Merck).   Racemic cyclohexylphenylglycollic acid (CHPGA) was a gift from Ciba-Geigy, Basel.   Cyclohexylphenylacetic acid (CHPAA) and mandelic acid (Janssen, Beerse, Belgium)
were used as received. Enantiomers of CHPGA were obtained by crystalli-
zation from the racemic acid [4].

For the synthesis of the HPLC stationary phase we used 5 μm
Lichrosorb Si60 (Merck) and *N*-[3-trimethoxysilyl]-propylethylene-
diamine, technical grade (Janssen).   β-Cyclodextrin was gifted by
Avebe (Veendam, The Netherlands).

Apparatus.- HPLC was performed with a Waters M45 solvent delivery
system or a Perkin-Elmer Series 10 pump, a Rheodyne 7125 sample injector
with a 20 μl loop, a Spectra-Physics 770 UV-detector operating at
205 nm, and an RDK B-161 recorder or a Kipp BD40 recorder.

Chromatographic conditions.- The chiral stationary phase containing β-cyclodextrin was synthesized according to Fujimura [5].
Silanol groups on the silica were derivatized [cf. J. Smith, A-3,
this vol.] with $(CH_3O)_3-Si-(CH_2)_3-NH-CH_2-CH_2-NH_2$ and the product was

coupled to the β-cyclodextrin. The columns, 175 or 250 mm ×4.6 mm i.d., were packed by a balanced density slurry method [6], and were thermostatted during runs by water circulating in a jacket. Mobile phases were mixtures of 0.1 M K phosphate buffer, acetonitrile and methanol. The flow rate was 1 ml/min.

RESULTS AND DISCUSSION

Petterson & Schill [7] separated enantiomeric amines by ion-pair chromatography using d-camphorsulphonic acid as a chiral counter-ion. Oxyphenonium, being a quaternary compound, was expected to form ion pairs with this chiral acid likewise. We failed to resolve racemic oxyphenonium using such a system (Nucleosil 5 CN column; hexane & halocarbons in mobile phase). Petterson likewise was unsuccessful in resolving the enantiomers of atropine using this system. This lack of separation may be due to the relatively long distance between the amine group and the chiral centre with its hydroxyl group, possibly preventing adequate ion-pair formation.

Another approach to separating enantiomers is the use of chiral stationary phases as described by Pirkle [8, 9]. Two phases, having (R)-dinitrobenzoylphenylglycine covalently or ionically bonded to silica gel, were synthesized. Bisnaphthol, a test compound, was separated quite well using these stationary phases and non-polar mobile phases; but neither oxyphenonium nor atropine could be resolved into their enantiomers. Here too, the distance between the chiral centre and the nitrogen may be unsuitable. A possibly more important factor is that the nitrogen in oxyphenonium and/or atropine may be too polar for effective interaction with these chiral phases, which so far have proved useful only for less polar compounds.

From these results, we concluded that another approach to the problem had to be adopted. We decided to try to separate the enantiomers of the acid part of oxyphenonium, cyclohexylphenylglycollic acid (CHPGA), which can be obtained very rapidly by acid hydrolysis. Some other aromatic carboxylic acids with similar structures and likewise related to anticholinergics were investigated too.

The potentialities of cyclodextrins for separating optical antipodes have long been known [10], but exploitation of this feature started only a few years ago, when cyclodextrins became available in quantity. β-Cyclodextrin has been used as a mobile-phase component in HPLC for the resolution of racemates (mandelic acid derivatives [11], 1-([2-(3-hydroxyphenyl)-1-phenylethyl]-4-(3-methyl-2-butenyl)-piperazine [12]). Fujimura et al. [5] used a covalently bonded β-cyclodextrin stationary phase in order to separate aromatic compounds not posessing optical activity, especially benzene derivatives, by HPLC. We felt that a combination of these principles might enable racemates to be separated by HPLC on a chiral stationary phase containing β-cyclodextrin. Advantages of a bonded β-cyclodextrin phase, as compared to a mobile phase containing this compound, are the easier isolation of the enantiomers without contamination by cyclodextrin in the eluate, and reduced consumption of the cyclodextrin which may be regarded as somewhat expensive.

Preliminary results with this chiral stationary phase demonstrated the feasibility of separating the enantiomers of some aromatic acids [13].

Compound structure and mobile-phase composition

The aromatic acids investigated were CHPGA, CHPAA, mandelic acid (acid moiety of homatropine) and tropic acid (e.g. contained in atropine, methylatropine and scopolamine).

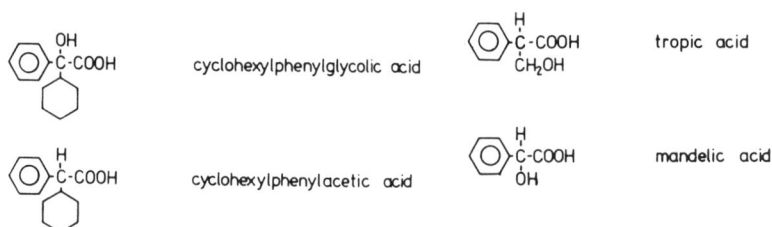

cyclohexylphenylglycolic acid

tropic acid

cyclohexylphenylacetic acid

mandelic acid

Fig. 1a illustrates some chromatograms obtained with our β-cyclo-dextrin-bonded stationary phase and an aqueous mobile phase. CHPGA and CHPAA can be separated into enantiomers with this system, whereas mandelic acid has a very small selectivity factor. Tropic acid is not separated at all. Obviously, the molecular structure determines the feasibility of resolving a racemate. The interaction of a compound with cyclodextrin is an inclusion process: β-cyclodextrin consists of a hydrophobic cavity and a hydrophilic exterior, hydroxy groups being on the rim of the cavity. The observation of enantioselectivity was explained by Hinze [14], in terms of the 'three-point attachment concept' [15].

CHPGA and CHPAA, both having a cyclohexyl group at the chiral centre, gave good separations, and we assume that this ring structure fits well into the cavity of the cyclodextrin molecule. There remain various possibilities for hydrogen bonding at the rim of the cavity. The phenyl group is somewhat smaller than the cyclohexyl group, which may result in a less tight fit with the cyclodextrin cavity. This can explain the lack of separation of tropic acid and the very slight separation of mandelic acid.

The influence of pH is demonstrated in Figs. 1a and 1b. The slight separation of mandelic acid obtained at pH 4.2 disappeared at pH 6.5. For CHPGA retention times were longer at pH 4.2, and for CHPAA they were longer at pH 6.5. These phenomena are difficult

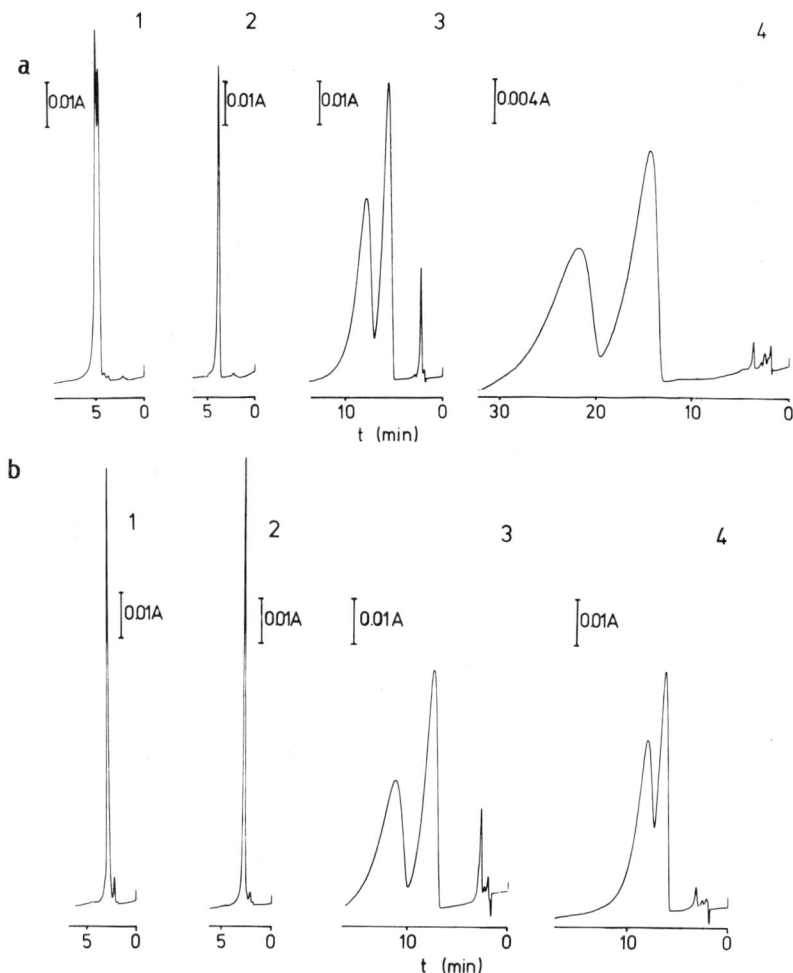

Fig. 1. Influence of pH on separation of the optical antipodes of aromatic acids: **a**, pH 4.2; **b**, pH 6.5;   1, mandelic acid (0.6 and 0.3 µg respectively); 2, tropic acid (0.3 µg load in each); 3, CHPAA (3 µg); 4, CHPGA (3 µg). Column, 175×4.6 mm; mobile phase, acetonitrile/phosphate buffer, 0.1 M (35:65 by vol.).

to explain. We may hypothesize that differences in dissociation that occur at pH 4.2 and pH 6.5 result in other modes of hydrogen bonding at the rim of the cavity, thus giving stronger interactions for mandelic acid and CHPGA at pH 4.2, but reduced interactions for CHPAA.

As alternatives to phosphate buffer we tried an acetate buffer, a $NaNO_3$ solution of comparable ionic strength, and water. These

variations resulted in very long retention times, and in some cases
the test compounds were not eluted at all. Tanaka et al. [16] observed
related phenomena. For the elution of aminobenzoic and nitrobenzoic
acids on β-cyclodextrin-bonded stationary phases they had to use
mixtures of methanol and phosphate buffer instead of methanol and
water. It is likely that this phenomenon is caused by masking of
underivatized silanol groups or —NH— groups of the spacer arm by phosphate ions. The findings described above make clear that the use of
phosphate buffer has a marked influence on the capacity factors of
these acids.

Recently Hinze and co-workers [14] published results achieved
with a new, commercially available β-cyclodextrin column (Cyclobond,
Astec), the cyclodextrin being bonded to silica through a spacer arm
that lacks nitrogen. When using a mobile phase without phosphate
buffer, these authors obtained reasonably small capacity factors.
This different behaviour could be explained by differences in synthesis and structure of the stationary phase material.

Since our main concern is with CHPGA, as the acid moiety of
oxyphenonium, we applied a modified simplex procedure [17] to obtain
the optimum mobile phase composition for separating the enantiomers
of this acid. Three variables were investigated: acetonitrile concentration, methanol concentration, and pH. This led to the following
optimum mobile-phase composition (v/v): 62.5% 0.1 M phosphate buffer
pH 4.2; 31.5% acetonitrile; 6.0% methanol. Further experiments were
done with this eluent.

Influence of temperature

With the above system we still observed a severe tailing. This
may be explained by the presence of non-derivatized silanol groups
on the silica gel and/or the presence of an amine function in the
spacer arm. However, another phenomenon can result in severe tailing
as well: slow mass transfer. We anticipated that tailing could be
reduced by increasing the temperature. Higher temperatures resulted
in shorter retention times, which is consistent with the observation
that the stability of various inclusion complexes in solution decreases
significantly as the temperature increases [18]. Fig. 2 shows the
dependence of retention time on column temperature. When ln k'
was plotted against the reciprocal of temperature, a straight line
resulted (r = 0.999), suggesting a linear relationship between ln k'
and $1/T$. This is explicable in terms of a thermodynamic approach to
liquid chromatography [19].

The influence on the separation factor ($\alpha = k'_1/k'_d$) is graphically
presented in Fig. 3. The factor α decreases with increasing temperature. However, the resolution defined as $Rs = (t_{R,1} - t_{R,d})/2(\sigma_1 + \sigma_d)$
[σ = S.D. of the eluite zone] was found to increase with temperature.

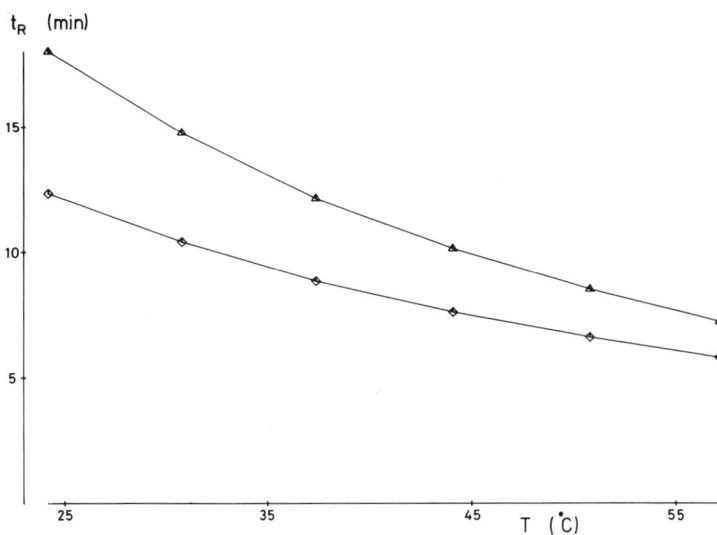

Fig. 2. Relation between retention time and column temperature for CHPGA. Load 3 µg (l, Δ; d, ◇). See below for conditions.

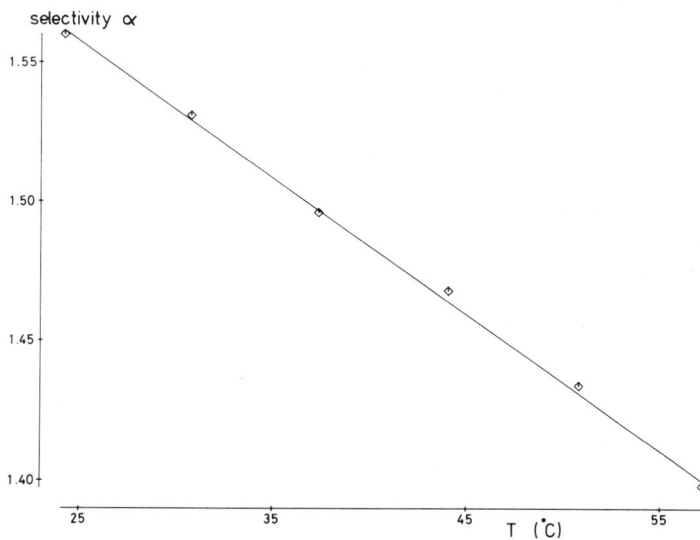

Fig. 3. Relation between selectivity and column temperature for enantiomers of CHPGA.
Applicable to both Figs.: column 175×4.6 mm; mobile phase: acetonitrile/methanol/K phosphate buffer (0.1 M) pH 4.2, 31.5:6.0:62.5 by vol.

We concluded that it is preferable to work at an elevated temperature. However, above 50° the stationary phase began to decompose as evidenced by a yellow colour of the column eluate. We therefore decided to do further work with this column at temperatures just below 50°. In Fig. 4, chromatograms at two different temperatures are shown.

Relation between sample concentration and retention

In preliminary studies we observed that retention time varied with the analyte concentration in the injected sample. To look into this phenomenon in more detail, different amounts of l- and/or d-CHPGA were injected into the system. Fig. 5 shows the dependence of retention times on concentration for samples having a 1:3 ratio of the enantiomers. Similar behaviour was seen with different ratios or on injecting only one enantiomer.

In the body of HPLC theory, attention has been paid to the dependence of retention time on the concentration in the sample. In the ideal case a linear isotherm is observed, the retention being independent of sample concentration. Variations of retention time with changes in injected sample amounts are explained by the occurrence of non-linear distribution curves. A convex isotherm causes a decreasing retention with increasing concentration in the sample, and a concave isotherm results in increasing retention with decreasing concentration; in both cases, retention should be nearly constant at low sample concentrations [20]. However, the occurrence of very long retention times at low sample concentrations cannot be explained by this theory. One can postulate irreversible adsorption of small amounts of analyte; but if this were true, the phenomenon should disappear after some injections of large amounts of sample - which was not the case. On the other hand, if competitive, reversible processes were involved one would anticipate that a large excess of the slower moving l-CHPGA would diminish the retention of small amounts of d-CHPGA. However, this was not observed when a 9:1 mixture of l- and d-CHPGA was used. An explanation of these phenomena is still lacking.

Quantitative evaluation

We had especial interest in the feasibility of analyzing the enantiomers side-by-side in bioanalytical applications, particularly stereoselective phenomena in pharmacotherapeutics. Accordingly, calibration plots for l- and d-CHPGA were determined, and good linearity was observed (r = 0.99). However, problems arose when both enantiomers were present in the sample. Notably, when the ratios of l- to d-acid in the investigated sample started to deviate from 1, differences in regression coefficients were observed. As shown in Fig. 5, resolution of the two enantiomers remained incomplete. This need not handicap quantitation if peak overlap is constant in the plot range used.

Fig. 4.
Chromatograms
of CHPGA at
different
temperatures.
Conditions as
in Fig. 2;
Fig. 5 likewise
for mobile phase.

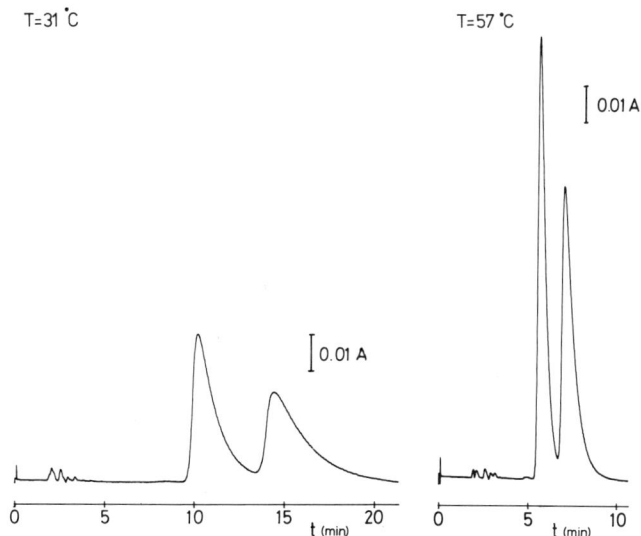

Fig. 5, *below.*
Relation between
retention time
and amount of
CHPGA injected:
l-, △, & *d*-, ◇;
3:1 in a, 1:3 in
b.   Column (250 ×
4.6 mm) at 47.2°;
20 μl injected.

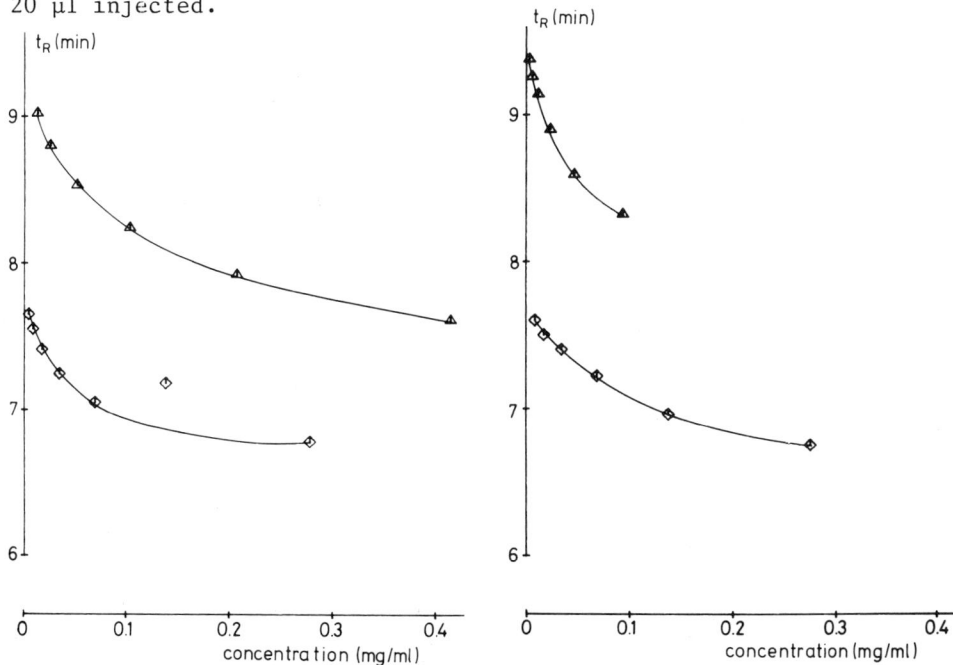

However, peak overlap will depend on the ratio of the enantiomers present in the sample, as can be concluded from Fig. 5.   This
behaviour is further demonstrated in Fig. 6, where *d*-CHPGA was kept
in constant amount but the *l*-acid was varied (the *l*-/*d*- ratios being
9:1, 1:1 and 1:9).   From these observations it is clear that quantitative determination of the two enantiomers side-by-side will be
very difficult if not impossible.

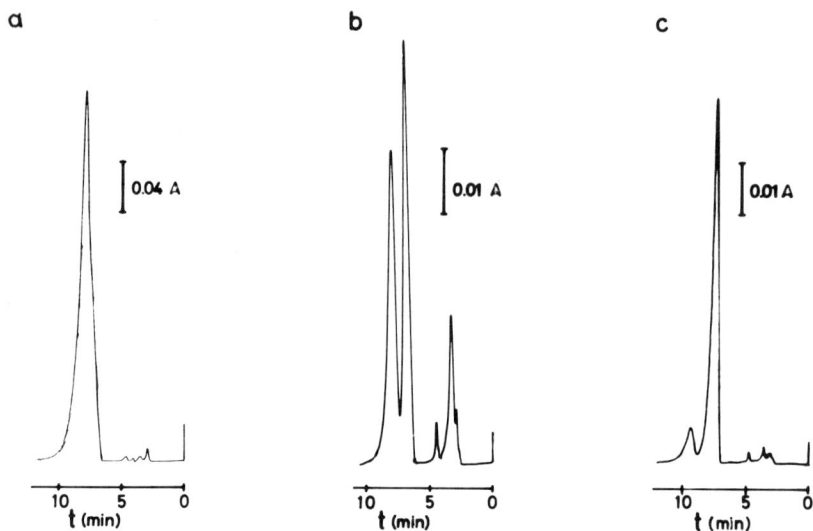

Fig. 6. Chromatogram of CHPGA enantiomers, with different ratios of *l*-acid to *d*-acid: a, 9:1; b, 1:1; c, 1:9, the concentration of the *d*-acid being constant (35 µg/ml). Other conditions as in Fig. 5.

CONCLUSIONS

The quantitative analysis of the enantiomers of CHPGA using this chiral-HPLC system was not possible, primarily because the overlap of the peaks varied with the ratio of enantiomers. Moreover, for concentrations that are of interest for bioanalytical purposes the retention times were rather long. The reasons underlying the phenomenon of increasing retention time with decreasing sample concentration are still unknown and require further studies.

Acknowledgements

We wish to thank Dr. C.J. Grol, D. Dijkstra and P. Tepper for assistance during the synthesis of the chiral stationary phase.

References

1. Cushny, A.R. (1904) *J. Physiol. 30*, 176-194.
2. Ellenbroek, B.W.J., Nivard, R.J.F., van Rossum, J.M. & Ariens, E.J. (1965) *J. Pharm. Pharmacol. 17*, 393-404.
3. Barlow, R.B., Franks, F.M. & Pearson, J.D.M. (1973) *J. Med. Chem. 16*, 439-446.
4. Ensing, K. (1984) *Thesis*, State University, Groningen.
5. Fujimura, K., Ueda, T. & Ando, T. (1983) *Anal. Chem. 55*, 446-450.

6. Kuwata, K., Uebori, M. & Yamazaki, Y. (1981) *J. Chromatog. 211,* 378-382.
7. Petterson, C. & Schill, G. (1981) *J. Chromatog. 204,* 179-183.
8. Pirkle, W.H., Finn, J.M., Schreiner, J.L. & Hamper, B.C. (1981) *J. Am. Chem. Soc. 103,* 3964-3966.
9. Pirkle, W.H. & Welch, C.J. (1984) *J. Org. Chem. 49,* 138-140.
10. Cramer, F. & Dietsche, W. (1959) *Chem. Ber. 92,* 378-384.
11. Debowski, J., Sybilska, D. & Jurczak, J. (1982) *Chromatographia 16,* 198-200.
12. Nobuhara, Y., Hirano, S. & Nakanishi, Y. (1983) *J. Chromatog. 258,* 276-279.
13. Feitsma, K.G., Drenth, B.F.H. & de Zeeuw, R.A. (1984) *J. High Resolu. Chromatog. Chromatog. Comm. 7,* 147-148.
14. Hinze, W.L., Riehl, T.E., Armstrong, D.W., DeMond, W., Alak, A. & Ward, T. (1985) *Anal. Chem. 57,* 237-242.
15. Dalgliesh, C.E. (1952) *J. Chem. Soc.* 3940-3942.
16. Tanaka, M., Kawaguchi, Y., Nakae, M., Mizobuchi, Y. & Shono, T. (1984) *J. Chromatog. 299,* 341-350.
17. Nelder, J.A. & Mead, R.A. (1965) *Comput. J. 7,* 308-313.
18. Hinze, W.L. (1981) *Separ. Purif. Meths. 10,* 159-237.
19. Horváth, C. & Melander, W.R. (1983) in *Chromatography, Fundamentals and Techniques, J. Chromatog. Libr. 22A* (Heftmann, E., ed.), Elsevier, Amsterdam, pp. A27-A135: see p. A54.
20. *as for* 19.: see p. A52.

#NC(C)

NOTES and COMMENTS relating to

SEPARATION TECHNOLOGY APPLICABLE TO VARIOUS DRUGS
AND TO ENANTIOMERS

Comments related to particular contributions

#C-1, C-2, and #NC(C)-6 to -8, p. 309
#NC(C)-9 and C-3, p. 314
#NC(C)-1 & -2, p. 315

'Chiral' material besides that in the first 4 'Notes' is to be
found on pp. 314-317.

#NC(C)-1

A Note on

SEPARATION OF FENFLURAMINE AND NORFENFLURAMINE
ENANTIOMERS BY DERIVATIZATION AND GC-ECD

[@]R.P. Richards, S. Caccia, A. Jori, M. Ballabio,
P. De Ponte and S. Garratini

Istituto di Richerche   [⊗]Servier Research and
  Farmacologiche 'Mario Negri'   Development
Milano, Italy   Fulmer Hall, Fulmer
                                    Slough SL3 6HH, U.K.

Fenfluramine is an anorectic agent which has been administered to obese patients during two decades. It undergoes extensive metabolism. One metabolite is norfenfluramine, which also has anorectic activity. Each molecule possesses one asymmetric carbon atom. It is the racemic form of fenfluramine that is currently used clinically.

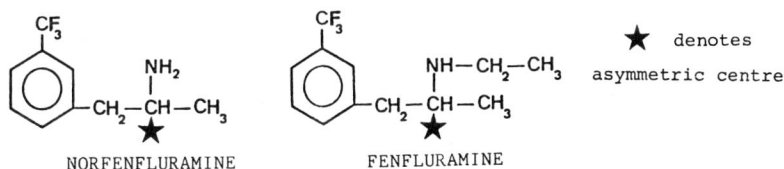

★ denotes asymmetric centre

NORFENFLURAMINE   FENFLURAMINE

Analytical methods are required for many purposes including pharmacokinetic analysis, dose-regimen determination, patient-compliance testing and pharmacodynamic/pharmacokinetic testing, i.e. establishing relationships between dose and blood levels of drugs and their pharmacological effect. Over the years various methods have been devised to measure fenfluramine and norfenfluramine in biological fluids. Being small and volatile, the molecules are well suited to GC. One early method [1] used FID and was only sensitive enough for urine analysis. ECD improved the sensitivity, but the method of Bruce & Maynard [2] was time-consuming. An improved extraction method enabled Campbell [3] to assay plasma samples rapidly. The assay was further improved by using nitrogen-specific detection [4]. There is also a rapid and sensitive GC-ECD procedure involving a derivatization step [5].

All these GC methods, however, suffer the drawback that they are not stereospecific. A stereospecific method is essential for meaningful analysis of racemic fenfluramine samples. When the pure active isomer of a drug is administered and there is no enantiomeric exchange, then a stereospecific assay is not necessary; but fenfluramine is used in its racemic form. Even so, if there is no stereoselectivity in the pharmacological action or toxicology of the compound, then measurement of the separated isomers offers no real advantage. The enantiomers of fenfluramine have been separated and examined for their individual pharmacology [6]. Fenfluramine showed stereoselective pharmacology to the extent that *d*-fenfluramine was anorectically active but the *l*-isomer appeared not to be. Also, the enantiomers of norfenfluramine showed different activities [7].

Even with stereoselective pharmacology, if there were no stereoselectivity in the kinetics and metabolism of the compound, then levels of each isomer could be predicted from a total racemic analysis. Studies with the radiolabelled isomers have shown that fenfluramine does exhibit such stereoselectivity [8]. A stereospecific analytical method was therefore developed [9] enabling the simultaneous separation and measurement of the optical isomers of both fenfluramine and norfenfluramine.

ASSAY PROCEDURE

Fenfluramine and norfenfluramine were derivatized with pentafluoropropionyl-*l*-prolyl chloride, allowing enantiomer separation on a packed GC column and providing a high ECD response. The derivatizing reagent was prepared by dissolving *l*-proline in pentafluoropropionyl anhydride at 0°, evaporating the excess anhydride and refluxing the residue with thionyl chloride. After evaporation of excess thionyl chloride, the reagent was dissolved in toluene [10].

Each plasma sample (0.1-0.5 ml) was spiked with internal standard (250 ng of amantidine), made alkaline with 0.2 ml 5 M NaOH and extracted by shaking for 15 min with 3 ml toluene. Derivatizing reagent (10 μl of the toluene solution) was added to the extract. After 30 min, finally shaking briefly with 5 ml 0.1 M NaOH, 1 μl aliquots of the organic phase were injected onto a 2 m × 4 mm i.d. column packed with 3% OV-225 on Chromosorb W (80-100) held at 190°. A ^{63}Ni ECD was used at 275° on the Carlo Erba Fractovap 2159 gas chromatograph.

The order of elution was *l*-norfenfluramine, *d*-norfenfluramine, *l*-fenfluramine, *d*-fenfluramine and then amantadine. As little as 10 pg of derivative injected on-column gave an ECD response, such that the assay detection limit is ~5 ng/ml using large plasma samples. Calibration curves were found to be linear between 30 and 300 ng/ml.

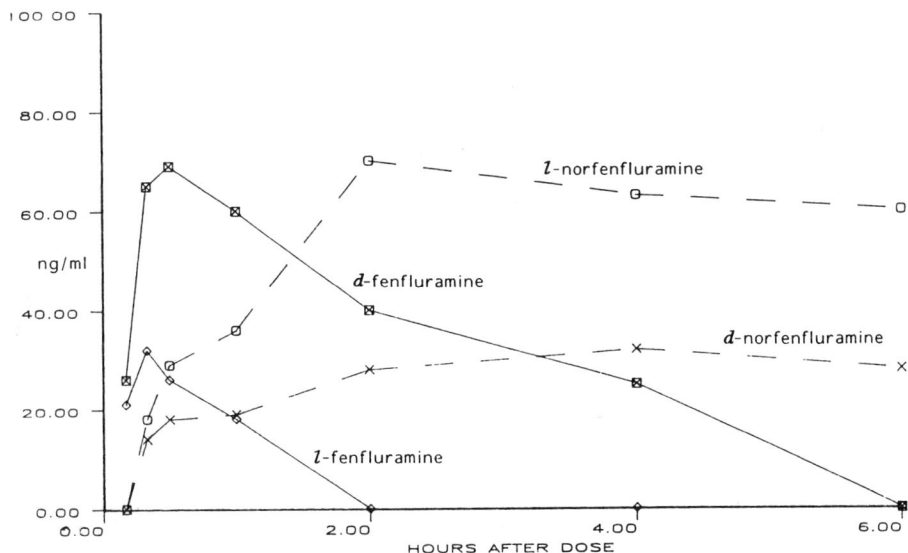

Fig. 1. Plasma concentrations of fenfluramine and norfenfluramine enantiomers in the rat after acute oral doses of fenfluramine as racemate (5 mg/kg).

APPLICATION OF THE METHOD

Mean plasma levels of d- and l-fenfluramine and norfenfluramine following a single dose of racemic fenfluramine to rats showed d- and l-fenfluramine peaking within 30 min after dosing; but d-fenfluramine concentrations were much higher (Fig. 1). Conversely, levels of l-norfenfluramine were higher than those of the d-isomer, indicating a stereoselectivity in the metabolic deethylation of fenfluramine to norfenfluramine.

The equivalent study in man showed no isomer difference for either compound. Thus a species difference became apparent through use of the stereospecific analytical method. Measuring total racemate levels, the differences in peak fenfluramine and norfenfluramine concentrations between rat and man would be obvious, as would the lower half-life of fenfluramine in the rat. However, without the stereospecific analysis there would have been no indication of the stereoselective differences seen in the rat that do not seem apparent in man.

However, radioactive studies in our own laboratory did show stereoselectivity in metabolism and kinetics in man. When plasma levels were measured in volunteers dosed daily for 10 days, stereoselective differences became apparent, different from that seen in the rat: for both l-fenfluramine and l-norfenfluramine the levels were higher than for the respective d-isomers. The clearance of d-fenfluramine exceeded that of the l-isomer.

Some clinical samples have shown up to 5 times as much *l*-fenfluramine as *d*-fenfluramine, the enantiomer with anorectic activity. This could explain why some patients have been unresponsive to the drug despite apparently adequate levels of racemic drug. It has proved more meaningful to relate the concentrations of *d*-fenfluramine than of racemic drug to pharmacological effects, e.g. weight loss. Moreover, *l*-fenfluramine is not totally inactive and may contribute to unwanted effects sometimes experienced with racemic drug. Hence patients exhibiting a marked stereoselectivity in clearance are likely to experience any unwanted effects of the *l*-isomer without the beneficial anorectic effect of the *d*-isomer.

References

1. Beckett, A.H. & Rowland, M. (1965)   *J. Pharm. Pharmacol. 17*, 59.
2. Bruce, R.B. & Maynard, W.R. Jr. (1968) *J. Pharm. Sci. 57*, 1173-1176.
3. Campbell, D.B. (1970) *J. Chromatog. 49*, 442-447.
4. Richards, R.P. & Gordon, B.G. (1986) to be published.
5. Midha, K.K., McGilveray, I.J. & Cooper, J.K. (1978) *Can. J. Pharm. Sci. 14*, 18-21.
6. Le Douarec, J.C., Schmitt, H. & Laubie, M. (1966) *Arch. Int. Pharmacodyn. Ther. 161*, 206-232.
7. Mennini, T., Caccia, S. & Garratini, S. (1985) *Psychpharmacology 85*, 111-114.
8. Richards, R.P. (1986) *Ph.D. Thesis, University of Surrey.*
9. Caccia, S. & Jori, A. (1977) *J. Chromatog. 144*, 127-131.
10. Wells, C.E. (1970) *J. Ass. Off. Agr. Chemists 53*, 113-115.

#NC(C)-2

A Note on

TOWARDS CHIRAL TLC PLATES: SOME PRELIMINARY STUDIES

Ian D. Wilson⊗

Department of Drug Metabolism
Hoechst Pharmaceutical Research Laboratories
Walton Manor, Walton
Milton Keynes, Bucks. MK7 7AJ, U.K.

For a number of reasons it is likely that, in the future, drug-regulatory authorities will require much more information on the fate of the individual components of drug racemates following dosing to man or experimental animals (cf. foregoing art. by I.W. Wainer). One important reason for this concern is the possibility that a pharmacologically inactive enantiomer may still contribute to, or indeed be the cause of, undesired side-effects and toxicity.

Gaining this information calls for rapid, efficient and reliable methods for separating enantiomers. Present-day procedures for resolving such mixtures involve either the production of diastereoisomers (by derivatization with chiral reagents) or the use of specially prepared chiral stationary phases (CSP's). Of these approaches the latter appears the most attractive for analytical purposes, as it avoids the need for optically pure reagents, high-yield derivatization procedures and also the potential requirement for extensive pre-chromatographic sample preparation.

At present the bulk of the research into CSP's is devoted to HPLC and GC, with few reports of work directed towards TLC [1, 2]. Here we describe the results obtained with a commercially prepared TLC-CSP and another described in a publication [1], and attempts to develop CSP's based on optically active ion-pair reagents or β-cyclodextrin.

TEST COMPOUNDS

The model compounds used included racemic mixtures of a variety of β-blockers, exemplified by propranolol, but also including several

⊗ Now at ICI Pharmaceuticals plc, Safety of Medicines Dept.,
  Mereside, Alderley Park, Macclesfield SK10 4TG

experimental drugs with the β-blocker chain, D(-)- and L(+)-mandelic acid and two non-steroidal anti-inflammatory drugs, isoxepac (itself optically inactive) and its analogue with a propionic acid side-chain. Isoxepac was used as a 'control', whereby an apparent separation of this optically inactive compound into 'enantiomers' would connote merely poor chromatography.

TRIALS WITH A COMMERCIAL 'CHIRAL PLATE'

Macherey-Nagel & Co. have recently marketed a product described as a 'chiral plate', designed for the separation of entantiomers. Manufacture entails treating C-18 bonded plates with a solution of copper acetate followed by (2S,4R,2'RS)-4-hydroxy-1-(2-hydroxy-dodecyl)proline [2]. The literature supplied by the company describes the separation of D- and L-amino acids but gives no guidance for method development (see, however, the recent paper by Brinkman & Kamminger [3]).

When the TLC of the β-blocking drugs was investigated with methanol/water mixtures as solvent, poor results were obtained (tailing spots). The addition of aqueous ammonia to the solvent, to suppress the ionization of the secondary amino groups on these compounds, failed to improve spot shape. No evidence was seen for the resolution of these β-blockers into enantiomers.

The mandelic acid enantiomers became strongly bound to the plates at the origin, giving rise to purple spots (the compounds themselves are not coloured). These remained at the origin irrespective of the eluotropic strength of the solvent (methanol/water mixtures).

Better results were obtained for isoxepac and the propionic acid analogue. Both chromatographed well on the 'chiral plate', the R_f values varying in a predictable way depending on the eluotropic strength of the solvent (Fig. 1). There was, however, no evidence for the separation of the racemate into two spots.

THE 'WAINER PLATE'

Wainer et al. [1] have described the preparation and use of an aminopropyl silanized silica-gel TLC plate coated with (R)-N-(3,5-dinitrobenzoyl)phenyl glycine for the separation of isomers ([1]; cf. foregoing art. on chiral HPLC). We attempted to apply this approach to the separation of our test compounds. The plates were prepared as described, but in our hands they very quickly became discoloured (oxidized?) and we were unable to obtain much useful information on their use. Further work will be necessary to determine whether this type of plate will be useful in this area, and to find ways of preventing their deterioration.

Fig. 1. Variations in the R_f values of isoxepac (●) and the racemate of its propionic acid analogue (o) on the 'chiral plate' with increasing methanol content (v/v). Note the absence of any separation of the propionic acid racemate into enantiomers.

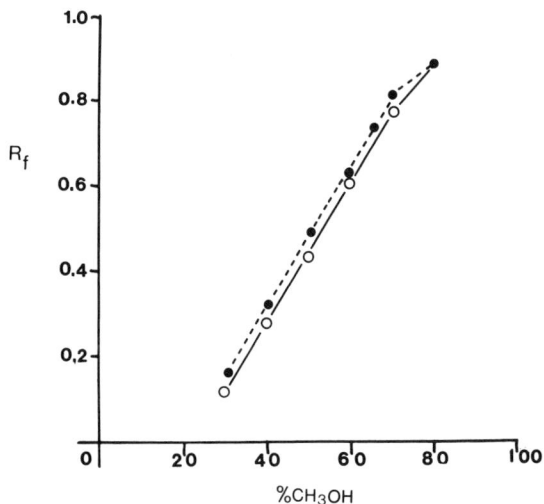

PLATES COATED WITH OPTICALLY ACTIVE ION–PAIR REAGENT

Petterson & Schill [4] have described the use of optically active ion-pair reagents (D-camphorsulphonic acid and quinine) in HPLC. Accordingly, silica gel TLC plates were coated with 2% (w/v) solutions of these reagents in ethanol, and dried. Separation of D- and L-mandelic acids was then attempted using methanol/water solvent systems. On the quinine sulphate-coated plates with methanol/water (10:90 by vol.) the mandelic acid enantiomers may have differed slightly in R_f, although the spots remained close to the origin. This provides good evidence for ion-pair formation, since in the absence of the reagent the test acids chromatographed close to the solvent front. However, an attempt to increase the R_f of the mandelic acid enantiomers in the hope of improving the separation was unsuccessful due to breakdown of the layer of ion-pair reagent. Interpretation of the results was also complicated by the high fluorescence background caused by the reagent itself. No success was obtained with camphorsulphonic acid-coated plates.

β–CYCLODEXTRIN–COATED PLATES

Several groups have developed HPLC separations based on the use of β-cyclodextrin, either in the mobile phase or chemically attached to the stationary phase (e.g. see K.G. Feitsma et al., this vol.). As β-cyclodextrin is commercially available (relatively cheaply) we decided to coat it onto silica-gel TLC plates.

A major problem in coating β-cyclodextrin onto TLC plates was its poor solubility in all the usual organic solvents. After considerable (and tedious) trial-and-error a 1% solution (w/v) of β-cyclodextrin in ethanol/dimethyl sulphoxide (80:20 by vol.) was obtained. Silica-gel TLC plates were dipped in this solution and allowed to

Fig. 2. Chromatography of D(+)- and L(+)-mandelic acid, with replicate spotting, on silica-gel TLC plates doubly coated with β-cyclodextrin as described in the text. Solvent: methanol/water, 1:1. Spots were visualized under UV light (254 nm).

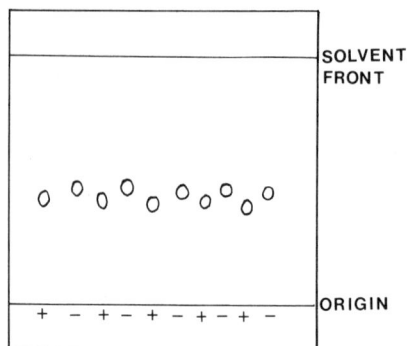

dry in a fume cupboard. To assess the effect of coating, a number of these plates were dipped in the cyclodextrin solution for a second and third time.

Development was then attempted using methanol/water solvent systems. For the β-blockers, isoxepac and its propionic acid analogue no satisfactory results were obtained; however, for D- and L-mandelic acids different R_f values were obtained. Further studies with these plates concentrated on this apparent separation. Firstly a clear relationship was established between the degree of coating of the plate and the R_f. Thus for D-mandelic acid with methanol/water (1:1) as solvent, a single coating of the plate gave an R_f of 0.82, double coating gave an R_f of 0.46 and a third coating an R_f of 0.1. Thereafter double-coated plates were used.

The next property to be investigated was the effect of the eluotropic strength of the solvent on R_f. Rather surprisingly, and contrary to all predictions, the percentage of methanol in the solvent could be varied from 0% to 100% without any change in the R_f of either D- or L-mandelic acid. As yet we are unable to explain this result. However, whatever the cause, it clearly limits the usefulness of the plate if the only way in which R_f may be altered is by varying the degree of coating with β-cyclodextrin.

A typical plate showing the chromatography of the individual mandelic acid isomers is shown in Fig. 2. An attempt to increase the separation between D- and L-mandelic acid by using multiple development in the same solvent system resulted only in both enantiomers eventually attaining the same R_f (after 3 developments in methanol/water, 1:1). Like the lack of variation in R_f with solvent composition, this is another surprising result which goes against generally accepted chromatographic principles.

An attempt to separate mixtures of the mandelic acid isomers was without success, giving a single spot with an R_f in between those of the pure isomers.

The properties of the plates are quite fascinating, and further studies are in progress in an attempt to determine whether useful chiral TLC plates can be developed from them.

CONCLUSIONS

It should be clear from our results that CSP's for TLC require much more development before a suitable product is available for general use. The fact that certain manufacturers are now showing an interest is encouraging and, even without active development by them, CSP's for TLC are likely to come as a spin-off from research on stationary phases for HPLC.

Our own studies, whilst having done little to advance development of this type of plate, have at least served to illustrate the difficulties involved in chiral TLC, and the results obtained with β-cyclodextrin merit further investigation.

Meanwhile, in the absence of satisfactory CSP's for TLC, the options seem to be limited to diastereoisomer formation, with all the problems that this implies.

Acknowledgements

Prof. U.A.Th. Brinkman and Dr. I.W. Wainer are thanked for their valuable comments.

References

1. Wainer, I.W., Brunner, C.A. & Doyle, T.D. (1983) *J. Chromatog.* *264*, 154.
2. Günther, K., Martens, J. & Schickendanz, M. (1984) *Angew. Chem.* *96*, 514-518.
3. Brinkman, U.A.Th. & Kamminga, D. (1985) *J. Chromatog. 330*, 375-378.
4. Petterson, C. & Schill, G. (1981) *J. Chromatog. 204*, 179-183.

#NC(C)-3

A Note on

RP-HPLC SEPARATION, AS DIASTEREOISOMERS, OF ACEBUTOLOL
AND RELATED COMPOUNDS

A.A. Gulaid,   O.R.W. Lewellen & ⊗A.R. Boobis

Biopharmaceutical Research, ⊗Department of Clinical
May & Baker Ltd.   Pharmacology
Rainham Road South   Royal Postgraduate Medical
Dagenham, Essex RM10 7XS   School, Ducane Road
U.K.   London W12 OHS, U.K.

Acebutolol and M&B 17,908 are β-adrenoreceptor blocking agents.
They are administered as racemic mixtures of two optical isomers.
Acebutolol is extensively metabolized to diacetolol, its acetamido
analogue.

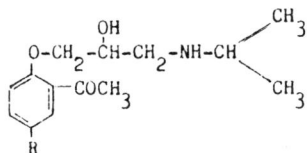

O-CH$_2$-CH(OH)-CH$_2$-NH-CH(CH$_3$)(CH$_3$)   acebutolol, R = -NH-CO(CH$_2$)$_2$CH$_3$

⎯COCH$_3$ diacetolol, R = -NH-COCH$_3$

R   M&B 17,764, R = -NH-COCH$_2$CH$_3$
                                   (i.s.)

Sensitive methods of assay, using HPLC, have been developed for
the determination of these three products in plasma.   The enantiomers of each have been resolved by HPLC after derivatization with
R-(+)-1-phenylethyl-isocyanate.   The methods have been evaluated
and applied to the determination of each compound in plasma obtained
after oral administration to humans and dogs. Stereoselective disposition was not apparent.

*Senior Editor's excerpts from a publication to which the foregoing
Forum abstract relates*

In the assay description for acebutolol and diacetolol [1],
reports are cited concerning biological activities of enantiomers
of this class of drug: cardiac β-blockage is generally greater for
S-(-)-, and membrane stabilization is found with *R*-(+)-enantiomers.
To form diastereoisomers for HPLC separation, *S*-(-)-*N*-trifluoro-
acetyl prolyl chloride (TPC) was used in the first instance [2];

but the commercial material is contaminated with up to 15% of the
(+)-enantiomer, and the reagent rapidly racemizes during storage.
Stability was better for the reagent adopted, R-(+)-1-phenylethyl-
isocyanate (PEIC), as used in J.A. Thompson's laboratory for resolving propranolol; it readily gave the urea (not carbamate) derivatives of each test compound and the internal standard (i.s.).

Plasma (1 ml) with NaOH added was extracted with diethyl ether,
and the residue from drying down (50°, N_2) was taken up in dichloromethane for treatment with PEIC in this solvent (30 min, room temp.).
The residue from re-evaporation was dissolved in the HPLC mobile
phase, viz. water/methanol/triethylamine (50:50:0.05 by vol.).
The column (250 × i.d. 4.6 mm) was packed with 5 μm ODS-2. The order
of elution was diacetolol, i.s. and acebutolol; the S-isomer of
each preceded the R-isomer. The detection limit (fluorescence,
238/450 nm) was ~0.05 μg/ml of human or dog plasma, adequate for
pharmacokinetic studies.

Reference

1. Gulaid, A.A., Houghton, G.W. & Boobis, A.R. (1985) *J. Chromatog.*
    318, 393-397.
2. Sankey, M.G., Gulaid, A.A. & Kaye, C.M. (1984) *J. Pharm.*
    Pharmacol. 36, 276-277.

#NC(C)-4

A Note on

SEPARATION OF CHIRAL DRUGS AND METABOLITES
BY CAPILLARY GAS CHROMATOGRAPHY

H. Frank

Institut für Toxikologie
University of Tübingen
D-7400 Tübingen, FRG/W. Germany

Certain chiral therapeutic drugs are administered as racemic mixtures. However, in respect of their biological activities optical antipodes should be regarded as different entities rather than as two faces of the same compound. For pharmacological evaluation of optically active compounds, efficient methods for stereochemical analysis are required. The recent development of chromatographic systems for direct enantiomer separation has notably extended our capabilities for separating chiral drugs and metabolites, especially through use of enantioselective stationary phases. There are two other approaches that suffer from certain limitations: derivatization with a stereochemically pure chiral reagent and separation of the resulting diastereoisomers by conventional GC or HPLC, or the employment of pseudo-racemic mixtures involving labelling of either enantiomer with a stable or radioactive isotope.

Whilst HPLC with chiral stationary phases plays an important role in our laboratory, it is not now considered in view of the foregoing survey by I.W. Wainer. For GC, the first chiral phases were synthesized by Gil-Av et al. [1]. Most of the early GC chiral phases had poor thermal stability; introduction of enantioselective silicone phases by Frank et al. [2] improved this situation considerably. In addition, silicones with different chiral selectors having distinct enantio-selectivities for various compound classes could be synthesized. In a Note that follows, the advantages of using capillary rather than traditional GC columns are brought out (glass in the present context).

The GC-phase Chirasil-Val has been employed for analysis of various chiral drugs, e.g. penicillamine, DOPA, *S*-carboxymethylcys-teine [3] or *N*-acetylcysteine [4], sympathomimetic drugs, β-blockers, chiral barbiturates and hydantoins [3, 5]. In general, the L-valine-t-

butylamide moiety is the optimum chiral selector;   but others (e.g.
L-valine-*R*-1-phenylethylamide) are preferable for certain structures.

Equally important for stereochemical analysis of chiral drugs in
biological samples is the fact that the low bleed of chiral silicone
phases allows stereochemical analysis by GC in combination with
MS [3] as a highly selective and sensitive detection mode.

References

1. Gil-Av, E., Feibush, B. & Sigler, R. Charles (1966) *Tetrahedron
    Lett.*, 1009-1015.
2. Frank, H., Nicholson, G.J. & Bayer, E. (1977) *J. Chromatog. Sci.*
    15, 174-176.
3. Frank, H., Nicholson, G.J. & Bayer, E.(1978) *J. Chromatog. 146*,
    197-206.
4. Frank, H., Thiel, D. & Langer, K. (1984) *J. Chromatog. 309*,
    261-267.
5. Wedlund, P.J., Sweetman, B.J., McAllister, C.B., Branch, R.A.
    & Wilkinson, G.R. (1984) *J. Chromatog. 307*, 121-127.

=============

*The foregoing adaptation of the author's Forum abstract
is reinforced by —*

SENIOR EDITOR'S SUPPLEMENT

From ref. 2:

In the context of separating amino acid enantiomers, using open-
tubular columns (pre-treated with colloidal silicic acid or aerosil),
improved stationary phases were developed in the author's laboratory.
The requisite thermal stability and low volatility was achieved
with a diamide such as *N*-n-docosanoyl-L-valine t-butylamide; but
above 140° (the allowable maximum being 190°) the baseline was prohibi-
tively high and column life was short.

Satisfactory behaviour was achieved with, as the chiral diamide
phase, *N*-propionyl-L-valine t-butylamide polysiloxane, possessing a
thermally stable backbone obtained by co-polymerizing dimethylsiloxane
and carboxyalkylmethylsiloxane. Such columns (coated with a chloroform
solution of the stationary phase by the static method) showed sustained
stability at 175°, and with programming from 90° to 170° gave enantiomer
discrimination when used for a mixture of *N*-pentafluoropropionyl-D,L-
amino acid isopropyl esters.

From ref. 4:

The aim was to measure *N*-acetyl-L-cysteine, particularly in
plasma where therapeutic levels are in the range 1-30 µM. A chiral-HPLC
approach was satisfactory for urine, but with plasma there were

Fig. 1. Separation of *N*-acetyl-*S*-methylcysteine methyl ester and its D-enantiomer (which served as internal standard) by GC with a 'Chirasil-Val' stationary phase. Injector at 250° (split injection); H_2 carrier. (a) Pure compounds (using FID).
(b) *N*-acetyl-L-cysteine in serum, by enantiomer labelling, using AFID (NPD). Estimated serum level = 12 µM (10 fmol injected).
(c) Similar to (b), with spiked control serum (L-, 0.6 µM; D-, 1.2 µM), but with MS detection at m/z 132 (only the relevant portion of the trace is shown).

From ref. [4], courtesy of Elsevier.

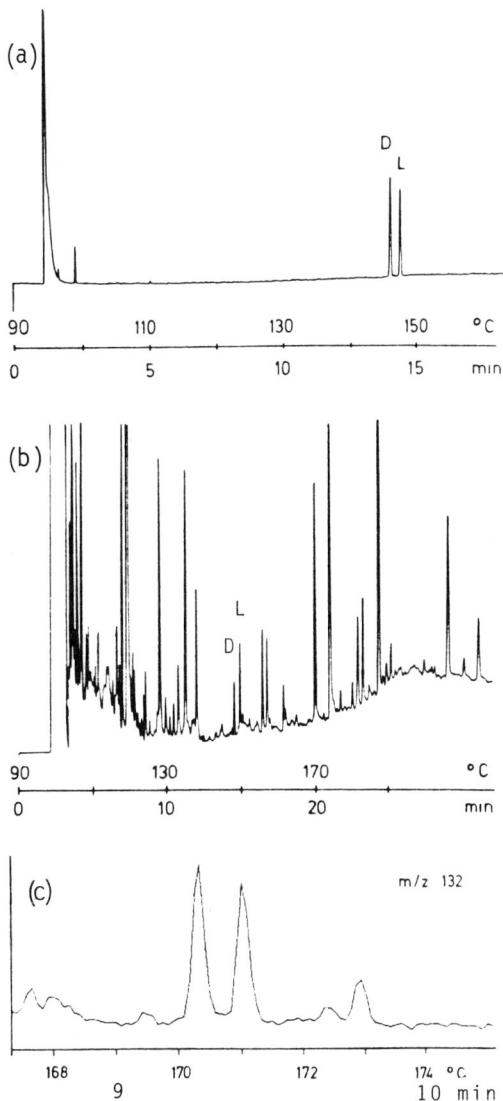

interferences varying from one patient to another. Better results for plasma were obtained by GC in conjunction with 'enantiomer labelling', the D-isomer being spiked into the plasma as an internal standard (Fig. 1). Sample preparation entailed acetone deproteinization, washing with hexane at pH 9, concentration of the aqueous phase, application to a Dowex-1 column, elution with M HCl, and treatment with diazomethane after drying down. With plasma, GC-MS (mass fragmentography; Fig. 1c) served better than GC-FID, which showed interferences, or GC-AFID (Fig. 1b) which gave a 'noisy' trace.

#NC(C)-5

A Note [*] *on*

PREPARATION, PROPERTIES AND USE OF
CAPILLARY COLUMNS FOR DRUG ANALYSIS

H. Frank

Institut für Toxikologie
University of Tübingen
D-7400 Tübingen, FRG / W. Germany

The invention of flexible fused-silica capillaries, the development of bonded phases and the commercial availability of standardized capillaries have been important pre-requisites for their introduction into routine drug analysis. While most users rely upon commercial suppliers, the capability of preparing one's own capillaries offers the advantage that columns may be tailored to the specific needs of a type of analysis or compound, besides being less costly. But even for the user of commmercial capillaries a knowledge of the chemistry and techniques of column preparation is important in order to be able to judge the performance of columns and to identify potential sources of inadequacies.

A number of aspects determine the overall procedure for preparation of a capillary, the most important being the compound of interest or the type of sample and, in consequence, the stationary phase. Usually fused silica is the preferred material. In some instances as with underivatized drugs of slightly basic character, soda-lime glass may offer advantages; but these generally exhibit poorer temperature stability.

The methods for surface pre-treatment and deactivation must comply with the specific requirements for satisfactory GC of the compounds or derivatives of interest. Different test mixtures have been introduced for checking the suitability of capillaries for specific compound classes [1-3]. Bonded phases are preferable, especially with biological samples containing large amounts of material that could contaminate a capillary, or where the concentration of the analyte is so low that injection must be split-less or on-column.

---

[*] Based (by Senior Editor) on Forum Abstract; see Vol. 7, this series, for pertinent arts. by B.S. Thomas and by K. Grob, jr.

The injection mode also determines the precision of quantitative determinations. The dimensions of the capillary are equally significant. For on-column injection or for GC-MS, wide diameters (~0.3 mm) are preferred, but for high-speed analysis short narrow-bore capillaries (≤100 μm) offer considerable advantages.

The decision on which mode of capillary GC is the most suitable for a certain application depends upon several interdependent factors. In order to adopt the most suitable procedure, careful consideration of various aspects is required: sample matrix, structure and stability of the compounds of interest, their concentrations, eventual derivatization, precision and accuracy of quantitative analysis, number of compounds to be analyzed, and cost and time required for sample pre-treatment. All these factors determine which type of capillary should be used, whether and how it should be deactivated, which stationary phase and which film thickness may be suitable, and whether a certain mode of injection or detection is preferable.

References

1.   Grob, K., Grob, B. & Grob, K., jr. (1981) *J. Chromatog.* *219*, 13-20.
2.   Donicke, M. (1973) *Chromatographia 6*, 190-196.
3.   Nicholson, G.J., Frank, H. & Bayer, E. (1979) *J. High Resolu. Chromatog. Chromatog. Comm. 2*, 411-415.

#NC(C)-6

A Note* *on*

GC ANALYSIS WITH A DEDICATED AUTOMATED DERIVATIZER

H. Frank, G.J. Nicholson and J. Gerhardt

Institut für Toxikologie and Institut für Organische
Chemie, University of Tübingen
D-7400 Tübingen, FRG / W. Germany

In chromatographic analysis a number of individual segments of the analytical train have been automated, such as sample injection, chromatography itself, detection, peak integration and data handling. However, automation of the most laborious and time-consuming segments, sample pre-treatment and derivatization, promises greater savings in time and considerably higher reproducibility, especially when large numbers of samples are to be analyzed. The specific conditions of chemical derivatization, mainly the involvement of aggressive, volatile, unstable and often toxic reagents, demand that release of these compounds into the atmosphere or access of humidity to the reaction mixture are kept to a minimum. This is difficult to achieve with the general laboratory robotics which are being introduced currently [1] (see also J.C. Pearce et al., this vol., #NC(C)-7).

We have constructed a dedicated automated derivatizer [2] which consists of a lever arm to transfer the sample vials, a movable heating/cooling block for temperatures between 10° and 180°, a transfer manifold for addition of reagents and gases, and three reagent/solvent-dispensing systems. The derivatizer repetitively performs all steps involved in chemical derivatization, such as reagent addition, heating, cooling, drying, solvent addition and sample transfers, in an automated controlled manner. At least 40 samples may be processed in one series and in step with chromatography; this notably contributes to the high precision achieved with the automated derivatizer. Since the reaction conditions such as temperatures, reaction times, volumes and reagents as well as the sequence of steps may be freely chosen, the instrument may perform any derivatization scheme involving up to three derivatization reactions.

[Refs. overleaf

---

* *Abstract of a Forum contribution by H. Frank.*

References

1. Hawk, G.L. & Strimaitis, J.R., eds. (1984) *Advances in Laboratory Automation*, Zymark Corporation, Hopkinton.
2. Gerhardt, J., Frank, H,, Nicholson, G.J. & Bayer, E. (1984) *Chromatographia 19*, 251-253.

#NC(C)-7

A Note on

ROBOTICS IN DRUG ANALYSIS

J.C. Pearce[1], M.P. Allan[2] and R.D. McDowall[1]

Departments of Drug Analysis[1] and Research Engineering[2]
Smith, Kline & French Research Ltd.
The Frythe, Welwyn, Herts. AL6 9AR, U.K.

Sensitive and specific assays for inotropic agents in plasma have been developed in our laboratories over the past three years. The methods incorporated a liquid-solid extraction step followed by automated HPLC with UV detection. Our early assays utilized C-18 bonded-phase extraction columns, but following the introduction of the Analytichem Automated Sample Processor (AASP) in 1983, the analyses were rapidly converted to take advantage of this new technology [1] (cf. foregoing art. by R.D. McDowall et al.). The injection of analytes by the AASP LC module is automatic but the off-line preparation of the sample cassette is a manual process. Accordingly, we have investigated the potential of robotics in sample preparation and specifically the automation of the AASP sample cassette preparation.

THE ROBOT

As we had no previous experience with robots we purchased a fully 'customized' assembly, a Zymate Laboratory Automation System (Zymark Corpn.). It combines a computer-controlled robot arm and, within its reach, commercially available laboratory 'stations'.

The system is programmed to mimic the operations carried out by a human analyst. Key components are shown in Fig. 1, notably (1) the arm of the robot having a suitable hand attached, capable of transferring samples and probes from station to station. The first step in the construction of a program is to move the arm manually, using the soft-keys of the controller (not shown), to the desired position and assign a unique descriptive name. This name and the Cartesian coordinates for that position are stored in the computer's memory. When a series of locations have been defined, they are sequentially listed to produce a sub-routine, which is itself given a unique name. A number of these sub-routines are then combined to formulate the final program.

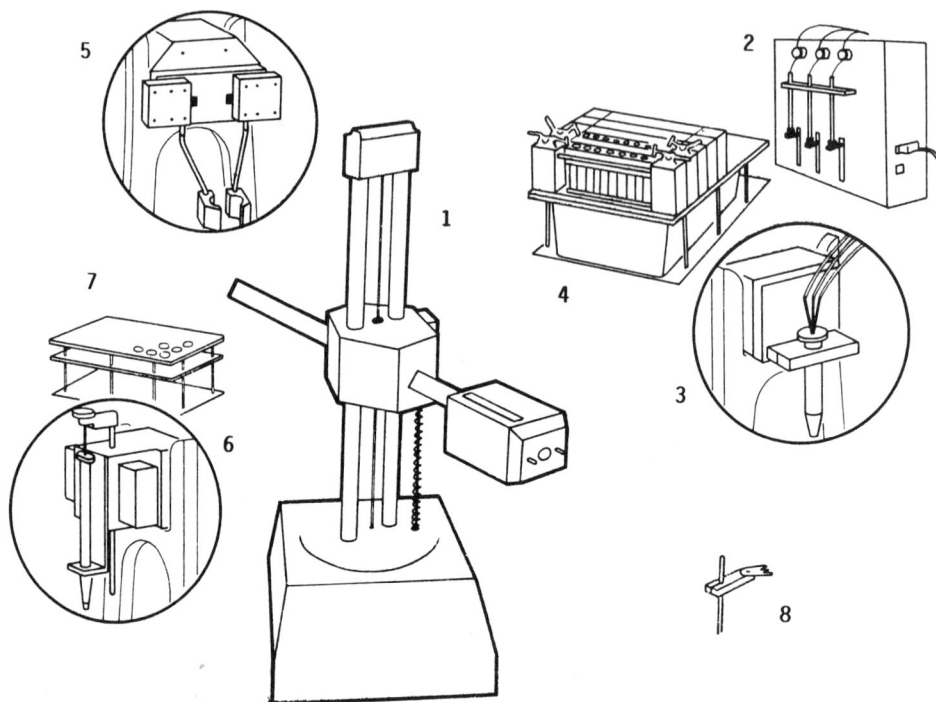

Fig. 1.   Some modules referred to in the text (with identifications).   *[The authors' fuller diagram showed the controller etc.-Ed.]*

The 'master laboratory station' (2 in Fig. 1) consists of 3 programmable stepper-motor driven syringes to dispense reagents (and
incorporates a 2-way gas valve).   Connected to the station is a
remote multi-tube dispensing nozzle (3), used to deliver methanol and
water to condition and wash the AASP casettes, 10 of which with
reservoirs, can be housed in the casette rack (4).   Interfaced between
the controller and external devices is a power- and event-control module
(not shown), providing DC and variable AC voltages, sensing of logic
inputs, an A/D converter and various relay contacts.   A gripper hand
for 1, used to transfer tubes and probes between stations, is shown
(5). Accurate transfer of samples and reagents is effected by a
syringe hand (6) in conjunction with pipette tips housed in a rack (7);
both 1 ml and 200 µl versions are provided.   A pipette tip ejector
(8) facilitates the removal of pipette tips from syringe hand into
waste container.   Pipette-tip racks have a verification switch to
ensure that a tip has been picked up; the status of the switch is
sensed by the power- and event-control module, which also powers
a vortex mixer for aggressive mixing of single tubes or vials.
All racks are firmly fixed to the work-surface to prevent any movement
which would render the system unusable.   The printer for providing
hardcopy listing of programs is not shown, nor the vital controller.

PROCEDURES FOR THE EXTRACTION OF PLASMA SAMPLES

This outline of the extraction procedure applies to both human and robot analysts except where otherwise indicated.

1. Thaw plasma samples and centrifuge to remove fibrous material, then pipette 100 μl into a 1.5 ml polypropylene centrifuge tube (effected manually whether or not the extraction will be by robot).

2. Add 100 μl of water and 500 μl of an internal standard (i.s.), and mix by vortexing.

3. Condition the AASP cartridges with 1 ml aliquots of methanol followed by 1 ml water (the column **must not dry out**).

4. Transfer 300 μl of the diluted plasma sample to a cartridge and apply compressed air to drive it through the sorbent bed (via the gas valve, connected to one delivery line, if by the remote nozzle hand).

5. Wash the cartridge with 1 ml water and then transfer the complete cassette to the AASP LC module for HPLC.

CALIBRATION STANDARDS AND VALIDATION

To 100 μl control plasma placed manually into a 1.5 ml polypropylene centrifuge tube are added 100 μl of the appropriate standard solution and the i.s.; vortex and extract as for test samples.

The precision and accuracy of the robot-operated syringes was tested with distilled water (10 determinations per value), with different aliquot sizes. *Italicized values* represent bias (% error).
- 250 μl syringe: **10** μl, C.V. 4%/*-1*; **50**, <1/<*+1*; **100**, <1/<*+1*.
- 1 ml syringe: **250** μl, <1/<*+1*; **500**, <1/<*+1*; **750**, <1/<*+1*.
- 10 ml syringe: **250** μl, <1/<*-1*; **500** μl, <1/*0*; **1000**, <1/<*-1*.

Evidently the syringes were very accurate and precise even at the lowest volumes, below what would normally be expected of them – a surprising finding. The ability of the arm to return to the same position within the x, y and z axes was within 0.5 mm in all planes of movement, adequate for all operations in the present application.

COMPARISON OF HUMAN AND ROBOT, AND BENEFITS OF AUTOMATION

The ability of the robot to carry out the sample preparation procedure (above) was evaluated with one series of spiked plasma samples prepared manually and another prepared by robot. The following results show that the robot was as good, if not slightly better, at achieving precise and accurate data (*italics* connote bias) for the stated concentrations (6 obs.) of the drug, viz. an inotropic agent:
- 25 ng/ml: **human**, C.V. 8%/*+4*;   **robot**, 2%/*-4*
- 50   :   2%/*+2*;   3%/*0*
- 75   :   6%/*-7*;   3%/*+1*
- 100   :   3%/*+2*;   5%/*+3*.

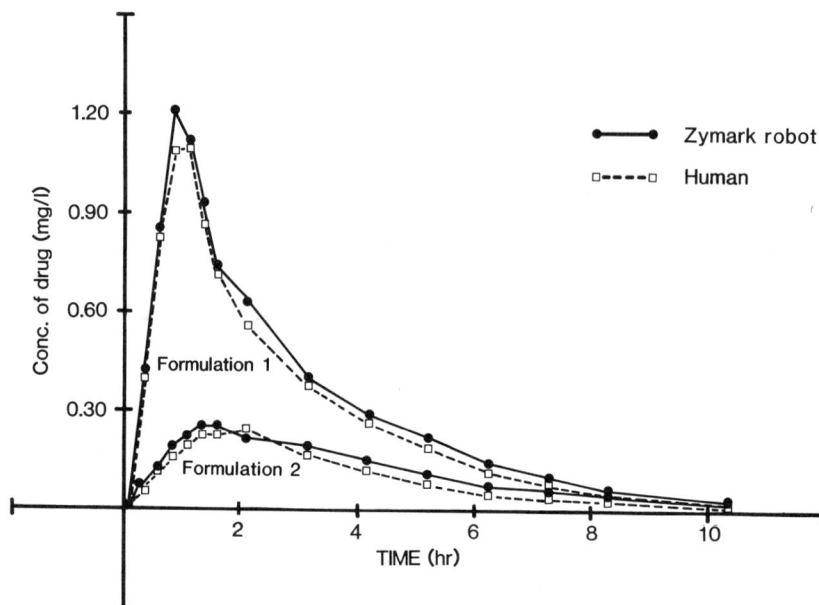

Fig. 2. Determination of an inotropic agent in plasma during a bio-equivalence study in the dog: human *vs.* robot.

In a bioequivalence study (Fig. 2), manual and automated methods of sample preparation showed excellent agreement in the assay values.

We regard the major benefits of using a robot system for sample preparation to be as follows:
1) unattended operation 24 h/day, thus freeing analysts to carry out more detailed evaluation of the data;
2) greater integrity of data: the robot will repeat procedures unaffected by distractions;
3) reduced handling of biological samples, and thus a reduction in the exposure of the analyst to a potential biohazard.

In the future we envisage a greater deployment of both flexible automation (robotics) and dedicated analyzers (e.g. AASP) for the analysis of drugs in biological fluids. These, together with Laboratory Information Management Systems (LIMS), will be conducive to increased sample throughput and improved integrity of the resulting data.

References

1. Pearce, J.C., Jelly, J.A., Fernandes, K.A., Leavens, W.J. & McDowall, R.D. (1986) *J. Chromatog. 353*, 371-378.
2. Hawk, G.L., Little, J.N. & Zenie, F.H. (1982) *Ind. Lab. (Engl. transl.) 12*, 48.

#NC(C)-8

A Note on

FLUORIMETRIC ASSAY OF AN ANTIHYPERTENSIVE DRUG
WITH AUTOMATED SAMPLE PROCESSING AND HPLC

P.R.J. Ceelen, H.M. Ruijten and H. de Bree

Duphar Research Laboratories
P.O. Box 2, Weesp, The Netherlands

Using an automatic sample processor (AASP-LC) we were readily able to develop a fluorimetric assay for DU 29373

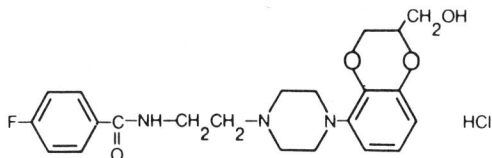

with an isomeric internal standard; after the plasma sample had been loaded off-line into a concentration cartridge, they eluted onto the analytical column as a narrow band. The detection limit was 10 ng/ml of plasma. Before loading into the C-18 cartridge, the plasma sample (1 ml) was made alkaline with ammonia (25% w/w; 0.5 ml).

After the loading, by cartridge loader, casettes containing 10 cartridges were processed simultaneously. With N_2 pressure the sample is forced through the cartridge at a flow-rate of 1 drop/sec. Salts, proteins, etc., are washed off by a 1 ml water rinse, and the casette is then placed in the processor. [*Editor's note*.- Earlier in this vol., art. C-2, R.D. McDowall et al. explain the nature of the equipment, with a company diagram identical with one furnished with the MS. of the present Note, and relevant to the following description.]

The instrument is equipped with a programmable purge function (and a 10-port injection valve), allowing venting-off of all compounds having a smaller k' value than the analytes, which are subsequently eluted onto the analytical column. After a short (pre-set) time the cartridge is by-passed, still holding compounds of higher k' value. Thereby the HPLC run time is minimized, being only 8 min/sample for DU 29373; the cartridge was purged 10 times with 25 µl of mobile phase before elution, which took 1 min (2 ml).

HPLC was performed with a Waters M-6000 pump and a Zorbax C-18 column (250×4.6 mm). The detector was a Shimadzu RF-530 fluoro-meter, set at 260 nm for excitation and 370 nm for emission. The mobile phase was water/acetonitrile/methanol (6:3:1 by vol.), con-taining 4 g/l of NH_4HCO_3. The flow-rate was 2 ml/min.

COMMENTS

It took only a month to develop the assay for this new drug. The C.V.'s were 4% and 6% for repeatability and reproducibility respectively. The overall analysis time is 20 min per sample.

The AASP-LC module enables sorbent-extracted samples to be automatically injected reproducibly. A batch of 100 (off-line) pre-concentrated samples can be processed without any attendance. Using the programmable purge function and 10-port valve it is possible to inject only the compounds of interest onto the analytical column, resulting in clean and relatively short chromatograms.

To avoid pressure build-up in the cartridges, we found it advisable not to exceed a sample volume of 2 ml plasma. The most serious problems encountered were between-batch variations in characteristics of the sorbent and (observed in a few batches) deformation of casette material.

#NC(C)-9

A Note on

HPLC SEPARATION OF MALOPRIM-RELATED ANALYTES, EXEMPLIFYING COMPUTER-GUIDED OPTIMIZATION

C.R. Jones and B.C. Weatherley

Wellcome Research Laboratories
Langley Court, Beckenham, Kent BR3 3BS, U.K.

When presenting one's scientific findings to an audience, one normally shows slides of tables and graphs and may forget that these are merely convenient shorthand forms which have had to suffice since the distant past. Using the computer, we are now in a position to illustrate data more directly, exemplified here by the influence of mobile-phase changes on the chromatographic behaviour of analytes relevant to the determination of Maloprim in plasma.

Maloprim is a combination of pyrimethamine (Pyr) and dapsone (DDS) used for prophylaxis against malaria. When examining extracts of plasma from patients we have to separate these from three other components – the added internal standard, metoprine (DDMP); monoacetyl dapsone (MADDS) which is a metabolite; and the inevitable caffeine (Caff).

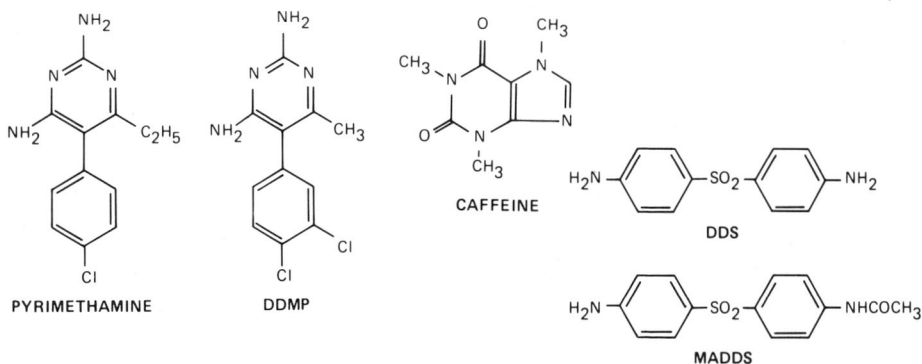

Our HPLC method is based on an earlier version [1] with a normal-phase (silica) column and a mobile phase consisting of an ether, methanol and a trace of aqueous ammonia. The method needed improvement.

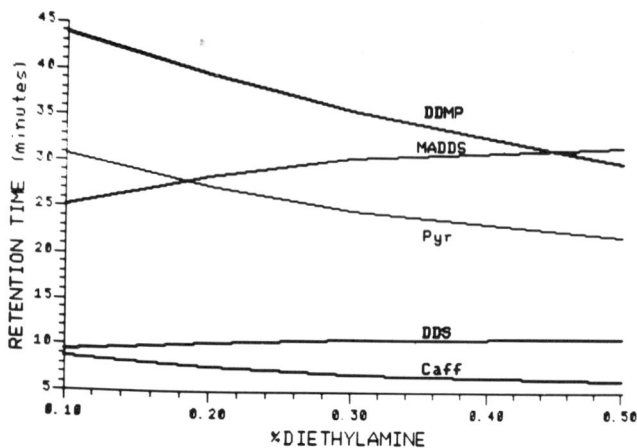

Fig. 1. Effect on retention time of increasing % diethylamine.

Firstly I tried a different ether (methyl tert-butyl); but this was too strongly eluotropic in itself. By diluting with hexane, the retentions of the 5 components were increased, but to different extents. The effects of partial replacement of methanol by acetonitrile were also examined, and also the aqueous ammonia was replaced by varying concentrations of diethylamine.

Each of these variables changed the elution order of the 5 components, so this information was fed into the computer when then produced the graph shown in Fig. 1. Thus, in effect, by changing the composition of the mobile phase, the peaks could be made to interchange and pass through one another on the chromatogram. We set out to illustrate this using a personal computer (IBM PC/TX) in which the chromatograms were simulated on the screen to fit the experimental data. The first programme was designed with the following objectives:
(1) to give the peaks different colours and make them gaussian in shape;
(2) to make peak heights fall and peak widths increase with retention time, by means of a quadratic function;
(3) to enable peaks to pass through one another without interacting in any way;
(4) to indicate by means of a symbolic thermometer the state of a given variable at any particular time.

Later a second programme was written in which the peaks were summed where they overlapped to give a more authentic effect. Clearly in both these programmes the chromatograms were an idealized representation of reality, no account being taken of peak symmetry or of changes in apparent column efficiency; but they did serve a useful purpose for illustration.

Limitations in memory capacity prevented direct animation of peak movements on the screen. Each chromatogram took ~15 sec to build up; hence a simple 8 mm cine camera was used in the single-frame mode to capture each completed chromatogram from the computer screen. The camera was operated directly by the computer so that the final film showed time-lapsed movements of peaks passing through one another and changing shape with time.

This exercise will be extended for training purposes to illustrate simple concepts such as the Van Deempter effect, and hopefully will be improved by the use of 16 mm cine, so as to avoid such problems as strobing with subsequent copying onto video tape.

No attempt to use this exercise for prediction has been made here; it simply clarifies presentation. However, by combination with a programme for mobile-phase optimization, a much better picture of the options available to a chromatographer could be obtained.

Reference

1.   Jones, C.R. & Overell, S.M. (1979) *J. Chromatog. 163, 179-185.*

#NC(C)-10

A Note on

BULKY ION-PAIR REVERSED-PHASE HPLC:

SOME APPLICATIONS IN BIOMEDICAL RESEARCH

Hermann–Josef Egger[†] and Guy Fischer

Biological Pharmaceutical Research Department
F. Hofmann–La Roche & Co. Ltd.
CH–4002 Basel, Switzerland

The simultaneous determination of substances with large chromato-graphic differences, e.g. parent drug and its more polar metabolites, may present difficulties [exemplified in Vol. 12, this series - *Ed.*]. The approach now outlined is an alternative to gradient elution and column-switching techniques. By ion-pairing between the different analytes and 'bulky' ion-pairing reagents, the contribution of the reagent can be such as to reduce the retention differences between the analytes. Thereby a group separation of the analytes from inter-fering substances and hence a decreased limit of determination may be achieved.

THE PROBLEM AND THE APPROACH

The starting point was the development of an analytical method for determining 5'-deoxy-5-fluorouridine (5'-dFUR) and its metabolite 5-fluorouracil (5-FU). Both substances are highly water-soluble and have to be extracted from plasma with a polar extractant such as ethyl acetate. Using 'conventional' RP-HPLC (C-18 silica; 0.1 M phosphate buffer pH 5.0 and 1-4% organic modifier), conditions for isocratic determination of both compounds could not be obtained due to the limited amount of organic modifier in the mobile phase (Fig. 1). Even gradi-ent-elution techniques failed, due to co-extracted interferences. Therefore we tried to achieve specific retardation of these compounds with respect to interfering compounds either via specific interactions (unpublished work by ourselves and by H-J. Egger & W. Bannwarth) or via ion-pair chromatography [1, 2].

Fig. 2 shows the basic principle. If, with great simplification, one considers only the ion-pair adsorption model (the formed ion-pairs

---

[†] now at Ciba-Geigy (Central Research), Basel

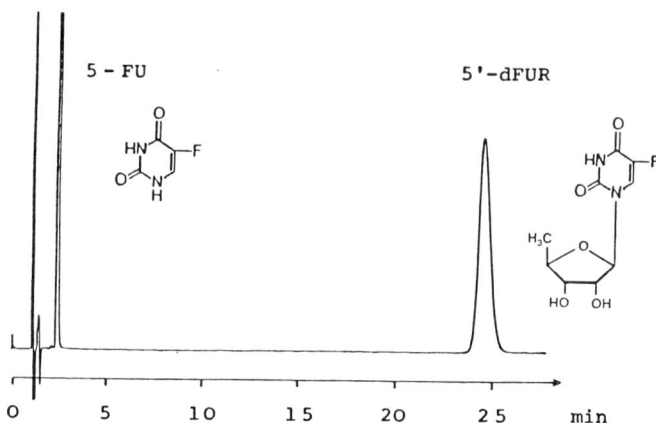

Fig. 1.   Separation obtained using conventional RP-HPLC.   Column: Hypersil ODS 5 μm, 125 × i.d. 4 mm.   Mobile phase: 0.1 M KH_2PO_4/ methanol (99:1 by vol.); 1 ml/min.   *From ref. [1], courtesy of Elsevier.*

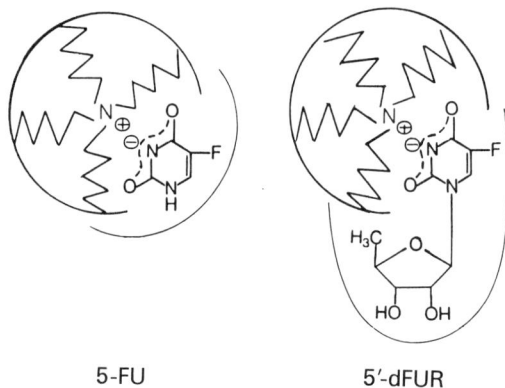

Fig. 2.   Reduction of retention differences between 5-FU and 5'-dFUR by ion-pair formation with bulky ion-pairs. *From ref. [3], courtesy of Elsevier.* [pKa 8.0 for FU, 7.7 for 5'-dFUR.]

5-FU   5'-dFUR

are retained by solvophobic interactions), the differences in k' between the nucleobase and the nucleoside (cf. Fig. 1) should shrink with lessening of the influence of the additional sugar moiety of the nucleoside in relation to the total size of the ion-pair formed, i.e. the more space-occupying, voluminous or 'bulky' the ion-pairing reagent is. Therefore the effectiveness, in reducing the k' differences, of 'bulky' ion-pairing reagents having more than one long aliphatic chain, e.g. tetraoctylammonium salts, will certainly exceed that of 'single chain' ion-pairing reagents such as n-alkyl-trimethyl-ammonium salts.

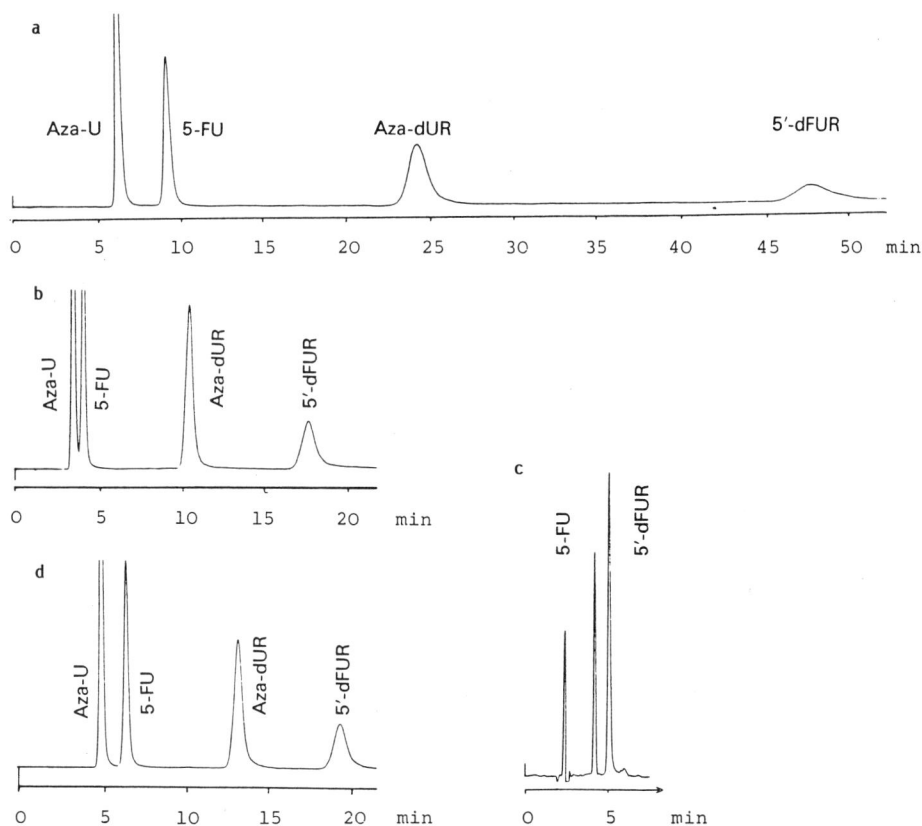

Fig. 3. Retention of two analytes (Aza–U = 6-azauracil, Aza–dUR = 5'-deoxy-6-azauridine) as affected by the ion-pairing reagent, single-chain - **a**, hexadecyl-trimethyl-ammonium bromide, or bulky: **b**, tetrabutyl-ammonium bromide; **c**, tetrahexyl-ammonium bromide; **d**, trioctyl-methyl-ammonium bromide. Column: Spherisorb ODS 2, 5 μm, 250 × i.d. 4 mm; 1 ml/min. Mobile phase: 5 mM phosphate buffer pH 8.5/acetonitrile - 95:5 or, for **d**, 70:30; 1 mM or, for **d**, 2.5 mM ion-pairing reagent. *From [1], courtesy of Elsevier.*

The influence of the type and size of the ion-pairing reagent is shown in Fig. 3, a-d. With bulky reagents such as trioctyl-methyl- or tetraoctyl-ammonium bromide, even baseline separations of 5-FU and 5'-dFUR can be obtained (Fig. 3d).

APPLICATIONS

Determination of 5–FU and 5'–dFUR.– A method for their simultaneous isocratic determination has been developed [3], with HPLC as shown in Fig. 4. By selective retardation of both compounds, the limit of

Fig. 4. Human blank plasma spiked with 50 and 100 ng/ml respectively of 5-FU and 5'dFUR, demonstrating the limit of determination. Column: Ultrasphere ODS, 5 μm, 250 × i.d. 4.6 mm. Mobile phase: 5 mM phosphate buffer pH 8.0/acetonitrile, (75:25) containing 5 mM tetraheptyl-ammonium chloride, apparent pH 8.4; 1 ml/min. *From [1], courtesy of Elsevier.*

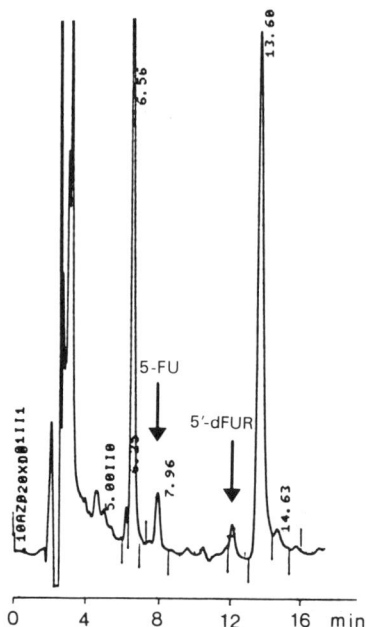

quantification could be reduced from 500 down to 100 ng/ml for the slower component; simultaneously 5-FU could be determined down to 50 ng/ml. Because of the high pKa values of 5-FU (8.0) and 5'-dFUR (7.7) the apparent pH of the mobile phase had to be adjusted to ~8.4. Although alkaline mobile phases had to be used, the column life was ~2 months. We assume that the silica surface is well covered by a layer of bulky ion-pairing reagent which prevents the direct attack of hydroxyl ions.

Separation of other nucleobases and nucleosides.- Using dioctyl-sulphosuccinate (20 mM), other nucleobases and nucleosides with an amino group could be separated [1]; thus a mixture of adenine, cytosine, guanine and the corresponding 2'-deoxy nucleosides separated on a column as in Fig. 3 (but 125, not 250 mm) with 70:30 20 mM phosphate pH 2.8/acetonitrile. Other 'bulky' ion-pairing reagents might be used, e.g. dialkylaminosulphonates (may be synthesized from the corres-poinding dialkylamines), or branched sulphonic acids [4,5].

Separation of an ester and its corresponding acid.- Using conventional RP-HPLC, the cephalosporanic acid and ester shown opposite are eluted with ~10% and ~30% organic modifier respectively, whereas baseline separation is obtainable by bulky ion-pair RP-HPLC (Fig. 5).

COMMENTS

Since the bulky trialkylmethyl- and tetraalkyl-ammonium salts tend to precipitate at alkaline pH, 5 and 20 mM respectively represent the concentration limits for the reagent and buffer. The precipi-

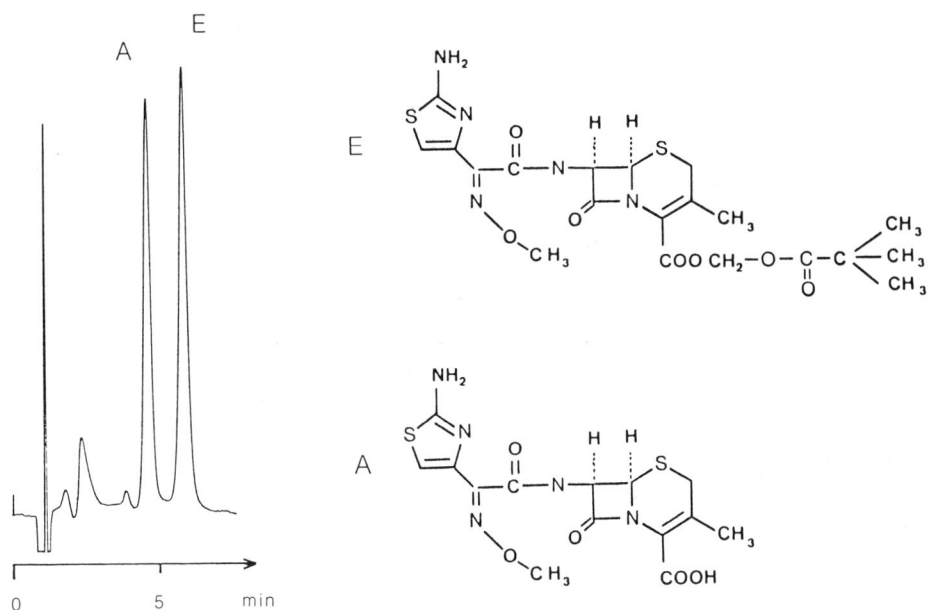

Fig. 5. Separation of a cephalosporanic acid (A) and its pivaloyl-methyl ester (E). Column: as for Fig. 3, but 125 mm. Mobile phase 10 mM phosphate pH 6.5/acetonitrile (70:30) containing 5 mM tetra-octyl-ammonium bromide; 1 ml/min.

tation is, of course, dependent on the amount of organic modifier used. At pH >10, precipitation generally occurs.

Subject to this limitation, with an appropriate choice of ion-pairing reagent conditions can be obtained which allow the simultaneous analysis of substances differing widely in k'. Thereby gradient elution and column-switching techniques can be avoided.

References

1. Egger, H-J. & Fischer, G. (1986) *J. Chromatog.*, submitted.
2. Egger, H-J. & Fischer, G. (1985) in *Vortrage anlässlich der Königsteiner Chromatographie-Tage* (Aigner, H., ed.), Waters (Millipore).
3. Egger, H-J. & Fischer, G. (1986) *J. Chromatog.*, submitted.
4. Vivian, D.L. & Reid, E.E. (1935) *J. Am. Chem. Soc.* 57, 2559-2560.
5. Freeman, F. & Angletakis, Ch.N.(1982) *J. Am. Chem. Soc.* 104, 5766-5774.

Comments on material in #C

Comments on #C-1, B. Caddy - NOVEL CAPILLARY-GC PHASES
   & #NC(C)- 6, H. Frank - GC DERIVATIZER

Remarks by R.A. de Zeeuw.- Although it cannot be denied that looking at novel stationary phases for capillary GC serves various purposes, its usefulness may be limited. If we look at the developments in GC, TLC and HPLC it becomes clear that despite many attempts to devise novel stationary phases, only a few have survived and are in common use today. However, even with these 'work-horses' such as OV-1, silica-gel G or RP-18, it remains a problem to put well-defined, reproducible batches on the market. Accordingly, analytical chemists should also be urged to devote time and effort to this problem of (non-)reproducibility in stationary phase material. This is of vital importance to the further advancement of chromatography even though such work is extremely time-consuming, is of repetitive character and is not very appealing from a so-called scientific point of view.

A. Hulshoff.- Stationary phases for capillary GC of carboxylic acids have been described. Why is it that almost everybody still derivatizes the carboxylic acids prior to GC? (Possibly the performance of these columns deteriorates when introducing 'real' samples.) **H. Frank, replying:** non-derivatization may be feasible for short-chain carboxylic acids, but there are problems with long-chain, particularly peak-height variability. **H. Frank, answering B. Gordon** who asked about carry-over problems in the auto-injection systems used routinely especially after derivatization.- No problems exist, as the derivatization takes place in individual vials and the derivatized sample does not come into contact with any part of the derivatizer or its reagent delivery system; however, as the automated derivatizer has just started to be employed on a routine basis in an outside pharmaceutical company, one has to wait for the results of real routine use during coming months.

Comments on #C-2, R.D. McDowall/J.G. Pearce - CARTRIDGE & 'AASP' USE
   & #NC(C)-7 - ROBOTICS;
   also #NC(C)-8 - C.R.J. Ceelen, H.M. Ruijten & H. de Bree - AN
   ASSAY WITH USE OF 'AASP' AND HPLC

Question by R. Whelpton to H. de Bree: have you linked an AASP to an EC detector? **Reply by de Bree:** I have not heard of any success with such a combination. **Comment by R.D. McDowall.-** After 6 months we gave up because of large baseline perturbation. K.C. van Horne from Analytichem International visited us and suggested   this problem was due to elution of silanes from the phenylboronic acid solid phase we were using. As a short-term remedy a dichloromethane or hexane wash prior to use might remove the problem; in the long term they would have to alter the method of synthesis of the phase. **R. Schmid suggested** that the EC baseline perturbation might be due to oxygen contained in the cartridge when compressed. **Reply.-** This seems not to be the case, since there was no improvement when we used the purge pump to pass through the cartridge up to 225 µl of mobile phase prior to elution. **Remarks by R. Schmid.-** Band broadening can occur if, as should never happen in off-line work, the column (cartridge) is allowed to dry out, resulting in non-wetting and irregular elution from the analytical column. Moreover, the AASP cartridges have a coarse packing, rather loose, and are only 3 mm diam. such that wall effects are manifest.

   Remarks by J.E.H. Stafford.- There is a risk that the amount of solid phase used may be inadequate to achieve quantitative extraction of a drug analyte (our experience at Searle with RP cartridges in the AASP system). With this in mind, we have used the Zymark robot system to automate the use of BondElut columns for drug extraction; the system has been use for 18 months already. **H. de Bree asked J.G. Pearce** whether with the robotics system there is any risk of carry-over between high-concentration samples and blanks? **Reply:** no; all parts that the sample touches are disposable.

Some citations contributed by Senior Editor

GC assays for various drugs

   Assay of **isosorbide dinitrate** and its mononitrate metabolites in plasma: GC-ECD methods have been reported besides those considered in Vol. 14 by A.J. Woodward et al. After adding $AgNO_3$ as stabilizer and extracting with chloroform, use of a conventional column enabled 1 ng/ml of drug to be measured [1]. Similar sensitivity was obtained by use of WCOT silica columns after solid-phase extraction [2].

   In determining **chloroquine** and metabolites (de-ethylated) in blood, plasma and urine with a silica capillary column, two types of stationary phase were investigated; the analytes, solvent-extracted at alkaline pH with a back-extraction into aqueous acid, were injected by the falling needle technique, and measured with a N-S thermionic detector [3]. A GC method, with a conventional column and AFID, has been described for **diethylcarbamazine** (an antifilarial), solvent-extracted from plasma at alkaline pH; 50 ng/ml was detectable [4]. 'Oltipraz', a new antishistosomal (a pyrazine with sulphur moieties), was solvent-extracted from blood and assayed by GC-FID with a conventional column (1-2 µg/ml detectable) [5]. GC-AFID served to determine **dicyclomine** [6] and **glycopyrronium** ([7]; capillary GC, with an 'ion-pair complex') after solvent extraction from plasma.

Besides the foregoing examples of GC assays, and the following exam-
ples of 'straightforward' HPLC assays, some are cited in a 'chiral'
or 'sample handling' context (below), and others are cited late
in #NC(D) at the end of section #D, e.g. where assay approaches were
compared or where HPLC entailed EC detection. Cf. #NC(B), CNS drugs.

HPLC assays for drugs detectable by UV or intrinsic fluorescence

RP-HPLC assays for **dipyrone** [8] and **bupranolol** [9] and their
respective metabolites have been described for plasma, solvent-extracted at an appropriate pH. Plasma and urinary levels of **verapamil**
and dealkylated metabolites have been measured, by fluorescence,
after ether extractions with a back-extraction [10]. For the anti-
inflammatory agent **nabumetone** [4-(6-methoxy-2-naphthyl)butan-2-one) a
C-18 HPLC method has been described, the drug and an acidic metabolite being detected by fluorescence; the respective sensitivities
were 0.25 and 0.1 µg/ml of plasma (which was solvent-extracted
initially) [11].

In the cancer chemotherapy context, methods have been developed
for the assay of **ceftriaxone** in serum and urine [12] and for **4'-epi-
doxorubicin** and its 13-dihydro derivative (fluorescence detection)
in plasma [13]. Another example is **'BCNU'** [1,3-bis(2-chloroethyl)-
1-nitrosourea], solvent-extracted from plasma for RP-HPLC [14].

Examples of drugs assayed by RP-HPLC without initial extraction
of the plasma are **phenprocoumon** (anticoagulant) [15] and (deproteinization by ethanol) **metronidazole** and **tinidazole** [16]. NP-HPLC was
used for **metronidazole** in membrane-filtered plasma or urine [17] and
for a quaternary ammonium ion, **prifinium** [18]. Besides RP-HPLC [19,
radial compression column; 20], NP-HPLC [20] has served in assaying
plasma and urine for **omeprazole** with its sulphone and sulphide. For
labetalol in plasma, solvent-extracted, the column packing was 'PRP-1'
[macroporous poly(styrene-divinylbenzene)]; detection was by fluorescence [21]. For pioneer studies by W. Dieterle & J.W. Faigle with
this type of packing, see Vol. 12, this series.

References

1. Morrison, R.A. & Fung, H-L. (1984) *J. Chromatog. 308*, 153-164.
2. Santoni, Y., Rolland, P.H. & Cano, J-P. (1984) *J. Chromatog.
   306*, 165-172.
3. Bergqvist, Y. & Eckerbom, S. (1984) *J. Chromatog. 306*, 147-153,
4. Nene, S., Anjaneyulu, B. & Rajagopalan, T.G. (1984) *J. Chromatog.
   308*, 334-340.
5. Ali, H.M., Bennet, J.L., Sulaiman, S.M. & Gaillot, J. (1984)
   J. Chromatog. 305, 465-469.
6. Beretta, E. & Vanazzi, G. (1984) *J. Chromatog. 308*, 341-344.
7. Murray, G.R., Calvey, T.N. & Williams, N.E. (1984) *J. Chromatog.
   308*, 143-151.
8. Katz, E.Z. & Grant, L. (1984) *J. Chromatog. 305*, 477-484.

9. Walmsley, R.M., Brodie, R.R. & Chasseaud, L.F. (1984) *J. Chromatog. 311*, 227-233.

10. Barbieri, E., Padrini, R., Piovan, D., Toffoli, M., Cargnelli, G. Trevi, G. & Ferrari, M. (1985) *Int. J. Clin. Pharmacol. 5*, 99-107.

11. Ray, J.E. & Day, R.O. (1984) *J. Chromatog. 336*, 234-238.

12. Salvador, R.P., Smith, G., Weinfeld, R.E., Ellis, D.H. & Bodey, G.P. (1983) *Antimicrob. Agents Chemother. 23*, 583-588.

13. Moro, E., Jannzzo, M.G., Ranghieri, M., Stegnjaich, S. & Valzelli, G. (1982) *J. Chromatog. 230*, 207-211.

14. Yeager, R.L., Oldfield, E.H. & Chatterji, D.C. (1984) *J. Chromatog. 305*, 496-501.

15. De Vries, J.X., Harenberg, J., Walter, E., Zimmermann, R. & Simon, M. (1982) *J. Chromatog. 231*, 83-92.

16. Mattilla, J., Mannisto, P.T., Mantyla, R., Nykanen, S. & Lamminsivu, U. (1983) *Antimicrob. Agents Chemother. 23*, 721-725.

17. Adamovics, J. (1984) *J. Chromatog. 309*, 436-440.

18. Tokuma, Y., Tamura, Y. & Noguchi, H. (1982) *J. Chromatog. 231*, 129-136.

19. Mihaly, G., Prichard, P.J., Smallwood, R.A., Yeomans, N.D. & Louis, W.J. (1983) *J. Chromatog. 278*, 311-319.

20. Lagerström, P-O. & Persson, B-A. (1984) *J. Chromatog. 309*, 347-356.

21. Alton, K.B., Leitz, F., Bariletto, S., Jaworsky, L., Desrivieres, D. & Patrick, J. (1984) *J. Chromatog. 311*, 319-328.

Sample handling: approaches, and the wherewithal (incl. automation)

Pre-HPLC extraction **by solid-phase or solvent approaches** was simple and effective for plasma **cortisol** [22] and (glassy-carbon EC detection) for an **amine-derived glycol**, 3-methoxy-4-hydroxyphenyl-glycol, in urine, plasma and brain [23]. Urine to be assayed for **aztreonam** was subjected to solid-phase clean-up; plasma was deproteinized with acetonitrile/dichloromethane [24].

Solid-phase extraction devices have been described: Pasteur-type pipettes as an alternative to cartridges [25], and vacuum-operated assemblies for multi-cartridge handling [26, 27]. An automated **HPLC column switching** assembly was devised for assaying a new **cephalosporin** in urine or deproteinized plasma [28]. The analyte-enriched eluate from an initial anion-exchange (DEAE) column was concentrated on a short RP column before analytical separation (C-18; 295 nm detection); 0.5 or (plasma) 0.05 µg/ml was measurable.

Robotics and automation, especially for performing HPLC, have been surveyed in a 1985 issue (No. 2 of Vol. 4) of *Trends Anal. Chem.* and in a sketch from a drug-company laboratory [29]. The Gilson system [30] provides for pre-HPLC steps such as sampling and derivatization, but not for extraction.

Capillary-GC sample introduction terminology and procedures have been discussed in the context of unfortunate ambiguities [31].

References

22. Hofreiter, B.T., Mizera, A.C., Allen, J.P., Masi, A.M. & Hicok, W.C. (1983) *Clin. Chem. 29*, 1808-1809.
23. Karege, F. (1984) *J. Chromatog. 311*, 361-368.
24. Mihindu, J.C.L., Scheld, W.M., Bolton, N.D., Spyker, D.A., Schwabb, E.A. & Bolton, W.K. (1983) *Antimicrob. Agents Chemother. 24*, 252-261.
25. Nicholls, C.R. (1985) *Lab. Pract. 34 (8)*, 68-69.
26. Wright, H., Smith, B.S.W. & Brown, K.G. (1985) *Lab. Pract. 34 (11)*, 78-79.
27. Brown, W.C.B. & Hyslop, W. (1984) *Lab. Pract. 33 (5)*, 83-84.
28. Tokuma, Y., Shiozaki, Y. & Noguchi, H. (1984) *J. Chromatog. 311*, 339-346.
29. Clarke, G.S. & Robinson, M.L. (1985) *Anal. Proc. 22*, 137-138.
30. Verillon, F.s & Glandian, S. (1985) *Int. Lab.*, Oct., 36-41.
31. Pretorius, V. & Bertsch, W. (1983) *J. High Resolu. Chromatog. Chromatog. Comm. 6*, 64-67.

HPLC packings and separation strategy or problems

In RP-HPLC, skewing of peaks was related, for **naproxen** assay in plasma, to strong binding to serum albumin [32], whereas distorted and multiple peaks were thought, in the case of **metronidazole**, to be due to disturbance of the mobile phase by organic solvents used to deproteinize the serum initially [33].

In an assay procedure for **oxmeditine** and metabolites (glucuronides of the drug and its sulphone) in biological fluids [34], an NP-HPLC system was developed for plasma, and an RP-HPLC system suited well for urine and bile, but with plasma was prone to blank interferences [35]. With a suitable mobile phase the drug and its sulphoxide could be distinguished. The initial step was n-octanol extraction at alkaline pH; glucuronides were hydrolyzed if the total amount of each compound was to be ascertained.) The urine assay went awry (skewed peaks, poorer resolution) when, as it turned out, an 'improved' factory process for 'end-capping' Ultrasphere ODS columns – abolishing free silanols – affected analyte chromatography. With a modified mobile phase the RP approach was restored to health and was applicable to plasma as well as urine, once a solution had been found to a new problem, viz. split peaks. Sample preparation had entailed adding acetonitrile and Na_2CO_3 to the octanol extract and recovering the analyte in an acetonitrile layer; use of ethanol instead of acetonitrile overcame the HPLC problem [35].

Use of **alumina as an HPLC packing** has been appraised [36]. Besides being a polar adsorbent by virtue of OH groups, as for silica, it can interact with basic solutes through nucleophilic interaction and can form charge complexes with electron-donor solutes, e.g. aromatic. With appropriate pre-washing, alumina can have cation- or anion-exchange properties in appropriate pH ranges; a particular pH, influenced by the buffer anion, represents the zero point of [net surface] charge ('ZPC'). Illustrative model compounds included procaine, codeine and morphine; applicability to proteins is also discussed.

For **salbutamol,** which is so hydrophilic that it cannot be solvent-extracted, an ion-pair reagent (Na heptane sulphonate) was used in the C-8 HPLC mobile phase and also the initial solid-phase extraction of the rabbit plasma [37].

References

32. Wahlund, K.G. & Arvidsson, T. (1983) *J. Chromatog. 282,* 527-539.
33. Wollard, G.A. (1984) *J. Chromatog. 303,* 222-224.
34. Lee, R.M, & McDowall, R.D. (1983) *J. Chromatog. 273,* 335-345.
35. Murkitt, G.S., Lee, R.M. & McDowall, R.D. (1984) *Anal. Proc. 21,* 246-248.
36. Billiet, H., Laurent, C. & de Galan, L. (1985) *Trends Anal. Chem. 4,* 100-103.
37. Kurosawa, N., Morishima, S., Owade, E. & Ito, K. (1984) *J. Chromatog. 305,* 485-488.

Comments (at the Forum) on #**NC(C)-9,** C.R. Jones, HPLC OPTIMIZATION

R. Whelpton, concerning film shown by C.R. Jones on HPLC optimi-zation.- Were you suggesting that peak area was better than peak height for overlapping peaks? Doesn't the area more or less double when the peak height doubles? **Reply.-** No! This is true only when one peak is centralized under the other. The film showed that when a small peak is only just obscured by a larger one, the peak height of the larger may be almost unchanged although the areas will be the sum of the two. **Remark by R. Schmid.-** If different modifications of the solvent system could be combined in a 3-D representation of the chromatogram, this would be informative and helpful.

Comments on #**C-3,** I.W. Wainer - CHIRAL HPLC

S. Fowles asked, concerning retention and selectivity (usually increase with decreasing temperature), what temperature gives best results with CSP's? **I.W. Wainer's reply.-** The optimum is ~20°; a lowered temperature may be advantageous when acidic mobile-phase additives are used, since pH lowering adversely affects selectivity and retention. **Wainer, in response to A.A. Gulaid** who had found a rather short column life with biological samples (as distinct from standards; maybe less prone to happen with BSA than with Pirkle-type CSP's): one can use a C-18 column for clean-up, then switch to the chiral column; the C-18 column can serve to separate the compounds of interest, and the chiral column for enantiomer separation.

R. Whelpton remarked: it is disappointing that good separation often calls for derivatization even with chiral HPLC columns. What are the possibilities for tertiary amines in very low concentration? **Reply:** tertiary amines can be chromatographed and resolved on Pirkle-type CSP's by use of naphthylchloroformate as a derivatizing agent. Concerning α-acid glycoprotein CSP's, **K.G. Feitsma asked** about biological applications. **Reply.-** We have no experience, but drug studies have been performed by Hermansson (cf. [43] in my art., above). This type of column may manifest concentration effects on k' and α; concerning possible low efficiency (**replying to query by A. Hulshoff**) plate heights ranged from 0.07 to 0.28 mm in drug-enantiomer separations (e.g. tocainide, ephedrine, metoprolol) at pH 6.6 (0.02 M phosphate, with or without 0.003 M tetrapropylammonium bromide). **Question by K.K. Midha.-** Does any racemization occur when d- or l-methamphetamine is derivatized with naphthylchloroformate? **Wainer's reply:** none has been observed.

Comments on #**NC(C)-1**, R.P. Richards - DERIVATIZED ENANTIOMERS BY GC & #**NC(C)-2**, I.D. Wilson - CHIRAL TLC TRIALS

B. Scales, to R.P. Richards concerning his GC-ECD assay of diastereoisomers: does urine give more interfering peaks than plasma? **Reply:** we have not tried assaying urine. **Remark by H. Frank to I.D. Wilson:** for mandelic acid I would employ chiral GC!

Remarks by U.A.Th. Brinkman to I.D. Wilson.- The manufacture of a 'chiral plate' is a sophisticated procedure, and the plate used for the two-stage treatment is not a normal-type Macherey-Nagel plate. For tertiary amines a chiral plate gives excellent separations. Concerning β-cyclodextrin plates, Armstrong (cf. ref. [30] in Wainer's art., above) has already used the HPLC-CSP material (available from Astec) to coat TLC plates, but for economic reasons they are not yet available commercially; separations are apparently good, but the fit of the molecule within the conical CSP molecule has to be rather tight, and the 'active' centre of the analyte should be at the outer rim. With the 'Wainer plate' the problem is that the coating reagent is easily oxidized in air, giving a rather dark (violet) place; besides, the intrinsic fluorescence severely handicaps screening for fluorescent derivatives as commonly employed. **Remark by A. Hulshoff.-** Your finding of R_f invariability with varying methanol concentration might be due to two opposing factors: stripping of the β-cyclodextrin from the plate at higher methanol concentrations (tending to lower the R_f), and the higher R_f usually obtained in the RP mode with higher methanol concentrations.

SOME CITATIONS contributed by Senior Editor

HPLC chiral separations with a CSP

For a 'DNBPG' **chiral phase** (Baker Chemical Co.; cf. foregoing art. by I.W. Wainer), a report from the company laboratory [1] deals with optimization of the mobile phase. The enantiomeric model compounds were mainly as used by other chiral HPLC investigators (cf. foregoing art. by I.W. Wainer): they included amphetamine, propranolol, a phenyloxazolidine, a benzodiazepinone, and a nitro-imidazole - generally with an introduced naphth(o)yl or naphthylamide group. An example of optimization for several enantiomers was substitution of t-butanol for 2-propanol or ethanol as the polar partner to hexane in a binary mobile phase.

D.R. Taylor [2] has summarized studies in his laboratory on **CSP development** and behaviour [e.g. 3], studied with model racemates: typically these were alkyl esters of *N*-acyl amino acids. (The *N*- and *O*-protection served to impart adequate solubility in non-polar solvents.) HPLC was performed mainly under NP conditions, with chiral packings comprising aminopropylated silica gel to which *N*-protected amino acid enantiomers were attached, particularly L-isoleucine. With formyl as the protecting group, separations were especially satisfactory. Similar packings developed elsewhere are considered.

GC experience led a Japanese group [4] to develop HPLC CSP's with the *s*-triazine derivative of a short peptide or α-naphthyl-ethylamine bonded to silanized silica. The model racemates tested, in *N*-substituted form, were representative alcohols, amino acids and other carboxylic acids, and amines of phenylethylamine type. In another laboratory [5], chiral analytes such as 2,2'-dihydroxy-1,1'-binaphthyl were resolved with amine-bonded silica (3-glycidoxy-propyltrimethyloxysilane as reactant). The overall picture is that the area of CSP development, dominated by amino acid resolutions, still has no new 'message' for drug-enantiomer determination as comprehensively surveyed by Wainer (#C-3, above).

Separations by GC or, for analyte diastereoisomers, by HPLC

Mephenytoin and its *N*-desmethyl metabolite were each resolved (underivatized) by capillary GC, with an acidic pH for blood or plasma extraction and with detection by NPD (AFID); the CSP was Chirasil-Val [6]. The following citations concern chromatography of **diastereo-isomers without a CSP**. Enantiomers of **propranolol** are separable by GC or HPLC after derivatization to give diastereomers [7]. **Tocainide** enantiomers, solvent-extracted from plasma and derivatized with a chiral reagent having ECD-responsive fluorines, have been separated by GC [8], this being an alternative approach to capillary GC with a CSP, Chirasil-Val, after non-chiral derivatization [9].

For resolution of **amphetamines by RP–HPLC** (detection at 220 or 254 nm), four chiral reagents were investigated [10]. The reagents included sugar isothiocyanates (with a base catalyst), and the test compounds included l-phenylethylamine and p-chloroamphetamine. The authors, who cite literature on analytes such as catecholamines, envisage applicability to biological samples, and note that <100 ng of derivative on-column is detectable. **NP–HPLC for an amphetamine** (2,5-dimethoxy-4-methyl-) in plasma, with fluorescence detection: diastereoisomer formation was done by use of D- or L-l-aminoethyl-4-dimethylamino-naphthalene in the presence of a water-soluble diimide as 'catalyst'[11]. **Indoprofen** [12] and **warfarin** [13] have been studied.

The following examples concern HPLC separation of **inherently diastereomeric analytes:** synthetic **angiotensin I's** (anion-exchange or RP-HPLC) [14]; a *cis* compound, **nadolol** (NP) [15]; and **temocillin** (RP) with investigation of configuration by NMR and of epimerization of each diastereoisomer in the natural mixture [16].

HPLC separations with a chiral eluent; also a 'kinetic' approach

For **a piperazine** analgesic, 1-[2-(3-hydroxyphenyl)-1-phenyl-ethyl]-4-(3-methyl-2-butenyl)piperazine, whose enantiomers differ in pharmacological activity, RP-HPLC separation was achieved by adding β-cyclodextrin to the mobile phase [17]. A laboratory which had already used this approach for mandelic acid has now explored the effectiveness of α- or β-cyclodextrin for separating isomers of **cinnamic acids,** including positional isomers [18]. Another study centered on model compounds (as distinct from drugs in plasma) made use of a copper complex of L-phenylalanine as the chiral component; besides tryptophan and hydroxytryptophan, the analytes included **methyldopa, thyroxine** and iodothyronine [19]. In contrast, enantiomeric iodinated thyronines in plasma and urine have been resolved by RP-HPLC after chiral derivatization (E.P. Lankmayr; Vol. 14, this series).

For studying the stereoselective metabolism of **dimethylpropion** and its desmethyl metabolite, Beckett & co-workers [20] applied an approach they had published in 1972 [21] based on differences in the rates at which isomers give rise to oxazolidines when reacted at acid pH with acetone. The metabolic investigation centred on a range of enantiomeric or diastereomeric **ephedrines** (also **diethylpropion**) and entailed use of a GC system appropriate to each separation. Separation of *threo* and *erythro* isomers was in fact achievable; but there were co-elution problems with metabolite peaks, hence the oxazolidine approach. Detection was by FID.

General survey of racemate resolution: see [22]; ion-pairing ref.: [23]. Drugs in biological matrices [24]: 538 refs. on **GC derivatization, incl. chiral.**

References

1. Zief, M., Crane, L.J. & Horvath, J. (1984) *J. Liq. Chromatog.* *7*, 709-730.

2. Taylor, D.R. (1984) *Anal. Proc. 21*, 199-200. See also ref. 22.

3. Akanya, J.N., Hitchen, S.M. & Taylor, D.R. (1982) *Chromatographia 16*, 224-227.

4. Ôi, N., Nagase, M. & Sawada, Y. (1984) *J. Chromatog. 292*, 427-431.

5. Sinibaldi, M., Carunchio, V., Corradini, C. & Girelli, A.M. (1984) *Chromatographia 18*, 459-461.

6. Wedlund, P.J., Sweetman, B.J., McAllister, C.B., Branch, R.A. & Wilkinson, G.R. (1984) *J. Chromatog. 307*, 121-127.

7. Thompson, J.A., Holtzman, J.L., Tsuru, M., Lerman, C.L. & Holtzman, J.E. (1982) *J. Chromatog. 306*, 470-475.

8. Sedman, A.J. & Gal, J. (1984) *J. Chromatog. 306*, 155-164.

9. Antonsson, A-M., Glyllenhaal, O., Kylberg-Hanssen, K., Johansson, L. & Vessman, J. (1984) *J. Chromatog. 308*, 181-187.

10. Miller, K.J., Gal, J. & Ames, M.M. (1984) *J. Chromatog. 307*, 335-342.

11. Goto, J., Goto, N., Hikichi, A. & Nambara, T. (1979) *J. Liq. Chromatog. 2*, 1179-1190.

12. Tamassia, V., Jannuzzo, M.G., Moro, E., Stegnjaich, S., Groppi, W. & Nicolis, F.B. (1984) *Int. J. Clin. Pharm. Res. 4*, 223-230.

13. Banfield, C. & Rowland, M. (1984) *J. Pharm. Sci. 73*, 1392-1396.

14. Margolis, S.A. & Dizdaroglu, M. (1985) *J. Chromatog. 322*, 117-128.

15. Piotrovskii, V.K., Zhirkov, Yu.A. & Metelitsa, V.I. (1984) *J. Chromatog. 309*, 421-425.

16. Bird, A.E., Charsley, C-H., Jennings, K.R. & Marshall, A.C. (1984) *Analyst 109*, 1209-1212.

17. Nobuhara, Hirano, S. & Nakanishi, Y. (1983) *J. Chromatog. 258*, 276-279.

18. Sybilska, D., Debrowski, J., Jurczak, J. & Zukowski, J. (1984) *J. Chromatog. 286*, 163-170.

19. Oelrich, E., Preusch, H. & Wilhelm, E. (1980) *J. High. Resolu. Chromatog. Chromatog. Comm. 3*, 269-272.

20. Markantonis, S.L., Kyroudis, A. & Beckett, A.H. (1986) *Biochem. Pharmacol. 35*, 529-532.

21. Testa, B. & Beckett, A.H. (1972) *J. Chromatog. 71*, 39-54.

22. Taylor, D.R. (1986) *Lab. Pract.*, January, 45-51.

23. Pettersson, C. & No, K. (1983) *J. Chromatog. 282*, 671-684.

24. Hulshoff, A. & Lingeman, H. (1984) *J. Pharm. Biomed. Anal. 2*, 337-380.

Solid-phase and HPLC separation of endogenous conjugates

Problems in assaying human bile for bile acid conjugates have been considered [25], with citation of past HPLC approaches (often at a low pH, detrimental to column efficiency). Satisfactory RP-HPLC separation of either glycine or taurine conjugates was achieved isocratically with methanol/pH 6 aqueous buffer containing octane-sulphonic acid. The two conjugated groups were pre-separated by differential elution (after initial C-18 extraction) from piperidinohydroxypropyl-Sephadex LH-20 (reacts with OH groups).

25. Campbell, G.R., Harriott, M. & Burns, D.T. (1986) *Anal. Proc. 23*, 33-34.

Section #D

APPROACHES TO ANALYTE DETECTION, IDENTIFICATION AND
MEASUREMENT

#D-1

THE APPLICATION OF HIGH RESOLUTION PROTON NMR SPECTROSCOPY TO THE DETECTION OF DRUG METABOLITES IN BIOLOGICAL SAMPLES

[1]J.K. Nicholson, [1]P.J. Sadler, [2]K. Tulip and [2]J.A. Timbrell

[1]Department of Chemistry
Birkbeck College
University of London
Malet Street
London WC1E 7HX

[2]Toxicology Unit
Department of Pharmacology
The School of Pharmacy
University of London
Brunswick Square
London WC1N 1AX

Recent developments in high-resolution ^{1}H NMR allow biological samples to be analyzed for certain low mol. wt. components with little or no sample pre-treatment. The ^{1}H NMR methods require only small sample volumes (0.3 ml), are non-destructive and usually give qualitative results within a few minutes if adequate steps are taken to reduce the intensity of the solvent water signal with an appropriate secondary irradiation field or pulse sequence. Notably, pre-selection of instrumental conditions to observe different classes of compound is not necessary, e.g. when studying compounds whose metabolic and excretory mechanisms are poorly understood.

The latter is the case for N-methylformamide (NMF), an experimental anti-tumour agent, but not for paracetamol. ^{1}H NMR has been applied to the detection and quantitation of urinary metabolites of these drugs. For paracetamol, the free drug and major metabolites (glucuronide, sulphate, cysteinyl and N-acetylcysteinyl conjugates) were all detected in untreated urine, and there was quantitative agreement with HPLC results. However, two-dimensional (2-D) NMR methods were required to separate the aromatic resonances of the cysteinyl conjugate and the free drug. For NMF, ^{1}H NMR measurements led to detection and identification of previously unknown metabolites including formic acid and a novel N-acetylcysteinyl derivative (N-acetyl-S-[N-methyl-carbamoyl]cysteine) as well as the parent compound and methylamine. Signals for various excreted compounds of endogenous origin are also manifest in ^{1}H NMR spectra of urine, so that information on the toxicological effects of drugs and xenobiotics can be obtained simultaneously with data on their metabolism.

In recent years, the rapid development of high-field Fourier transform NMR spectrometers with increased sensitivity, resolution and dynamic range has made possible the analysis of complex mixtures of low mol. wt. compounds in biological samples and non-invasive metabolic studies of intact biochemical systems. However, in comparison with most other spectroscopic techniques, sensitivity is relatively low (detection limit ~50 μM) even with ^{1}H NMR (protons being the most readily detectable magnetically-active nuclei). Nevertheless there are a number of intrinsic advantages that make the NMR approach to the detection of endogenous and drug metabolites worthy of more widespread attention. Previous studies have shown that ^{1}H NMR can also provide quantitative information on the concentrations of many low mol. wt. compounds present in plasma, urine, cells and cell extracts [1-6]. This method has advantages over HPLC and GC in that little or no pre-treatment of samples is required and a wide screen of many ^{1}H-containing metabolites in the mM range can be run within a few minutes.

Unlike most other techniques employed in biochemical analysis, NMR requires no instrumental pre-selection of analytical conditions (cf., in chromatography, the need to choose column size, packing material, eluent, flow rate and detector). Furthermore, the sample requirement is small (0.3 ml), and the technique is non-destructive and does not perturb equilibrium mixtures of compounds. These features are of great value in metabolism studies on small animals, where only limited volumes of sample are available that must serve for a number of biochemical assays, or in experiments that deal with unstable metabolites which would decompose under conventional sample 'clean-up' or isolation procedures.

INSTRUMENTAL REQUIREMENTS

^{1}H NMR spectroscopy of biological materials is hindered by three types of problem: (i) peak overlap due to large numbers of biomolecules appearing in a relatively narrow chemical shift range; (ii) dynamic range problems due to the intense (110 M) proton signal from solvent water; (iii) low sensitivity relative to chromatographic (e.g. HPLC) techniques and other spectroscopic techniques.

Problems (i) and (iii) can be minimized by using spectrometers of very high field strength. To date most of our work has involved the use of spectrometers with superconducting magnets of 9.5 T or 11.75 T field strength operating at proton resonance frequencies of 400 and 500 MHz respectively. For most purposes 400 MHz observation is adequate, but the combination of higher sensitivity and extra signal dispersion given by the 500 MHz instrument may be necessary, particularly when signals from structurally similar metabolites need to be distinguished or when concentrations are low. In some instances even 500 MHz measurements are insufficient to separate signals from related drug metabolites in biological fluids, e.g. those of paracetamol [5]. In such cases 2-D NMR experiments (e.g. homonuclear correlated spectroscopy, COSY; see below) can greatly increase the amount of useful spectral information, and resonances that are extensively over-lapped in the 1-D spectrum are easily resolved and identified [7].

The most important problems in the ^{1}H NMR measurement of metabol-ites in untreated biofluids concern dynamic range as affected by the presence of water. These can usually be overcome by applying a secondary irradiation field, continuous or gated (off during acquisi-tion), at the water resonance frequency, as done in the studies described below. The water signal may also be attenuated by use of efficient solvent-suppression pulse sequences, e.g. the 'DANTE' pulse train centered on the water signal [4] or by binomial pulse-sequences [8]. The use of water suppression is *essential* for obtaining good signal-to-noise levels for resonances of biomolecules in untreated biological fluids. These procedures are usually straightforward in modern NMR spectrometers, and may achieve solvent-suppression factors of up to 10^3. In very dilute solutions these solvent-suppres-sion methods may still be inadequate, and the residual water peak may give rise to a severe dynamic range problem.

Spectrometers with 16-bit digital-to-analogue converters rather than the standard 12-bit word-length offer a further improvement, as this minor hardware alteration immediately results in a 2^4-fold increase in dynamic range [4]. In samples containing high concentra-tions of macromolecules, e.g. plasma or cell suspensions, besides water suppression, spin-echo pulse sequences are required to eliminate broad overlapping resonances on the basis of their short T_2 relaxation times [2, 3]. In urine samples protein concentrations are rarely high enough to necessitate such measures, except in cases of severe glomeru-lar disease. It is, of course, possible to freeze-dry urine samples and redissolve in a reduced volume of ^{2}H$_2$O which largely eliminates dynamic range problems and increases the concentration of metabolites of interest. Obviously, however, such action may result in the loss of volatile or unstable metabolites and in selective deuteration of metabolites possessing exchangeable protons.

EXAMPLES PRESENTED

We now illustrate uses of high-resolution proton NMR in drug metabolism and excretion studies by reference to a widely used drug, paracetamol, which is excreted rapidly in the urine and whose metabolism is well understood, and an experimental anti-tumour agent, *N*-methyl-formamide, whose metabolic profile has been only partly elucidated. The aim of the paracetamol study was to compare quantitative NMR results obtained from human subjects with data obtained by other workers using HPLC for detection and quantitation [9]. The aim of the NMR study was to ascertain whether NMR could give any new insights into the metabolism of this compound in the rat.

METHODS

^{1}H NMR spectroscopy.- Bruker WH400 and AM500 NMR spectrometers were used in these studies, operating at 400 and 500 proton resonance frequencies respectively. All spectra were recorded at ambient probe temperature (typically 25°). For each sample 32-64 free induction decays were collected into 16,384 data points, using 45-60° pulses and a pulse repetition rate of ~5 sec. The water resonance was suppressed by continuous or gated irradiation at the water resonance frequency. Before Fourier transformation, the aggregated free induction decays were zero-filled to 32,768 data points, to improve digital resolution, and an exponential function corresponding to a line broadening of 1 Hz was applied. ^{2}H$_2$O was added to each urine sample (to 10% v/v) to provide an internal field-frequency lock. Chemical shifts were referenced internally to the singlet resonance of sodium 3-(trimethyl-silyl)[^{2}H]$_4$ propanoate (TSP, δ = 0 ppm, which was added at known concentration in the ^{2}H$_2$O). NMR spectral data for pure paracetamol metabolites have been reported previously [4].

COSY (2-D; see above) was also used on certain samples where there was extensive overlap of drug-metabolite resonances in urine samples; this gives correlation peaks for protons on adjacent carbon atoms that exhibit scalar J-coupling. This type of spectroscopy is a very important new tool for studying complex mixtures of structurally similar metabolites containing spin-spin coupled protons, as resonances with multiple overlaps can be analyzed

The pulse sequence used in this COSY investigation [7, 10] is:
$$[90° - t_1 - 90°- \text{collect}(t_2) - \text{relaxation delay}$$
where the initial 90° preparation pulse perturbs the magnetization from equilibrium into the xy detection plane. This magnetization precesses during the evolution period t_1, and the individual vectors become separated according to their appropriate Larmor precession frequencies (chemical shifts) and couplings. The second 90° pulse, the 'mixing' pulse, transfers magnetization between the various transitions of the coupled spin-systems, and the resulting magnetization that is collected during the acquisition time, t_2, depends both on the observed nucleus and on those coupled to it. For an uncoupled nucleus, U, magnetization transfer occurs only between transitions of that nucleus and thus results in a peak in the 2-D matrix at the chemical shift, d_U, in both of the frequency domains, F_1 and F_2, i.e. at $d_U d_U$ (on the diagonal). However, for a coupled spin-system, e.g. AX, magnetization transfer can also occur between transitions of the separate nuclei, and this results in signals (cross-peaks) at the coordinates $d_A d_X$ and $d_X d_A$ (i.e. off the diagonal) as well as at $d_A d_A$ and $d_X d_X$.

For 2-D spectroscopy, sequential runs are carried out, incrementing the evolution time t_1. All 2-D spectra were generated using quadrature detection and phase cycling to select negative modulation

frequencies [10,11]. Completed data matrices were then zero-filled in
both dimensions. Fourier transformation was performed after the application of sine-bell or sine-bell-squared functions in both dimensions.
Prior to plotting, spectra were also mathematically symmetrized
about the diagonal. Exact details of 2-D spectral parameters are
given elsewhere [7].

Drug dosing and urine collections.- The excretion of paracetamol
and its metabolites was studied in male subjects after ingestion of
two 500 mg tablets (Paracetamol BP). Urine samples were collected
hourly for the first 6 h after drug ingestion, and the total urine
collected in the 6-24 h period was pooled. Analyte concentrations were
determined by comparing computer-integrated peak area or heights for
the urinary metabolite resonances with those of an added standard.
For NMF experiments, in rats (Sprague-Dawley, 200-250 g males),
urine was collected for 24 h before and 7-24 and 24-48 h after treatment
with NMF (1000 mg/kg, i.p.).

RESULTS FOR PARACETAMOL AND ENDOGENOUS CONSTITUENTS

Fig. 1 shows a typical ^{1}H NMR spectrum of untreated normal
human urine. Reasonable signal-to-noise ratios were usually obtained
with 48 accumulations, but very dilute urine samples required more.
Despite a long T_1 relaxation delay between pulses, spectra could often
be obtained within 5 min without sample pre-treatment. Resonances from
a wide range of endogenous compounds were observed and identified by
making standard additions of candidate compounds and by considering
their chemical shifts and coupling patterns [4]. Many of these
compounds are of considerable physiological importance and furthermore
their urinary concentrations often reflect the metabolic status of
the subject.

Fig. 2 shows a typical 500 MHz ^{1}H NMR spectrum of urine collected
6 h after paracetamol ingestion, and serves for discussion of the peak
assignments. These were aided by first recording and assigning peaks
for paracetamol and its major metabolites (Fig. 2). A major advantage
of NMR is that 'fingerprints' of molecules often consist of more
than one resonance, each with characteristic chemical shifts, relative
intensities and sometimes spin-spin coupling patterns. In favourable
cases this allows unambiguous identification of the substance. This
is in contrast to effluent traces in HPLC, obtained with absorption or
fluorescence detectors which give only a single peak for each metabolite. The acetanilide *N*-acetyl groups of the metabolites all gave sharp
signals in the narrow range from 2.13 to 2.19 ppm. These were well
resolved at 400 or 500 MHz if the resolution were enhanced by application of a Gaussian function to the free induction decay before
Fourier transformation.

Paracetamol metabolites have other characteristic ^{1}H NMR resonances [4]; thus, the aromatic ring protons give rise to resonances with

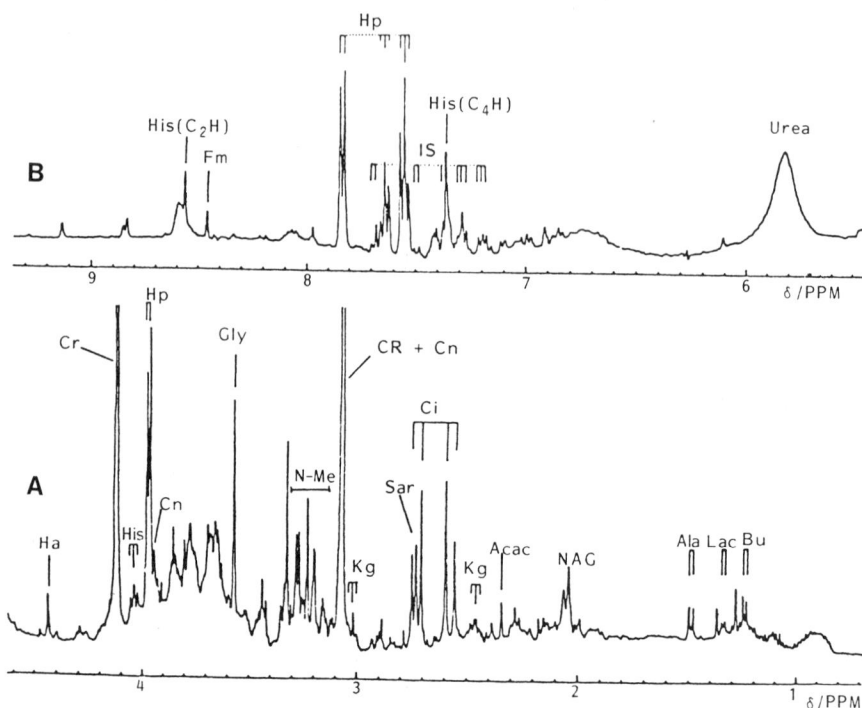

Fig. 1. Normal human urine: 400 MHz ^{1}H spectrum, aliphatic (**A**) and aromatic (**B**) regions. Cn, creatinine; Cr, creatine; Ci, citrate; Hp, hippurate; Gly, glycine; Bu, 3-D-hydroxybutyrate; Acac, acetoacetate; Ala, alanine; Lac, lactate; His, histidine; IS, indoxyl sulphate; Fm, formate; Hg, dihydroxyacetone; Kg, ketoglutarate; Sar, sarcosine; NAG, *N*-acetyl signals from glyco-proteins. *Modified from ref. [4].*

clearly identifiable coupling patterns spread over about 0.6 ppm (Fig. 2). In the case of the glucuronide, the β-anomeric proton of the sugar ring has a further characteristic doublet resonance at 5.11 ppm (J = 6 Hz) and also resonances between 3.6 and 3.9 ppm corresponding to other sugar-ring protons. An additional assignment aid for the *N*-acetyl-L-cysteinyl conjugate was the sharp singlet for the side-chain *N*-acetyl group at 1.84 ppm.

This analysis clearly indicated that ^{1}H NMR might be used to study quantitatively the urinary excretion of paracetamol and its major metabolites. The addition of standard solutions of paracetamol metabolites to 5 replicate urine samples showed that the analytical recovery of total paracetamol metabolites was good (97.7 ±2.4%). The calculation of the relative proportions of each metabolite is subject to an error (possibly up to 10% on some individual samples)

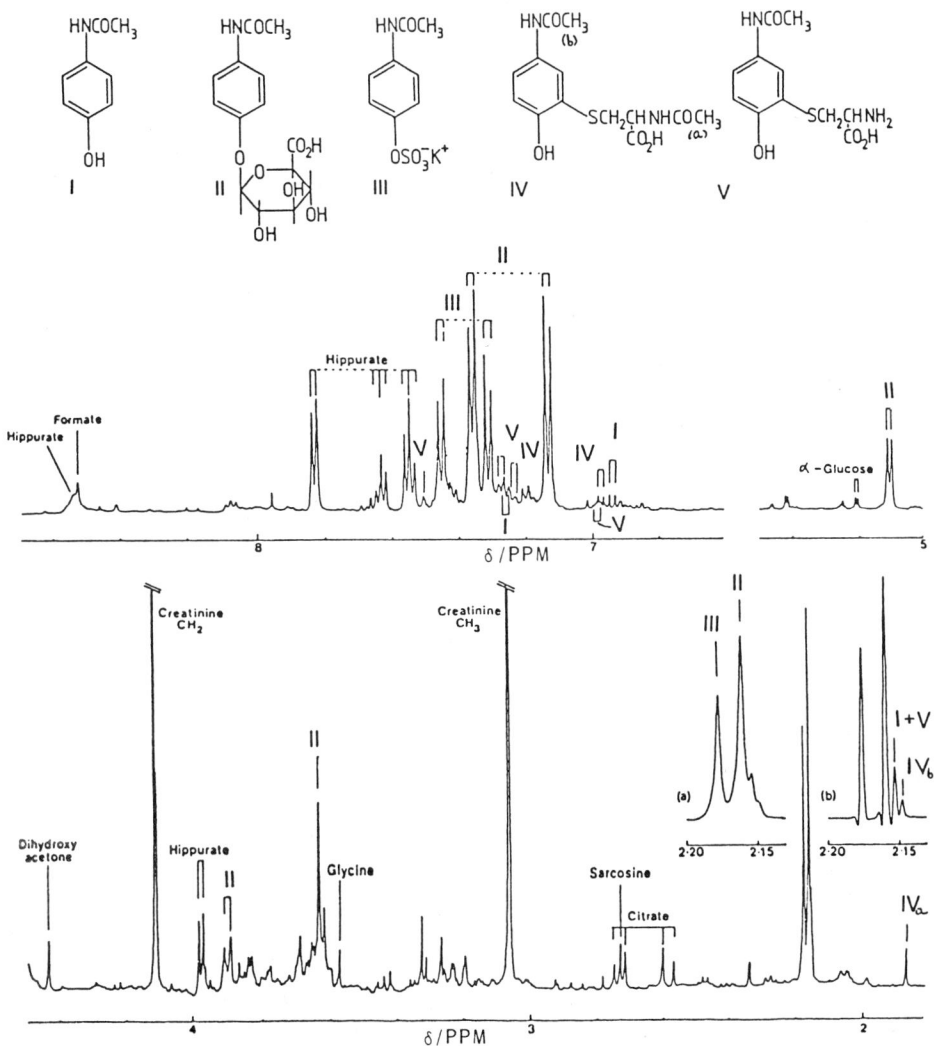

Fig. 2. Urine collected 6 h after paracetamol ingestion: ¹H NMR spectrum, aliphatic (**A**) and aromatic (**B**) regions. Shown in (**C**): structures of paracetamol (**I**; *N*-acetyl-4-aminophenol, acetaminophen) and its metabolites: 4-glucuronosido-acetanilide (**II**), *N*-acetyl-4-aminophenol sulphate (**III**), *N*-acetyl-2-(*N*-acetyl-L-cysteinyl)-4-aminophenol (**IV**), and *N*-acetyl-2-(L-cysteinyl)-4-aminophenol (**V**). *Modified from ref. [5].*

Fig. 3. Mean distributions (% of total amount of drug + metabolites at each time interval) for urinary excretion of paracetamol and its major metabolites as determined by ^{1}H NMR spectroscopy. Values were calculated from integrations of the *N*-acetyl signals. Error bars represent the S.E.M., for 6 subjects. *Modified from ref. [5].*

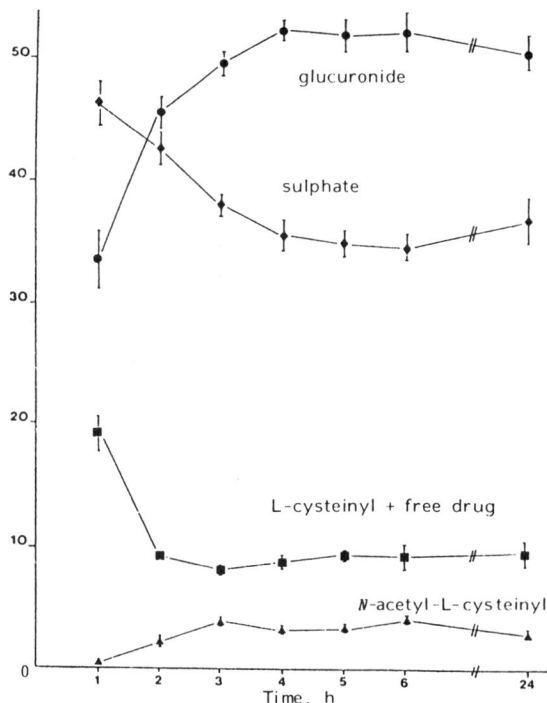

related to partial overlap of resonances; however, this can be improved considerably by use of mathematical resolution-enhancement techniques as in Fig. 2. In view of the overlapping *N*-acetyl signals from/of free drug and L-cysteinyl conjugate, their combined values were estimated.

The excretion patterns of paracetamol and metabolites now determined by ^{1}H NMR spectroscopy (Fig. 3) agreed well with those reported by earlier workers using other methods [9, 12]. Agreement between NMR and HPLC measurements [9] was also good with respect to the amounts and ratios of metabolites excreted during 24 h, the relative proportions (%) being as follows.- Glucuronide by NMR, 49.9 (±4.6 S.D., 5 subjects) *vs.* 54.7 by HPLC; sulphate, 37.6 (±4.6) *vs.* 32.3 by HPLC; *N*-acetyl-L-cysteinyl, 3.0 (±1.4) *vs.* 4.0 by HPLC; L-cysteinyl, 9.5 (±2.6) *vs.* 5.0 by HPLC; free drug, 5.0.

^{1}H 'COSY' (2-D) spectra as an identification aid

Even at 500 MHz (currently the highest commercially available spectrometer frequency) resonances for paracetamol and its *N*-acetyl-L-cysteinyl conjugate are overlapped. Clearly this places limitations on the application of conventional 1-D NMR spectroscopy to the identification of drug metabolites in untreated urine samples, particularly if the xenobiotic under consideration has a poorly understood metabolic profile. However, 2-D NMR spectra can now be obtained routinely from such samples. Fig. 4 shows, as contour 'maps', the aromatic

Fig. 4. The aromatic
regions of 500 MHz 2-D
^{1}H shift-correlated
(COSY) NMR spectra of:
(**A**) a model mixture of
paracetamol (I) and its
major metabolites (II-V);
(**B**) a control sample of
human urine;
(**C**) a urine sample
collected 4 h after
ingestion of 1 g of
paracetamol.
Modified from ref. [5].

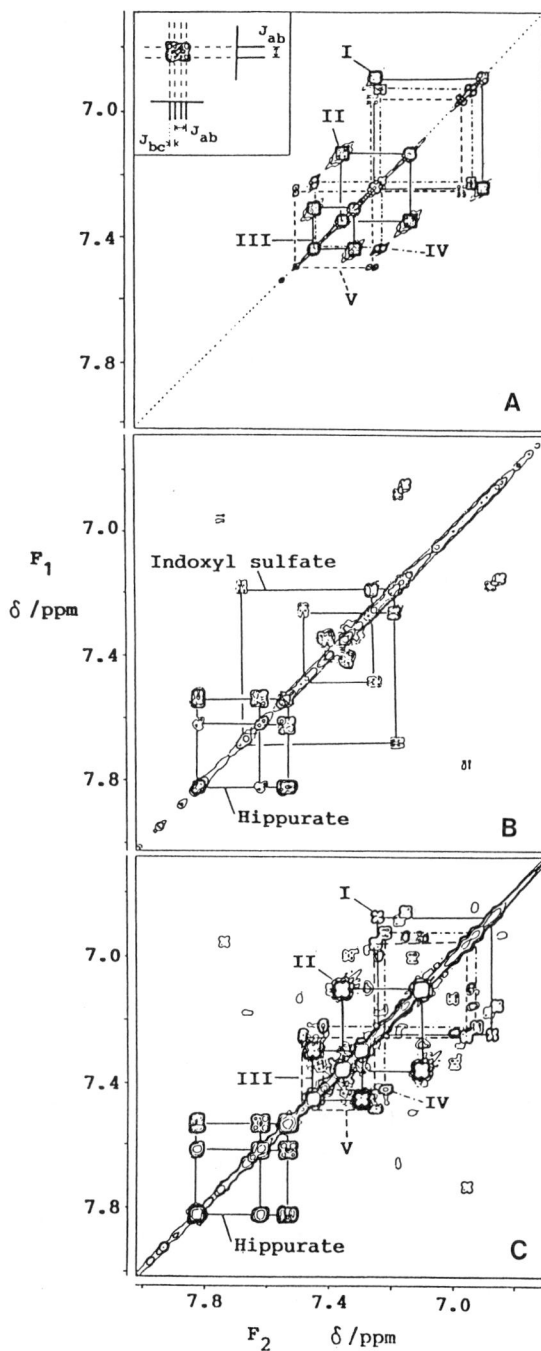

regions of ^{1}H COSY spectra for paracetamol and metabolites in pure solution, for control urine, and for urine which had been collected 4 h after paracetamol ingestion and then freeze-dried and redissolved in ^{2}H$_2$O (this latter step is not obligatory if water suppression is used as well as the 2-D pulse sequence). The 'normal' spectra or projections onto the X axis lie along the diagonals (bottom-left to top-right) of the contour map. For the model solution (Fig. 4A) there are 12 multiplet resonances in this region of the spectrum. Peaks off the diagonal (cross-peaks) indicate which of these multiplets are spin-spin coupled, and therefore a characteristic pattern is obtained for each metabolite. There are 7 cross-peaks symmetrically positioned on each side of the diagonal. Paracetamol and its glucuronide (II) and sulphate (III) each give rise to a pair of doublet resonances in the aromatic region of the 1-D spectrum, and these give only a single pair of cross-peaks in the 2-D map, i.e. they appear as a square pattern with corners at the chemical shifts of the individual multiplets.

The ring-substituted cysteinyl (V) and the *N*-acetyl-L-cysteinyl (IV) conjugates of paracetamol each have 3 non-equivalent aromatic protons that give rise to distinct resonances. These metabolites both give rise to a figure-of-eight pattern in the aromatic region of the 2-D map. The two pairs of symmetrical cross-peaks arise because H$_a$ is coupled to H$_b$, which in turn is also coupled to H$_c$, but the coupling between the distant H$_a$ and H$_c$ protons is weak.

It is also possible to analyze the fine structure of the cross-peaks to determine the magnitude of the coupling constants, and although the digital resolution of the 2-D spectrum may limit the accuracy of such estimates, it is often impossible to measure them from the overlapped 1-D spectrum alone. For example, the cross-peak at 6.96 (F$_1$)/7.24 (F$_2$) ppm (see inset in Fig. 4A) shows multiplet structure arising from H$_a$ and H$_b$ of IV. There are two rows of four cross-peaks which correspond to the various possible energy transitions of, and magnetization transfer between, the nuclei involved.

The inset in Fig. 4A also shows more clearly how the individual components of the cross-peak are related to projections of the 1-D multiplet patterns. Fig. 4B shows the same region of a 2-D COSY NMR spectrum of control urine. The characteristic connectivity patterns have been unambiguously assigned to the aromatic protons of endogenous hippurate and indoxyl sulphate. The contour plot for a urine sample taken 4 h after paracetamol ingestion (Fig. 4C) clearly shows the connectivity patterns both for these endogenous metabolites and for those of paracetamol. In particular it can be seen that the resonances from the free paracetamol and the cysteinyl derivative, that cannot be resolved in the 1-D experiment, can now be readily distinguished.

RESULTS FOR *N*-METHYLFORMAMIDE (NMF)

The ^{1}H NMR spectra (1-D) of urine from control and NMF-treated rats are shown in Figs. 5 & 6.   In addition to the resonances from endogenous components (which are both qualitatively and quantitatively different from those of human urine), several resonances from NMF and its metabolites were also clearly resolved.   Strong signals from the *N*-methyl and formyl protons from both *syn* and *anti* isomers of NMF were observed (Fig. 5).   Proton resonances for methylamine (δ = 2.61 ppm) and formate (δ = 8.45 ppm) were well resolved in the spectra of urine from NMF-treated animals (Fig. 5).   Although these metabolites are present in normal urine samples, they are present in much greater quantities after NMF treatment.

The major *N*-methyl resonance of NMF (δ = 2.77 ppm, *anti* isomer) appeared as a doublet (J = 4.88 Hz) due to spin-spin coupling to the adjacent slow-exchanging NH protons; this coupling disappeared in samples that had been made slightly alkaline or that had been freze-dried and reconstituted with ^{2}H$_2$O. A similar pattern of behaviour was displayed by another doublet resonance (J = 4.39 Hz; 0.02 ppm to high frequency) of the major NMF *N*-methyl signal when samples were made alkaline or deuterated, indicating that these protons were in a very similar chemical environment to those of the parent compound. The intensity of this N-CH$_3$ resonance was particularly strong in samples collected 24-48 h after NMF treatment (Fig. 6A), and computer integrations measured on several samples revealed good intensity correlations between this (3H) and those of new multiplets centered at 3.40 (CH$_2$) and 4.42 (CH) and a singlet (CH$_3$CO) at 2.03 ppm. COSY 2-D spectra (not shown) confirmed that the multiplets were spin-spin coupled, giving an ABX spin-system the chemical shifts of which are consistent with those of a cysteinyl or *N*-acetylcysteinyl derivative.

Extraction of urine samples (24-48 h) with ethyl acetate under acidic conditions was performed in order to separate *N*-acetylcysteine conjugates.   TLC of these extracts (silica gel; development with CHCl$_3$/methanol/acetic acid, 80:20:2 by vol.) gave a radioactive band, R$_F$ ~0.2, which gave a positive reaction for divalent sulphur when sprayed with potassium dichromate reagent [13]. After alkaline hydrolysis of these extracts, sulphydryl groups were detected with Ellman's reagent. ^{1}H NMR spectra of the material in these ethyl acetate extracts (Fig. 6B) when redissolved in ^{2}H$_2$O and corrected to pH 7 showed resonances for NMF itself and very strong signals for the *N*-acetylcysteinyl derivative, with shifts and splitting patterns similar to those seen in the unextracted urine samples.

These data are consistent with the presence in the urine of *N*-acetyl-*S*-(*N*-methyl-carbamoyl-)-L-cysteine (Fig. 6C), a new metabolite of NMF discovered primarily by NMR spectroscopy. We postulate that this metabolite arises after oxidation of the nitrogen centre of NMF to

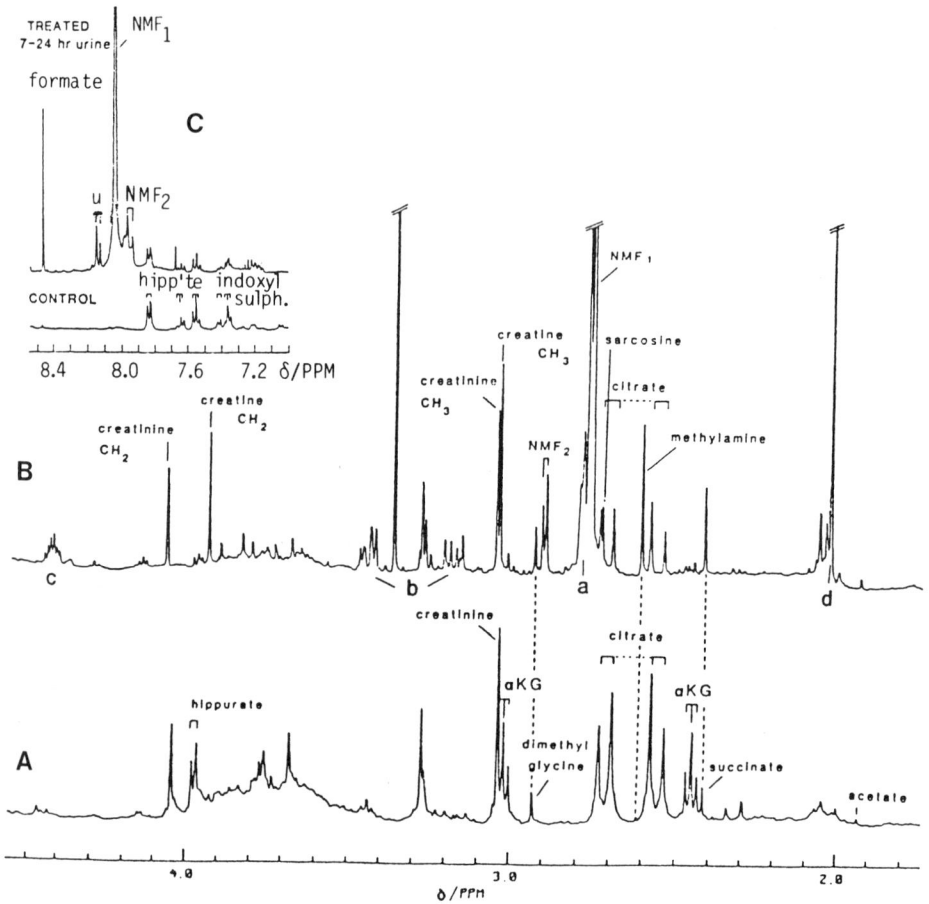

Fig. 5. Urine from control (**A**) and NMF-treated (**B**) rats: 400 MHz NMR spectra, and (**C**) comparison of the aromatic regions. Assignments a, b, c, d refer to the NMF metabolite N-acetyl-S-(N-methyl-carbamoyl)cysteine (see Fig. 6C). NMF$_1$ = syn, NMF$_2$ = $anti$.

give an intermediate which either reacts with glutathione or yields methyl isocyanate after dehydration. Methyl isocyanate itself is highly reactive towards free SH groups including that of reduced glutathione, which if conjugated could then be cleaved from the glycinyl and glutamyl residues to give a cysteinyl derivative which is then N-acetylated. The formation of this metabolite is probably involved in the depletion of liver glutathione which may be related to the hepatotoxicity of NMF [13].

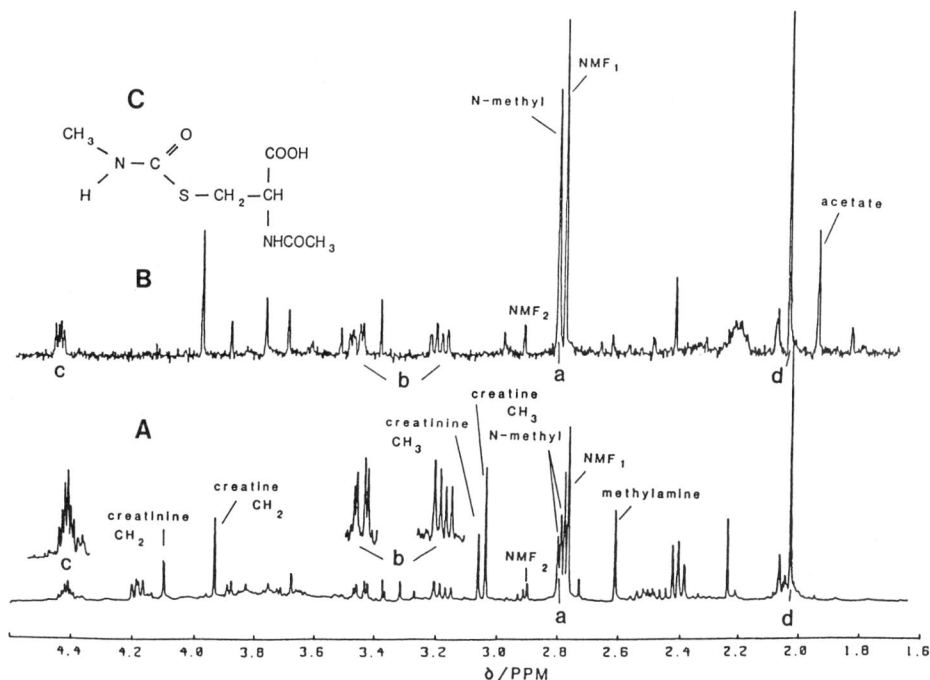

Fig. 6. Urine from an NMF-treated rat (24–48 h): 400 MHz ^{1}H spectra for (**A**) urine examined direct, and (**B**) an ethyl acetate extract, the residue from freeze-drying having been redissolved in ^{2}H$_2$O whereby the N-CH$_3$ peaks appear as singlets (NH coupling removed). Also shown (**C**): the structure of the novel NMF metabolite *N*-acetyl-*S*-(*N*-methylcarbamoyl)cysteine.

DISCUSSION AND CONCLUSIONS

These studies clearly indicate that there is great potential for applications of high-resolution ^{1}H NMR in studies of drug metabolism and excretion. Other workers have recently shown that these techniques can be applied to study completely different classes of drugs such as metronidazole [14] and penicillins [15]. In the latter case Everett and co-workers were able to identify a previously unknown metabolite of the β-lactam ampicillin, viz. diketopiperazine, using mainly spin-echo Fourier transform methods to analyze untreated urine samples. This group has also demonstrated the utility of combining ^{19}F and ^{1}H NMR methods to analyze untreated samples containing metabolites of fluorinated drugs such as flucloxacillin [16]. NMR is does not perturb equilibrium and is non-invasive, and so is uniquely suited to the study of drug metabolism in isolated but intact biochemical systems [17].

2-D COSY NMR is a powerful method for assigning resonances of both drug-derived and endogenous metabolites in biological materials. Quantification of metabolites from their 2-D NMR spectra may prove to be feasible, but this aspect of ^{2}D-NMR has yet to be explored (it would be much more complex than quantitation from 1-D spectra). At present the main limitation of using 2-D NMR spectroscopy is that it very demanding on computer time and memory, for data accumulation, processing and storage. The *minimum* time for obtaining a 2-D COSY spectrum of untreated urine with acceptably low signal-to-noise and digital resolution is at present ~1 h. Accordingly, this technique will be most useful for selected samples in which the identification of unknown drug metabolites is important and 1-D spectra show coupled signals that are severely overlapped.

At present NMR spectroscopy is an insensitive technique when compared with chromatographic analysis methods. Hence urinary drug excretion studies by NMR are limited to compounds that are administered in fairly large amounts and excreted rapidly. However, a major advantage in using ^{1}H NMR as a tool for directly analyzing the low mol. wt. compounds in biological materials is that toxicological information of mechanistic significance can be obtained, by interpreting the changing patterns and concentrations of endogenous metabolites in response to a xenobiotic challenge. This situation is well illustrated by reference to our ^{1}H NMR work on the effects of mercuric chloride on the composition of rat urine [6]. In this study it was possible to use NMR as a multi-parametric indicator of acute nephrotoxicity that besides being at least as sensitive as conventional biochemical measurements also gave information on basic mechanisms of mercury toxicity, particularly those relating to inhibitory effects on citric acid-cycle enzymes.

Finally, it should be stressed that NMR spectroscopy is a technique that is still developing rapidly. Major advances in the methodology, in particular data processing, are occurring in quick succession, so that the range of NMR applications in drug metabolism and toxicity studies will be expected to widen in the next few years.

Acknowledgements

We are grateful to the National Kidney Research Fund, the S.E.R.C. and the M.R.C. for financial support for this and related work.

References

1. Bock, J.L. (1982) *Clin. Chem. 28*, 1873-1877.
2. Nicholson, J.K., Buckingham, M.J. & Sadler, P.J. (1983) *Biochem. J. 211*, 605-615.

3. Nicholson, J.K., O'Flynn, M., Sadler, P.J., Macleod, A.F., Juul, S.M. & Sonksen, P.H. (1984) *Biochem. J. 217*, 365–375.
4. Bales, J.R., Higham, D.P., Howe, I., Timbrell, J.A. & Sadler, P.J. (1984) *Biochem. J. 217*, 426–432.
5. Bales, J.R., Sadler, P.J., Nicholson, J.K. & Timbrell, J.A. (1984) *Clin. Chem. 30*, 1631–1636.
6. Nicholson, J.K., Timbrell, J.A. & Sadler, P.J. (1985) *Mol. Pharmacol. 27*, 644–651.
7. Bales, J.R., Nicholson, J.K. & Timbrell, J.A. (1985) *Clin. Chem. 31*, 757–762.
8. Hore, P. (1983) *J. Magn. Reson. 55*, 283–300.
9. Prescott, L.F. (1980) *Br. J. Clin. Pharmacol. 10*, 291S–298S.
10. Bax, A., Freeman, R. & Morris, G. (1981) *J. Magn. Reson. 41*, 496–501.
11. Nagayama, K., Bachmann, P., Wuthrich, K. & Ernst, R.R. (1978) *J. Magn. Reson. 31*, 133–148.
12. Forrest, J.A.H., Clements, J.A. & Prescott, L.F. (1982) *Clin. Pharmacokinet. 7*, 93–107.
13. Tulip, K., Timbrell, J.A. & Nicholson, J.K. (1986) *Chemical and Biological Reactive Metabolites (Proc. 3rd Int. Symp.)*, Plenum, New York, in press.
14. Coleman, M.D. & Norton, R.S. (1986) *Xenobiotica 16*, 69–77.
15. Everett, J.R., Jennings, K., Woodnut, G. & Buckingham, M.J. (1984) *J. Chem. Soc., Chem. Comm.*, 894–895.
16. Everett, J.R., Jennings, K. & Woodnut, G. (1985) *J. Pharm. Pharmacol. 37*, 869–873.
17. Nicholson, J.K., Timbrell, J.A., Bales, J.R. & Sadler, P.J. (1985) *Mol. Pharmacol. 27*, 634–643.

#D-2

DETECTION, IDENTIFICATION   AND QUANTITATIVE ANALYSIS
OF DRUGS BY ^{1}H NMR

*Ismail M. Ismail and ⊗IanD. Wilson

Hoechst Pharmaceutical Research Laboratories
Walton Manor, Milton Keynes
Bucks. MK7 7AJ, U.K.

The application of high-resolution proton NMR spectroscopy to the measurement of drugs and their metabolites in biological fluids is of increasing interest to analytical chemists and toxicologists. Much of the pioneering work in this area has used very high magnetic field strengths (400 and 500 MHz). This article concerns the use of a 250 MHz NMR spectrophotometer in the detection and quantification of metabolites of the drug oxpentifylline in freeze-dried, reconstituted urine. The values obtained were within 10% of those from a specific HPLC method. The criteria necessary to obtain successful results using this technique are briefly discussed.

A number of studies have demonstrated the feasibility of using proton NMR to obtain qualitative and quantitative information on small molecules, e.g. drugs and their metabolites, in unprocessed biological fluids such as plasma and urine ([1-4], & preceding art. by J.K. Nicholson et al.). An attractive feature of this approach is that there may be little or no need for initial sample processing, whereas with other analytical methods this is often complex and tedious. However, almost invariably such studies have required the use of NMR spectrophotometers operating at very high magnetic field strengths, e.g. 9.4 or 11.75 Tesla corresponding to 400 and 500 MHz ^{1}H resonance frequencies. Whilst such instruments are becoming more common, 200-250 MHz instruments are even more likely to be available for routine analysis of biological specimens.

In exploratory studies with a 250 MHz instrument, we have examined the urine of volunteers dosed orally with the drug oxpentifylline, and urine samples spiked with the anti-inflammatory drug isoxepac.

Present addresses: *Glaxo Group Research, Ware, Herts. SG12 ODJ;
⊗ICI Pharmaceuticals, Mereside, Alderley Park, Macclesfield SK10 4TG

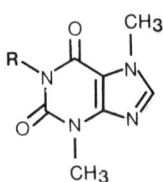

	R	
a.	$CH_3CO(CH_2)_4-$	parent drug (Trental®)
b.	$HOOC(CH_2)_3-$	metabolite **V**
c.	$HOOC(CH_2)_4-$	metabolite **IV**

Oxpentifylline (R = **a** above) is used extensively in the treatment of vascular disease. Studies on its metabolic fate (J. Chamberlain & co-workers, to be published) have shown it to be well absorbed, extensively metabolized and rapidly excreted, mainly in the urine. The major urinary metabolite, **V**, comprising ~50% of the total, has been identified as 1-(3-carboxypropyl)-3,7-dimethylxanthine. A similar acidic metabolite, **IV**, 1-(4-carboxybutyl)-3,7-dimethylxanthine, accounted for a further 10%. Oxpentifylline itself was not detectable in urine.

Preliminary NMR studies on virtually untreated urine samples revealed that the 250 MHz instrument was unsuitable for such material. Apart from its inherently lower sensitivity compared to 400/500 MHz instruments, we were unable to suppress the large signal due to water protons; hence we could not obtain good spectra of any metabolites present at the mM level (i.e. there was a severe dynamic range problem). However, the signals resulting from the proton at position 8 and from the *N*-methyls at 3 and 7 did seem to be present (Fig. 1). This encouraged us to continue our studies.

USE OF FREEZE-DRIED SAMPLES

By freeze-drying the sample and then reconstituting it in ^2H_2O, we largely eliminated the swamping by water protons of the signals from the compounds of interest. This simple pre-treatment also enabled us to improve our effective sensitivity by concentrating the urine. The following procedures were adopted.- Urine samples (5 ml) were freeze-dried and the residue redissolved in 1 ml of ^2H_2O. The ^2H_2O also contained 3.07 mM 'TSP', viz. 3-(trimethylsilyl)[^2H]$_4$propane sulphonate (δ = 0 ppm), as a reference compound in respect of internal chemical shift and concentration. With instrumental conditions as stated below, quantification was achieved by integrating signals from either the proton at position 8 or those of the *N*-methyls at 3 and 7 (Fig. 2) and comparing them with the TSP -Si(Me)$_3$ proton signal.

Legends for Figs. opposite

Fig. 1. Urine sample containg oxypentifylline metabolites: spectrum obtained using a 250 MHz spectrometer with instrumental suppression of the water signal. The arrowed signal loci refer to the proton at position 8 and the *N*-methyls at 3 and 7 respectively.

Fig. 2. As for Fig. 1, but freeze-dried urine reconstituted in ^2H_2O.

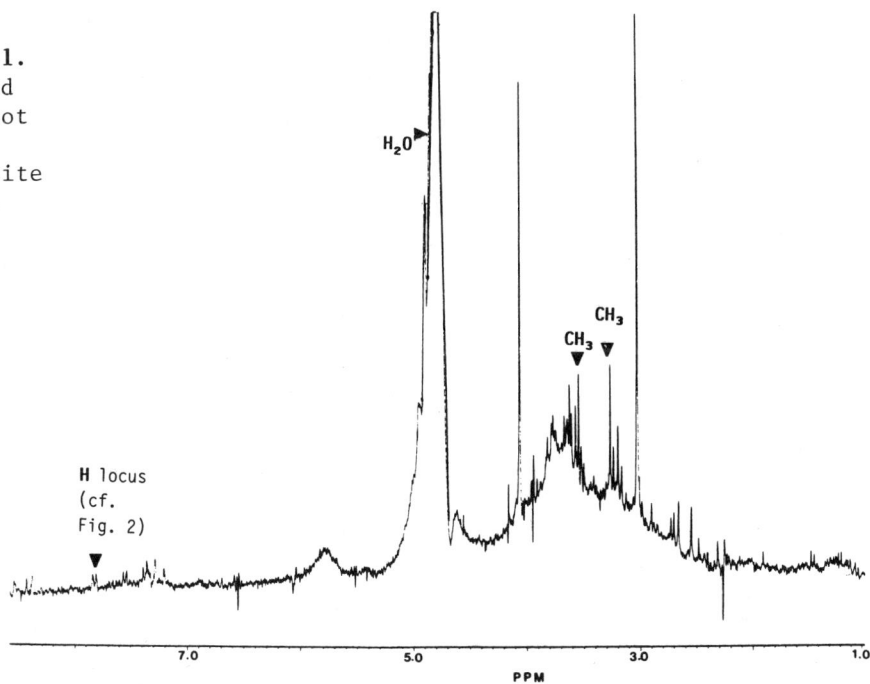

Fig. 1.
Legend
at foot
of
opposite
page.

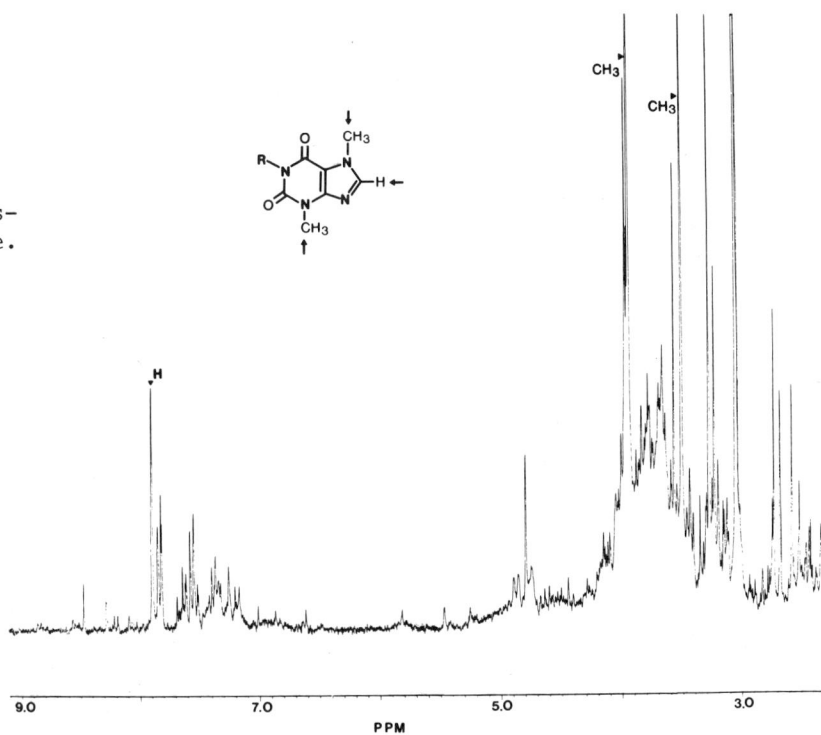

Fig. 2.
Legend
at foot
of oppos-
ite page.

The proton NMR spectra were obtained with a Bruker WM 250 NMR Spectrometer. All spectra were measured at ambient probe temperature (25 ±1°) using 16K data point over 3401.36 Hz sweep width and an acquisition time of 2.40 sec. The spectra were the result of collecting 640 free induction decays using 90° pulses and a delay of 5 sec between pulses, giving a recycle time for the experiment of 7.4 sec. The H_2O signal was 'suppressed' by application of a secondary irradiation field at the water resonant frequency, the decoupler being gated-off during acquisition to minimize break-through (cf. preceding article by J.K. Nicholson et al.).

Quantitative analysis of the freeze-dried samples for metabolites was also performed using a specific HPLC method [5]. Briefly, 1 ml samples were supplemented with internal standard and then acidified with 1 M HCl (1 ml), extracted with dichloromethane (6 ml), and centrifuged. The organic layer was evaporated to dryness with a N_2 stream. The residue was redissolved in 1 ml of HPLC mobile phase (0.02 M orthophosphoric acid/methanol, 71.5:28.5 by vol.), and aliquots taken for analysis. The column, 15 cm × 3 mm i.d., was packed with 5 μm ODS-Spherisorb; the flow-rate was 1 ml/min, and detection was at 274 nm. Distinct peaks were obtained for the drug, **IV** and **V**.

The outcome of examining the ^{1}H NMR spectra was most encouraging. Thus, whilst the water signal was not entirely eliminated it was substantially attenuated. This allowed a more effective use of the intrinsic dynamic range of the instrument (dependent on the computer word length of the digital-to-analogue converter, which in this case was 12 bits). Resonances from metabolites present at low concentrations could thus be observed more easily. Scrutiny of the spectrum (Fig. 2) clearly showed the presence of the signals from the proton at position 8 and the *N*-methyls at 3 and 7 of the oxypentifylline metabolites. The signal from the position-8 proton is well separated from those of endogenous compounds such as hippurate, and can readily be used for quantification purposes. The methyl resonances, whilst appearing in a region of considerable 'chemical noise', are nevertheless visible, providing additional evidence that the signal at 7.89 ppm is indeed due to the position-8 proton. Surprisingly, when used for quantification they gave similar results to those of the position-8 proton. The presence in the spectrum of these three signals, all of which may be used for identification and quantification, provides a triple check on metabolite concentration. A comparison of the results obtained by ^{1}H NMR and HPLC (metabolites **IV** and **V** conjointly) showed them to be very close (within 10%).

Thus, the simple procedure of freeze-drying the samples to reduce troublesome water signals, and concentration to improve sensitivity, enabled us to assess qualitatively and quantitatively the combined oxpentifylline metabolites using a 250 MHz NMR spectrometer.

The technique entailing freeze-drying and reconstitution in ^2H_2O may be used for other drugs. Fig. 3 shows its application to the determination of the anti-inflammatory drug isoxepac. For quantification the readily observable signals due to the methylene protons in the oxepin ring suit well; aromatic ring proton signals verify identity.

CONCLUDING COMMENTS

These results, and those of other authors [1-4], demonstrate that for suitable compounds ^1H NMR spectroscopy provides a relatively simple method of analysis for drugs and metabolites in urine. However, it should be noted that NMR is an inherently insensitive technique and that certain limitations to its use apply. Thus, to be a candidate for analysis using NMR, a compound should be present in the sample at reasonable concentrations ($\mu g/ml$ rather than ng/ml) and have signals which are not subject to interference by those of endogenous components. In this respect the metabolites of oxpentifylline are particularly advantageous in that they provide three 'handles' for the analyst to use, and enable the results for one signal to be checked against

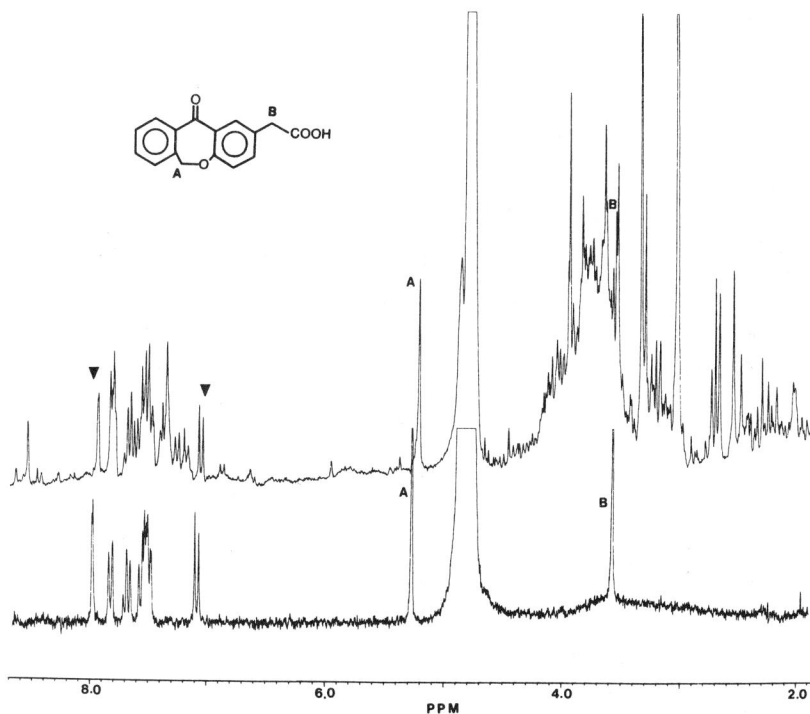

Fig. 3. *Upper spectrum:* urine containing 1 mg/ml of isoxepac, freeze-dried and reconstituted in ^2H_2O. *Lower spectrum:* pure isoxepac in ^2H_2O. A and B = side-chain and ring CH_2's; aromatic protons also marked.

those of another.   The analysis of drugs which are given in low
dose, and which are subject to extensive metabolism (to a large
number of metabolites), poses problems that are best solved by other
methods.

Whilst we have successfully used a 250 MHz spectrometer, there
is no doubt that the use of a higher field strength (e.g. 400 or
500 MHz) does provide certain benefits.   Thus, spectra are acquired
more rapidly as the instruments are more powerful, and the greater
dispersion of the signals resolves signals which at 250 MHz overlap.
Thus, the resonances of the side-chain methylene groups of the acidic
metabolites of oxpentifylline, which are lost in the 'chemical noise'
at 250 MHz, can be readily observed at 400 MHz (J.K. Nicholson, unpublished work).   Whilst not important for quantitative analysis, this
additional information might be very useful in a study of the metabolism
of a compound.   However, as our results show, the lack of a 400
or 500 MHz NMR facility does not preclude the type of assay described
above if a 250 MHz spectrometer is available and if each metabolite
need not be individually distinguished.

Acknowledgement

The help and advice of Dr. J.K. Nicholson is gratefully acknow-
ledged.

References

1. Nicholson, J.K., Buckingham, M.J. & Sadler, P.J. (1983)
    Biochem. J. 211, 605-615.
2. Bales, J.R., Migham, D.P., Howe, J.K., Nicholson, J.K. &
    Sadler, P.J. (1984) *Clin. Chem. 30*, 426-432.
3. Bales, J.R., Sadler, P.J., Nicholson, J.K. & Timbrell, J.A.
    (1984) *Clin. Chem. 30*, 1631-1636.
4. Bales, J.R., Nicholson, J.K. & Sadler, P.J. (1985) *Clin. Chem.
    31*, 757-762.
5. Bryce, T.A., Burrows, J.L. & Jolley, K.W. (1985) *J. Chromatog.
    334*, 397-402.

#D-3

PRE-COLUMN (HPLC) FLUORESCENCE LABELLING OF GLUCURONIDES

H. Lingeman[⊗], G.W.M. Meussen, C. van der Zouwen,
W.J.M. Underberg and A. Hulshoff

Pharmaceutical Laboratory
Department of Analytical Pharmacy
State University of Utrecht
Catharijnesingel 60
3511GH Utrecht, The Netherlands

A selective and sensitive HPLC method has been developed for the determination of glucuronides in plasma and urine. Prior to chromatography the carboxylic acid function of the glucuronic acid moiety is converted into a fluorescent amide by a method selective for the carboxyl group. The acidic function is first activated with 2-bromo-1-methylpyridinium iodide and then reacted with the fluorescence label [N-(1-dimethylaminonaphthalenesulphonyl)cadaverine or N-(1-naphthyl)ethylenediamine] to yield the amide. The derivatization products are separated by a two-column system in combination with a column-switching technique. For α-naphthyl-β-D-glucuronide, β-oestradiol-17-β-D-glucuronide and some other glucuronides, consideration is given to chromatographic properties, intrinsic fluorescence sensitivities (both of reagents and of derivatives) and clean-up procedures.

Conjugation with glucuronic acid by UDPglucuronosyl transferase is an important detoxifying system for the elimination of endogenous and exogenous organic compounds, especially phenols. Different types occur: $O-$, $S-$, $C-$ and N-glucuronides. They are more water-soluble than the parent compounds and are eliminated mainly by the kidneys and/or via the bile.

Specific and selective analytical methods are required for the investigation of glucuronidation *in vivo*. Techniques based on the enzymatic or chemical hydrolysis of the glucuronides, followed by the analysis of the parent compounds, may miss important information about metabolic pathways (i.e. changes in type or site of conjugation) [1]. Moreover, these methods may lack sufficient selectivity or sensitivity [2], particularly when the compound is metabolized into more than

---

⊗ See end of art. for present address.

one glucuronide [3]. Some of the parent compound may remain unmetabo-
lized, and be of interest, in the sample under investigation, and in
large excess may cause serious problems [4]. The stability of the
parent compound in the reaction medium is not always sufficient to
allow chemical hydrolysis [5]. Enzymatic hydrolysis is often influenced by the presence of inhibitors in urine [6] or by acyl rearrange-
ments of ester glucuronides [7, 8]. [See Vol. 12, this series, for
information on glucuronide types and behaviour, especially pp. 267-
268; Sect. C gives examples of intact glucuronide separations.-Ed.]

Consequently, specific quantitation methods based on the analysis
of the intact glucuronides are preferable. A general HPLC method
focused on the only constant moiety of the conjugate, the glucuronic
acid part of the molecule, should be of considerable interest. Because
the glucuronic acid function possesses no useful UV absorption, electrochemical (redox) or fluorescent properties, the use of a derivatization technique to improve the sensitivity of detection is indicated.

A number of derivatization techniques have been described for GC
as well as HPLC to convert the carboxylic acid function, for different
detection methods. Most of the reported derivatization reactions are
non-specific. Other functional groups, e.g. phenols, thiols and
imides, are also derivatized; some methods do not allow sufficiently
sensitive detection, others are not quantitative or require high
temperatures or long reaction times [9, 10]. [For a fluorescent
coumarin derivative, see W. Dünges et al. in Vol. 7, this series.-Ed.]

To overcome these limitations a pre-column HPLC derivatization
method has been developed that is selective for the carboxylic acid
function [11, 12].

MATERIALS

N-(1-Naphthyl)ethylenediammonium dichloride (NED.2HCl), triethylamine and tetramethylammonium bromide (TMABr) were obtained
from E. Merck (Darmstadt). Ammonium mentholglucuronate, sodium α-
naphthyl-β-D-glucuronate (NG), p-nitrophenyl-β-D-glucuronic acid, Na
β-oestradiol-17-β-D-glucuronate (17-EG), Na testosterone-17-β-D-glu-
curonic acid, diethylstilboestrol-monoglucuronic acid, Na D-glucuro-
nate and N-(1-dimethylaminonaphthalenesulphonyl)cadaverine (dansyl-
cadaverine, DC) came from Sigma (St. Louis). α-Oestriol-16-β-D-
glucuronic acid, etiocholanolone-3-α-glucuronic acid and androster-
one-3-α-glucuronic acid were purchased from Ikapharm (Ramat-Gan,
Israel). Tetrabutylammonium bromide (TBABr) and tetrahexylammonium
bromide came from Fluka (Buchs, Switzerland). Disodium citrate was
obtained from Brocacef BV (Maarssen, The Netherlands). Acetonitrile,
chloroform, dichloromethane, diethyl ether, dimethyl formamide (DMF),
absolute ethanol, ethyl acetate, hexane and methanol were obtained from
J.T. Baker Chemicals (Deventer, The Netherlands).

All these reagents and solvents were of analytical reagent grade. The solvents were further purified by distillation from glass. Anthracene, NED.2HCl and DC were recrystallized twice from absolute ethanol and stored over P_2O_5. Amberlite XAD-2 (Fluka) and the BondElut C-18 cartridges (Analytichem, Harbor City, CA) were thoroughly washed with 3 vol. of methanol followed by 3 vol. of distilled water.

2-Bromo-1-methylpyridinium iodide (BMP) was synthesized as previously described [11]. NED was extracted from 1 M NaOH, containing 1 mg/ml purified NED.2HCl, by 3 successive extractions with equal volumes of dichloromethane. After evaporation of the combined organic phases to dryness, the residue was dried over P_2O_5. 2-Dansyl-ethanol, 3-dansyl-1-propanol and 3-dansylamino-1-propanol were synthesized by Goya and co-workers and gifted by Dr. A. Takadate [13]. 2-Dansyl-amino-1-ethylamine was synthesized similarly [13]. Etoposideglucuronide was isolated from patients' urine (cf. Holthuis et al., in this vol.). Other chemicals came from various commercial sources and were used as received.

INSTRUMENTATION

The HPLC apparatus consisted of two Model 6000 A pumps and two U6K injectors (Waters Assoc.), equipped with a Perkin-Elmer Model 650 fluorescence detector (slit width 10 nm; 150 BC xenon power supply) and a Model M 440 absorbance detector (Waters Assoc.). A 30 cm × 3.9 mm i.d. steel column, slurry-packed with LiChrosorb Si 60 (10 μm particles; E. Merck), was used as the pre-column in a two-column switching device, in combination with a slurry-packed Lichrosorb RP-18 (10 μm particles; E. Merck) analytical column of the same dimensions. The Lichrosorb columns were maintained at 25±1°. The column switching (Fig. 1) was performed with a nitrogen-activated 7000 psi sample injection valve (Valco Insts. Co., Houston) controlled by a digital valve interface (Valco) and a SP 4000 central processor (Spectra Physics, Santa Clara, CA).

Excitation and emission spectra were obtained with a Perkin-Elmer Model 204 fluorescence spectrophotometer. Fluorescence quantum yields were determined with reference to anthracene in ethanol at ambient temperature [11, 14]. UV absorption spectra were recorded on a SP 8-400 UV/Vis spectrophotometer (Pye Unicam, Cambridge).

DERIVATIZATION PROCEDURE

With DC and NED.2HCl as the fluorescence-introducing agents the test compound was NG. The reaction is based on activation of the carboxylic function with BMP [11, 12]. Without activation of either the carboxylic acid or the amine (reagent) function, only minute amounts of the amide are formed under the mild reaction conditions used in this study. Instead of an amine reagent it is

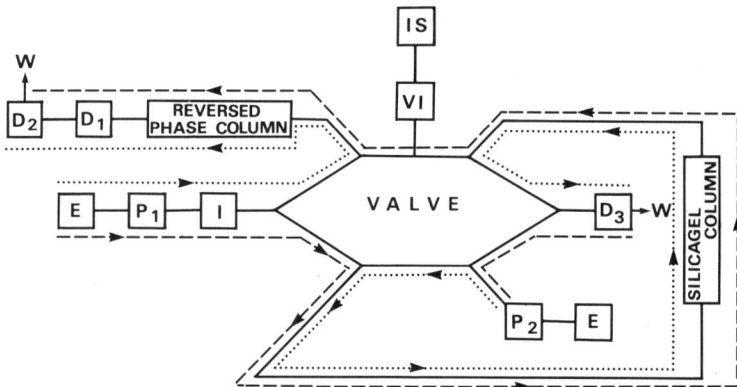

Fig. 1. Two-column system: —————, pathway during injection;
·········, pathway during elution; D_1, fluorescence detector; D_2, D_3,
UV detector; E, solvent reservoir; I, injector; IS, integrator;
P_1, P_2, high pressure pumps; VI, digital valve interface; W, waste.

also possible to use a primary alcohol as the labelling reagent [11].
The BMP method as developed by us is based on the work of Saigo et al.
[15]. The influence of the solvent and the choice of label on the
derivatization yield and the selectivity of the method towards the
carboxylic acid function was discussed in an earlier paper, where it
was concluded that only the carboxylic acid function is derivatized
by this method [12].

The reactions were performed in stoppered 1.5 ml polypropylene
tubes. To a solution of 1-1000 ng of the glucuronide in 40 μl DMF
(containing triethylamine, 2% w/w), 10 μl of BMP solution (10 mg/ml
in acetonitrile), 40 μl of DC solution (label; 2 mg/ml in dichloromethane) and 60 μl dichloromethane were added. After vortex mixing
for 30 sec the mixture was allowed to stand for 15 min at 25° and evaporated to dryness under a stream of nitrogen. The residue was dissolved
in 50-500 μl HPLC solvent (depending on the amount of the glucuronide)
and 10 μl portions were analyzed.

When NED.2HCl was used as the fluorescence label a suspension of
2 mg/ml NED.2HCl in dichloromethane containing 2 mg/ml triethylamine
was used instead of the described DC solution.

If instead of the protonated glucuronides the corresponding salts
were analyzed, the triethylamine was omitted.

HPLC ANALYSIS

The mobile-phase solvents were deaerated ultrasonically and
delivered at a flow-rate of 1 ml/min. For the analysis of the non-

Fig. 2. HPLC patterns
after derivatization of 1 µg
of NG with DC to give the
amide (x in B; A = reagent
blank). See text for
conditions.

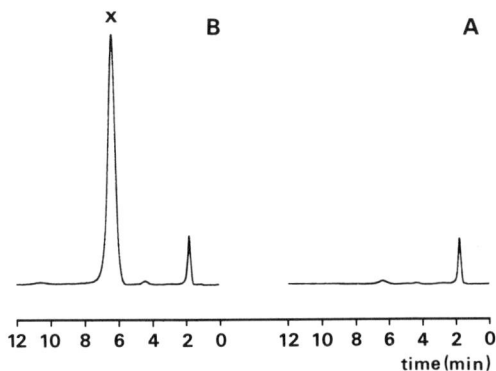

Fig. 3. As for
Fig. 2, but
NED.2HCl in
place of DC.

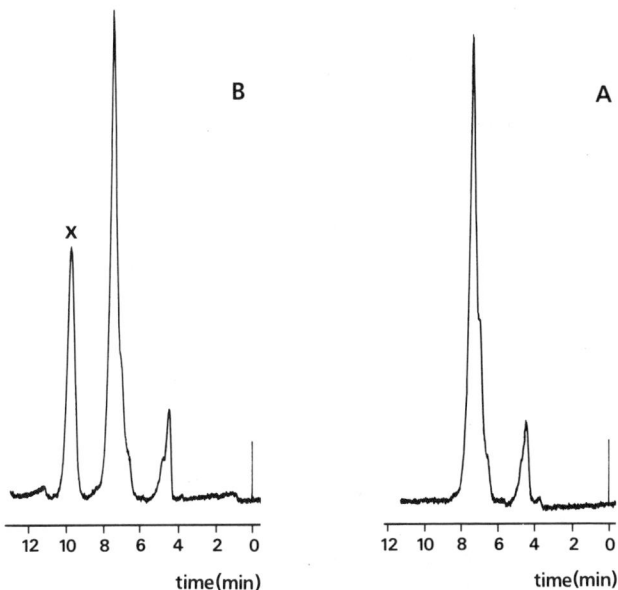

derivatized glucuronides the mobile phase (eluent-I) consisted of
methanol/water (4:6 by wt.) with 0.002m TBABR and 0.002 m$^{\otimes}$ Na$_2$citrate at
pH 5.4. The wavelengths for excitation/emission were 295/335 nm.
For the NG–DC amide the methanol/water ratio was 7:3 and the pH 5.1
(eluent-II); the wavelengths were 355/520 nm. For the NG–NED and
17-EG–NED amides the methanol/water ratio was 7:3 (eluent-III) or
6.5:3.5 (eluent-IV) and the pH 5.3; the wavelengths were 335/415 nm.

Representative HPLC patterns for the derivatization mixtures
are shown in Fig. 2 (eluent-II) with DC as the label and in Fig. 3
(eluent-III) with NED.2HCl as the source. Because of the strongly
tailing peaks obtained with the amine reagents (present in large excess)
with the usual RP column packings, the derivatives could not be
analyzed on a single column, and the following approach was used.

$\otimes$ m = mol/kg

With ion-exchange (IE) as one approach, a 2-column system (IE/RP) was developed. A non-modified silica gel column in the IE mode as described elsewhere [16] was used to retard the excess of the amine. The derivatives, however, being neutral compounds were not retained on this bare silica column; they are analyzed with the RP column which is coupled to silica gel column. For both columns the same eluent was used for injection and elution. The citrate buffer in the mobile phase is needed to preserve a pH value at which the amines are protonated, because only positively charged molecules can be retained on the silica gel column by an IE mechanism. The TBA$^+$ or TMA$^+$ ions added to the mobile phase act as competing ions and thus influence the retention of the cations (reagent) on the IE column.

Injection is performed with the two columns coupled (Fig. 1, ----), and the derivative is eluted from the silica gel column onto the RP (analytical) column, whereupon the valve is switched so that the derivative is eluted while the excess of the amine is washed off the silica gel column. No improvement in detection sensitivity was observed when the mobile phase was deoxygenated by flushing with N$_2$ rather than ultrasonically.

Calibration curves showed good linearity. Thus, after analyzing 10 samples containing NG (0.1-1.5 µg) as described with DC as the fluorescent label, the calibration line equation was y = (1.05±1.15)x + 4.24±0.23 (r = 0.997; S.D.'s denoted ±). With the conditions used the detection limit for the NG-DC amide was found to be 100 fmol (signal-to-noise ratio = 3); 100% conversion of NG to NG-DC was achieved. When NED.2HCl was used as the fluorophore source, 94% conversion was achieved, as estimated from the incomplete disappearance of the NG from the chromatogram (eluent-I). Instead of using NED.2HCl it was possible to derivatize with the free base NED, but it is rather unstable in contact with air and sometimes leads to ghost peaks evident in the blank chromatograms.

For some other glucuronides that were tested, the derivatization yields with NED.2HCl were of the same magnitude as found with 1 µg quantities of NG. HPLC was performed by IE followed by RP with eluent-IV. Steroid glucuronide derivatives usually separated well (k' values given parenthetically; 0.66 for glucuronic acid). Thus, it was possible to separate oestradiol glucuronides from one another, viz. 3- (2.71), 17- (3.96) and 3,17-di- (4.98). However, the two isomers androsterone- and etiocholanolone-glucuronide (10.64, 10.88) could not be separated. Four other steroid monoglucuronides were tested: testosterone-17- (4.04), oestriol-16- (1.90), diethylstilboestrol- (2.48), and hexoestrol- (3.00). Four non-steroid glucuronides were also tested: β-naphthyl- (2.11), menthol- (9.57), p-nitrophenyl- (1.99), and etoposide- (1.17).

Table 1. UV absorption and fluorescence data for dansyl derivatives. Anthracene serves as the reference compound. All measurements are performed at 20 ±1°. See text for terms used.

R	Solvent	ε_{355}	Q_f	BW (cm^{-1})	IFS
[Anthracene	methanol	7574	0.28	1390	1.53]
$-(CH_2)_2-OH$	methanol	3919	0.12	2960	0.16
$-(CH_2)_3-OH$	methanol	3955	0.13	2995	0.17
$-NH-(CH_2)_3-OH$	methanol	3434	0.17	3200	0.18
$-NH-(CH_2)_2-NH_2$	acetonitrile	3338	0.25	3140	0.27
	methanol	3062	0.17	3150	0.17
	water	2184	0.01	2210	0.01
$-NH-(CH_2)_5-NH_2$ (DC)	methanol	3246	0.17	3175	0.17

FLUORESCENCE SENSITIVITY

The detection sensitivity of a fluorescing compound is determined not only by its retention behaviour (k' and peak shape) and by instrumental factors, but also by its molar absorptivity, ε, at the excitation wavelength, its quantum yield of fluorescence, Q_f, and the width of the emission band (BW) at half peak height. The intrinsic fluorescence sensitivity (IFS) is a suitable parameter for evaluating the detection sensitivity of labelled compounds [11, 14, 17]; by definition, IFS = $\varepsilon.Q_f/BW$ (BW expressed in wave-numbers).

Table 1 gives these values for some dansyl derivatives, evidently almost independent of the substituent attached to the sulphonyl group. Other notable conclusions are that the fluorescence in water is almost completely quenched and that the fluorescence in acetonitrile is 50% higher than in methanol. Therefore the highest sensitivity can be obtained with high concentrations of organic modifier in the HPLC eluents. Although the IFS value of DC in methanol (0.17) is not very high, e.g. in comparison with the reference compound anthracene (1.53), the sensitivity of the method is satisfactory.

The advantage of DC for labelling (giving the NG-DC amide which has comparable fluorescence data) is the high emission wavelength, 520 nm, which offers a high degree of selectivity. However, problems arise due to the limited photostability of the label. The calibration line sometimes deviates from the origin due to a decomposition-product peak co-eluting with NG-DC. This can be avoided by using recrystalized DC, kept in the dark. Furthermore, the fluorescent transition of the dansyl nucleus is of $\pi-\pi^*$ type, resulting in an almost completely quenched fluorescence in water-rich media.

Table 2. UV absorption and fluorescence data for NED and α-naph-thyl-β-D-glucuronate. Measurements at 23 ±1°; otherwise as for Table 1 heading. The tabulated eluent was eluent-III (but pH of aqueous phase was 5.4).

Compound	Solvent	ε_{355}	Qf	BW (cm^{-1})	IFS
[Anthracene	ethanol	2671	0.28	2479	0.30
	methanol	2638	0.26	2511	0.27]
NED	0.1 M NaOH	4219	0.08	3835	0.09
NED.H$^+$	ethanol	6037	0.55	3776	0.88
	methanol	5913	0.50	3861	0.77
	water	5274	0.70	3857	0.96
	eluent		0.73		
NED.2H$^+$	0.5 M H_2SO_4	3122	0.08	3797	0.07
	hexane	2615	0.02	3447	0.02
NG–NED	eluent		0.31		

If the NED nucleus with a n-π* type emission transition was used instead of DC, a 100-fold increase of the IFS value was seen in water (Table 2) as compared with DC. As expected, the quantum yield of fluorescence in hexane (apolar solvent) was very low. Using NED.2HCl as the reagent, precautions have to be taken with respect both to eluent pH and to organic modifier concentration. The pH of the eluent's aqueous phase must be chosen between 4 and 10 because the NED nucleus fluoresces very poorly in acidic or alkaline aqueous solutions (Fig. 4). If the methanol percentage of the eluent was kept below 70% (w/w) only a slight variation in the IFS values was observed (Fig. 4). The advantage of NED as the fluorescence label is the 2-fold increased IFS value for the NG–NED amide as compared with NG–DC. The detection limit for NG–NED was found to be 50 fmol with a signal-to-noise ratio of 3 under these conditions. NED derivatization leads, however, to a poten-tially interfering peak in the chromatogram - a disadvantage of NED.

THE ANALYSIS OF GLUCURONIDES IN PLASMA AND URINE

The potential of derivatization with NED.2HCl for determining plasma and urinary glucuronides was investigated with NG and 17-EG as test compounds. Several methods have been described for isolating glu-curonides from biological fluids [18-22] (see also J. Tomašič in Vol. 12, this series.-Ed.). In this study, poor recoveries and very 'noisy' chromatograms resulted from the extraction modes tried: liquid-liquid (diethyl ether, ethyl acetate), ion-pair (THAB⊗) and liquid-solid (Amberlite XAD-2); also they were tedious to perform. A pre-extraction wash-step with dichloromethane followed by a liquid-solid extraction with a C-18 cartridge gave good results for plasma as well as urine samples (Fig. 5).

⊗ tetrahexylammonium bromide

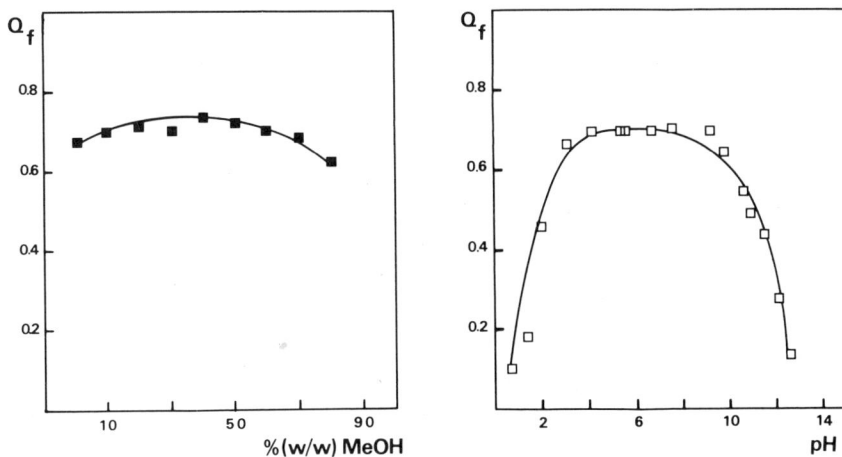

Fig. 4. Quantum yield of fluorescence of NED.2HCl *vs.* % (w/w) of methanol in a mixture otherwise as for eluent-I, pH 5.4 in aqueous phase *(left)*, and *vs.* pH of aqueous solutions *(right)*.

Fig. 5. Chromatograms obtained after derivatizing 17-EG with NED.2HCl, following isolation with a C-18 cartridge from a 100 µl plasma sample containing 1 ng (× in B denotes the amide derivative; A = plasma blank).

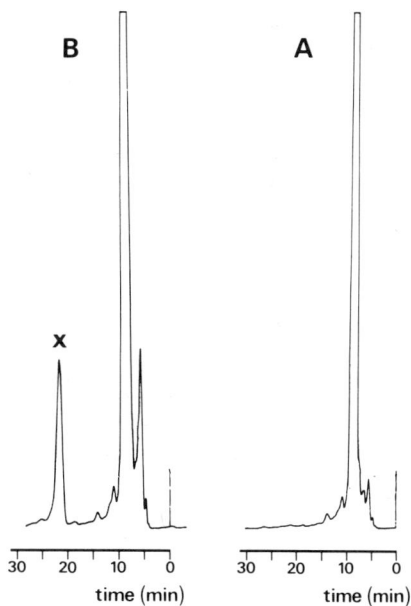

The procedure was as follows. Human plasma and urine samples, 100 µl, spiked with 1–1000 ng of glucuronide (or its Na salt) were mixed with 100 µl water and extracted by shaking for 2 min with 1.0 ml dichloromethane. After centrifugation (5 min) the resulting water fraction was transferred to a C-18 cartridge. After washing it with 200 µl 3% (w/w) acetic acid, the glucuronides were eluted with 1.0 ml of methanol/water (7:3 by wt.). The eluate was evaporated by a N_2 stream at ambient temperature. The residue was dissolved in 40 µl DMF containing triethylamine and derivatized as described above but with 100 instead of 10 µl of the BMP solution.

Calibration curves with this clean-up procedure showed good linearity: thus for 8 plasma samples spiked with 0.1–1.0 µg NG and with NED.2HCl as the reagent, $y = (39.9\pm1.6)x + 0.14\pm0.92$ ($r = 0.992$). With urine as starting sample the minimum amount of NG-NED that could be detected was 100 fmol, compared with 50 fmol for plasma samples. This difference, notwithstanding good separation of the NG-NED peak from the reagent blank peak, was due to incomplete separation from small peaks originating from urine constituents. Comparable calibration curves with excellent linearity were obtained for the determination of 17-EG in plasma and urine samples; here a detection limit of 50 fmol could be achieved.

CONCLUDING COMMENTS

The methods now developed with a derivatization procedure for the carboxylic acid functional group of glucuronides allows their detection at 10–20 pg/ml concentrations in urine and plasma. Sensitivity and specificity are achieved by clean-up followed by RP-HPLC with fluorescence detection of products that are pre-formed in the easy derivatization.

References

1. Kawasaki, T., Maeda, M. & Tsuji, A. (1982) *J. Chromatog. 233*, 61–68.
2. Takashi, U., Shigeru, A. & Kazuaki, K. (1983) *J. Chromatog. 277*, 308–313.
3. Colombo, T., D'Incalci, M., Farina, P., Rossi, C., Quatani, A., Bartosek, I., Benfenati, E., Fanelli, R. & Garratini, S. (1983) *Proc. Am. Ass. Cancer Res. 24*, 292.
4. Veenendaal, J.R. & Meffin, P.J. (1981) *J. Chromatog. 223*, 147–154.
5. Veenendaal, J.R. & Meffin, P.J. (1984) *J. Chromatog. 307*, 432–438.
6. Fenselau, C. & Johnson, L.P. (1980) *Drug Metab. Disp. 8*, 274–283.
7. Hasegawa, J., Smith, P.C. & Benet, L.Z. (1982) *Drug Metab. Disp. 10*, 469–473.
8. Blanckaert, N., Compernolle, F., Leroy, P., von Houtte, R., Fevery, J. & Heirwegh, K.P.M. (1978) *Biochem. J. 171*, 203–214.

9. Lingeman, H., Underberg, W.J.M., Takadate, A. & Hulshoff, A. (1985) *J. Liq. Chromatog. 8*, 789-894.
10. Hulshoff, A. & Lingeman, H. (1984) *J. Pharm. Biomed. Anal. 2*, 337-380.
11. Lingeman, H., Hulshoff, A., Underberg, W.J.M. & Offermann, F.B.J.M. (1984) *J. Chromatog. 290*, 215-222.
12. Lingeman, H., Haan, H.B.P. & Hulshoff, A. (1984) *J. Chromatog. 336*, 241-248.
13. Goya, S., Takadate, A. & Iwai, M. (1981) *Yakugaku Zasshi 101*, 1164-1169.
14. Parker, C.A. & Rees, W.T. (1960) *Analyst 85*, 587-600.
15. Saigo, K., Usui, M., Kikuchi, K., Simada, E. & Mukaiyama, T. (1977) *Bull. Chem. Soc. Jpn. 50*, 1863-1866.
16. Lingeman, H., Munsler, H.A. van, Beynen, J.H., Underberg, W.J.M. & Hulshoff, A. (1986) *J. Chromatog.*, in press.
17. Lloyd, J.B.F. (1979) *J. Chromatog. 178*, 249-258.
18. Meffin, P.J. & Zilm, D.M. (1983) *J. Chromatog. 278*, 101-108.
19. Musson, D.G., Lin, J.H., Lyon, K.A., Tocco, D.J. & Yeh, K.C. (1985) *J. Chromatog. 337*, 363-378.
20. Fransson, B. & Schill, G. (1975) *Acta Pharm. Suec. 12*, 107-118.
21. Svensson, J-O., Rane, A., Saewe, J. & Sjoeqvist, F. (1982) *J. Chromatog. 230*, 427-432.
22. Kawahara, K. & Ofuji, T. (1982) *J. Chromatog. 231*, 333-339.

Present addresss of first author (H. Lingeman): Division of Analytical Chemistry, Center for Bio-Pharmaceutical Sciences, Gorlaeus Laboratories, State University of Leiden, P.O. Box 9502, 2300 RA Leiden, The Netherlands.

#D-4

PHOTODIODE ARRAY HPLC DETECTORS IN METABOLIC PROFILING AND OTHER ANALYTICAL SCREENING TECHNIQUES

Rokus A. de Zeeuw

Department of Analytical Chemistry and Toxicology
State University
A. Deusinglaan 2, 9713 AW Groningen, The Netherlands

A new generation of UV-visible spectrophotometers has appeared in which a compound's absorption spectrum is depicted in a fraction of a second by a multichannel photodiode array system. These detectors can record a series of spectra of very low intensity and store the data in their own memory and/or in external devices such as magnetic tapes or discs. These properties give diode array detectors (DAD's) great potential as on-line detectors in HPLC.

We have evaluated two commercially available DAD's for use in drug metabolite profiling and systematic toxicological analysis. The combined HPLC-DAD system proved to be very useful, comparable in potential to a GC-MS or LC-MS combination yet much cheaper. However, limitations became apparent, particularly in the area of data generation, storage and retrieval. Some of these may be inherent in the technique; others may be obviated when the technique is further developed.

HPLC has proved to be a powerful technique in quantitative analysis. Yet when it comes to qualitative analysis, in which screening for unknown compounds is the major aim, no universal detection mode is available. This has led to a situation where most people use HPLC combined with conventional UV detection at low wavelengths for screening purposes; but where the UV absorption properties of the substances that one is looking for are unknown, this brings the risk that they will go unnoticed.

In recent years, however, multichannel diode array spectrophotometers (DAD's) have come on the market that are capable of recording the absorption spectrum of an HPLC eluate in <1 sec, covering the the range 190-600 or 190-800 nm. The heart of these instruments is a series of light-sensitive diodes etched onto a silicon chip. After passage of the light beam through the sample cell it is dispersed through a grating system and then monitored by the diode array, so that each diode monitors a given wavelength with 1-2 nm band width. As compared to conventional, single wavelength detection, it is evident that diode-array detection provides many advantages in screening analysis. Indeed, HPLC-DAD may yield two identification parameters in one run, namely the retention parameter (capacity factor or relative retention time) and the UV-VIS absorption spectrum.

Here we report on our experiences in two areas where screening for unknown compounds is of paramount importance, namely in drug metabolite profiling and in systematic toxicological analysis.

DRUG METABOLITE PROFILING (DMP)

DMP - the analysis of excretory fluids such as urine and bile to establish the metabolic fate of a particular drug - aims to give a complete qualitative picture of all metabolites therein. In general metabolites are quite polar and/or are conjugated, and HPLC is therefore the separation technique of choice, with an increasing role for DAD where the drug manifests some UV-VIS absorption.

Use of HPLC and DAD in combination is now exemplified by studies on the metabolism of butoprozine, an indolizine derivative with anti-anginal properties. Fig. 1 shows its structure and UV spectrum, and the experimental set-up, viz. (HP = Hewlett-Packard, Palo Alto, CA):- an SF-770 variable single-wavelength detector, A (Schoeffel, Westwood, NJ); an HP-8450A multi-channel diode array UV-VIS spectrorophotometer, B, equipped with an M-178.32 QS flow-through quartz cell C (8 µl; Hellma, Mühlheim Baden, W. Germany); an HP-9875A tape cartridge using a dual tape drive, D; an HP-9872A graphics plotter, E; an Apple II plus (64K) computer with a video display (F & G); a stainless steel column, H (150×4.6 mm i.d.) packed with 5 µm LiChrosorb RP-8 (Merck) or Nucleosil C-18 (Machery, Nagel & Co.); a WISP-710B autoinjector, two M-45 pumps and an M-720 solvent programmer (Waters).

The columns were packed by means of a balanced density slurry method specially developed for the ammoniacal elution system. Gradient elution was performed with 5 mM ammonia/methanol using linear and/or stepwise gradient programmes, usually starting with 5 mM ammonia and introducing methanol; the final elution was with 100% methanol. The flow-rate was 1 ml/min. The solvents were pre-saturated with He, and a He atmosphere was maintained in the eluent reservoirs.

The spectrophotometer B used as an HPLC detector was originally developed for UV-VIS spectroscopic analysis only, and was now adapted by replacing the sample cell with a flow cell. When the spectra are stored in its memory, consecutive spectra can be recorded with a time

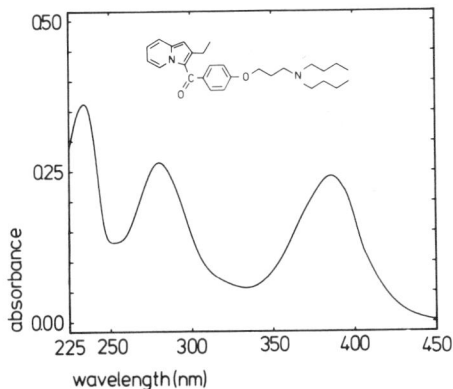

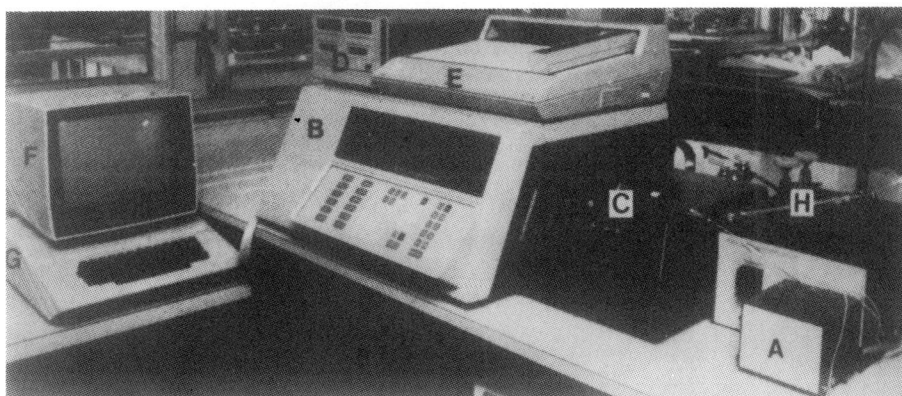

Fig. 1. Structure and absorption spectrum of butoprozine and the experimental set-up used for its metabolic profiling. For explanations see text.

interval of 1 sec. However, because of the limited storage capacity only 35 spectra could be thus stored, usually insufficient for a run on a biological sample. Also, because of the large amount of information generated by the detector, the data have to be written into a memory device, precluding direct data plotting during analysis. To overcome these limitations the data were transferred to an external storage device (tape or disc). This was found to require at least 3 sec per spectrum, which we found to be no handicap. During a run a built-in monitor in the detector can provide either the full spectra that are being recorded or a portion thereof, or the chromatographic trace at a single, pre-selected wavelength. Comprehensive access to the stored data and plotting thereof, e.g. in 3-D spectrochromatograms or in reconstructed, single-wavelength chromatograms, is possible after the run.

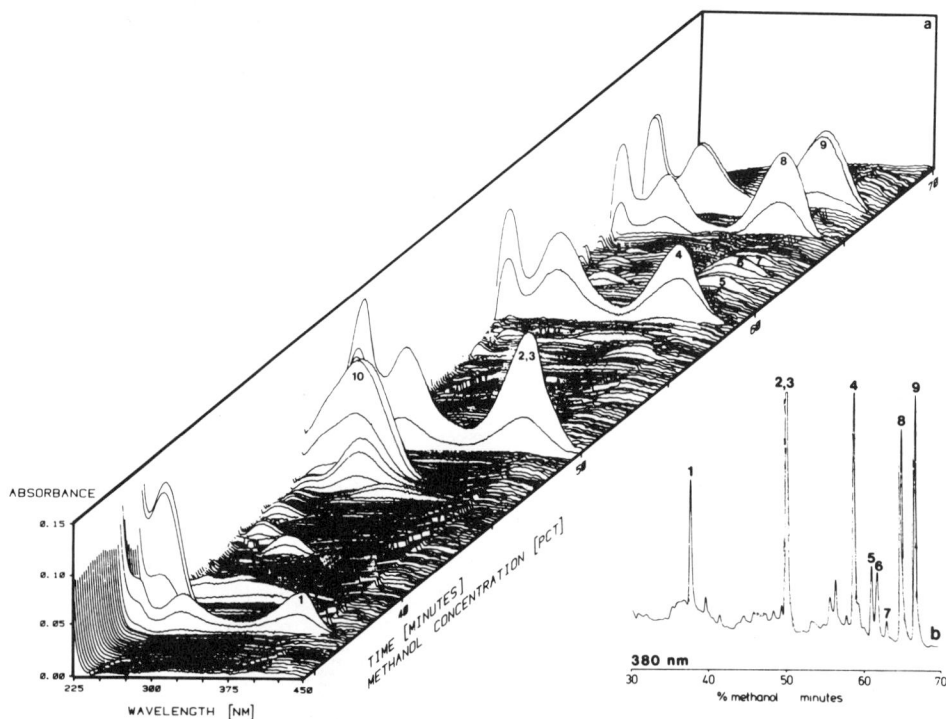

Fig. 2. *Left*, **a:** Spectrochromatogram of dog bile after administration of butoprozine. *Right*, **b:** Conventional, single wavelength chromatogram of the same fraction as in **a**, recorded at 380 nm.

In our experiments the DAD was connected in series with a conventional single-wavelength detector (**A**, Fig. 1), in order to compare the potential of the two detectors. This also had the advantage that, during a run, a display of the absorption spectra of the eluting components via the monitor of the DAD and the recording of the chromatogram at a single wavelength via the conventional detector was feasible. This set-up proved to be highly useful when dealing with complex materials in relatively long runs. Thus the conventional chromatogram, recorded at a wavelength at which we anticipated that most of the compounds of interest would be detectable, served as a lead to recall relevant data obtained by the DAD from the memory after the run, for further examination, manipulation and plotting.

The potential of DAD *versus* conventional, single-wavelength detection is shown in Fig. 2, which illustrates the analysis of dog bile after intravenous administration of butoprozine. The conventional chromatogram shows the absorption at 380 nm; the 3-D one, which we prefer to call a spectrochromatogram, depicts absorbance *versus* time over the range 225–450 nm as would seem to be relevant for butoprozine metabolites. For the latter chromatogram, spectra were taken every

8 sec, stored on tape during the run and then recalled for plotting after completion of chromatography. Comparison of the two chromatograms clearly shows the dramatic gain in selectivity and information provided by the multi-channel detector in a single run.

Recognition of butoprozine structural analogues against the background can be made immediately, based upon the absorption spectrum of the parent drug (metabolites 1-9). A spectrochromatogram of blank bile (not shown) is of further help. Structure elucidation studies showed that the above metabolites have an intact aromatic system but that hydroxy and/or methoxy groups had been introduced. Peak '10' apparently contained a compound different in spectrum from butoprozine and so undetected in the conventional chromatogram; it had to be a metabolite - as established by comparisons with chromatograms of blank bile.

HPLC-DAD proved to be most effective in certain human studies where where the use of radiolabelled drugs was precluded and the screening studies had to rely on UV-VIS absorption. Fig. 3 shows data obtained with human bile [2, 3]. In each 100 min run, with a linear gradient (5 mM ammonia to methanol without ammonia), spectra were recorded every 12 sec, resulting in 500 spectra each with 400 absorption points. For reasons of time (fully 7 h to print out fully) and simplicity, only the 225-500 nm range has been plotted; the 500-800 nm region was not of interest as none of the eluting compounds showed absorption there.

Comparison of the two 'straight' chromatograms (consecutive spectra corresponding in sequence to the time sequence) in Fig. 3, centre and (blank) right, readily shows the presence of (a) 3 main endogenous components - E_1, E_2 and E_3 - in the blank and after treatment, their concentrations changing with post-treatment time, and (b) one main metabolite, M, after treatment. Even though the plotting of spectrochromatograms is time-consuming, DAD provides a dramatic gain in time, by as much as 90% compared with the classical UV approach (off-line determination of spectra). Peak recognition is based on retention-time comparison (provided by the high reproducibility of the separation system) and spectra comparison (provided by the highly informative detection system). Also, the spectrochromatograms can give direct structural information. Thus, the metabolite M has a similar UV spectrum to the parent drug but very different chromatographic behaviour (eluting with ~60% methanol, *versus* ~90% for the parent drug), This indicates the introduction of a polar group in M, in an otherwise intact aromatic system. Structure elucidation has revealed the introduction of one hydroxyl at the 1-position of the butoprozine molecule [3].

With all the absorbance data on a tape or disc, plotting the data points as well as connecting them can be done in various ways, provided that the requisite computer programs are written for each purpose. Time, wavelength and absorbance axes can be varied in magnitude,

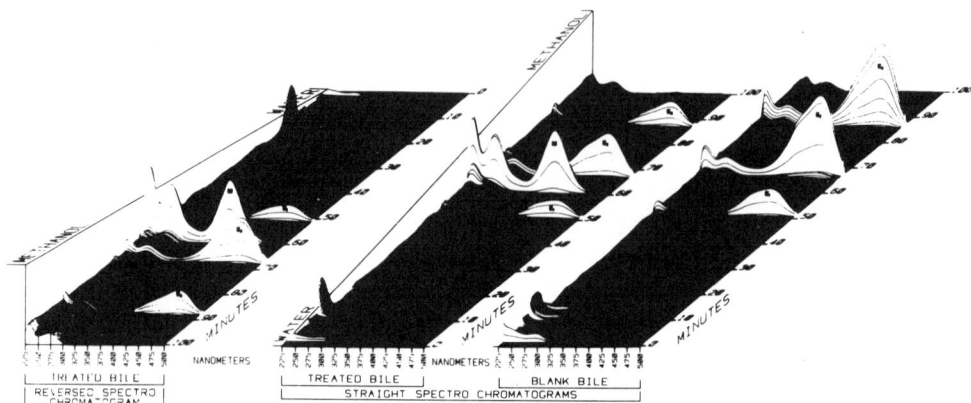

Fig. 3. Spectrochromatograms (225 to 500 nm) of human bile taken during 6 h following butoprozine administration ('treated bile') compared with bile taken during the hour preceding administration ('blank bile'), to allow differentiation between metabolites and endogenous components. The run time (MINUTES axis) was 100 min. 'Straight' is explained in the text.

direction and angle, as in the left-hand spectrochromatogram in Fig. 3 where the time axis has been reversed so that we are 'going back in time'. This reversed spectrochromatogram allows us to see what is present behind a peak. Detailed comparison of this and the 'straight' chromatogram and the blank chromatogram shows the possible presence of other minor butoprozine metabolites just before and just after the main metabolite M. Now the presence of the minor metabolites a, b, c and d can be better observed. However, because we instructed the computer not to plot in the shadow of a peak, Figs. 3 and 4 do not reveal what is present between M and E_2. To observe this, the spectra 41→50 were plotted (Fig. 5). Now the minor metabolite d can be better observed.

In the gradient runs performed, an increasing background can be seen in the wavelength region 225-310 nm when going from water to methanol. Such a background or a contribution from an overlapping peak can readily be subtracted (see later).

With the data from the entire run stored on tape or disc, one is able to examine carefully all areas in the chromatogram so as to gain the maximum amount of information, as indicated by Figs. 4 & 5 and reinforced by Fig. 6 – which demonstrates that conventional single-wavelength detection does not disclose the minor metabolites a-d. Fig. 7 further exemplifies the utility of DAD in establishing peak purity. This can be done by taking the recorded spectra in sequential order and computing their absorption ratio at two wavelengths [4].

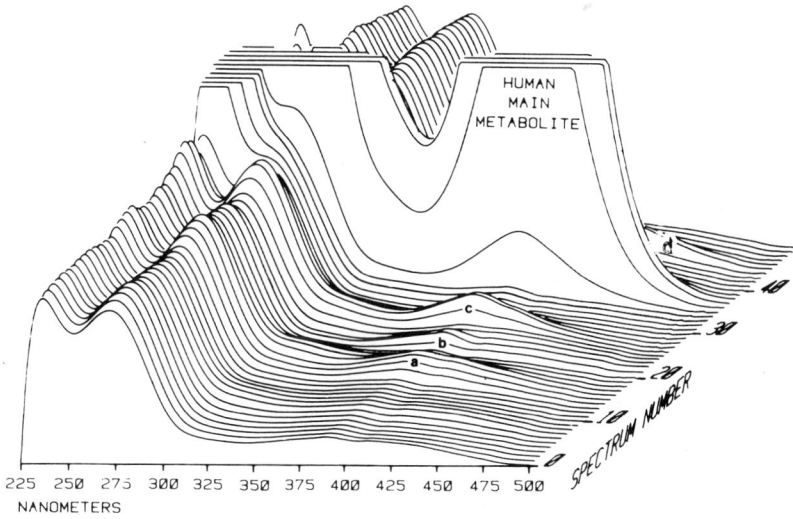

Fig. 4. Part of the 'TREATED STRAIGHT' chromatograms (cf. Fig. 3), now plotted at higher sensitivity and showing the individual spectra taken to allow detection of minor metabolites.

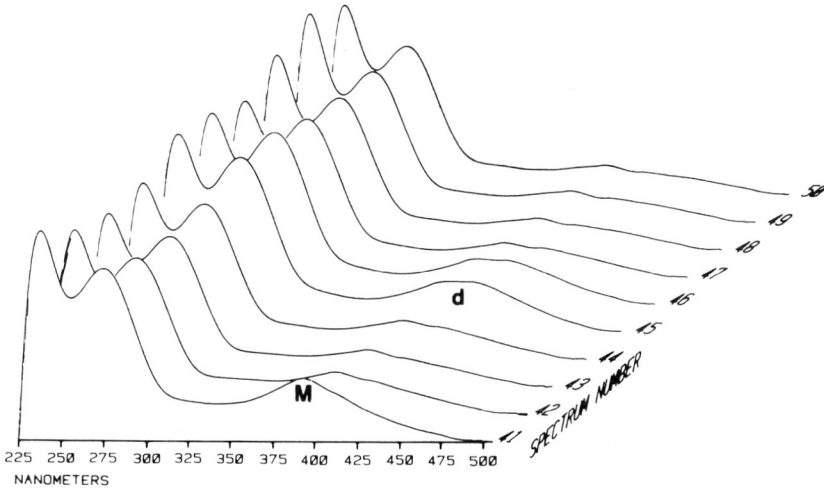

Fig. 5. Plots of spectra 41-50 in Fig. 4, just behind the main human metabolite: metabolite d now completely viewable.

In Fig. 7a the 2-D elution profiles of a mixture of drugs are given for absorption *versus* time at 230 and 240 nm, respectively, whereas in Fig. 7b the absorption ratio A_{230}/A_{240} is plotted *versus* time. If no peak is eluting, a horizontal line is obtained. If a peak elutes

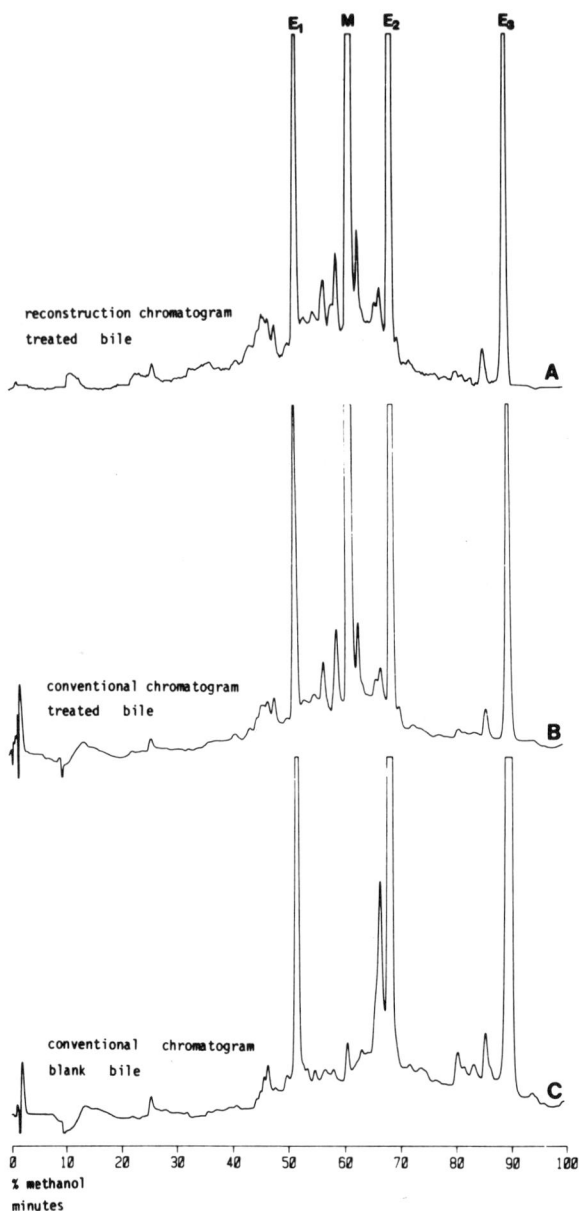

Fig. 6. Comparison of 2-D chromatograms of human bile after butoprozine administration: **A,** reconstructed from data obtained by DAD; **B** & **C,** recorded by a conventional single-wavelength detector at 380 nm.

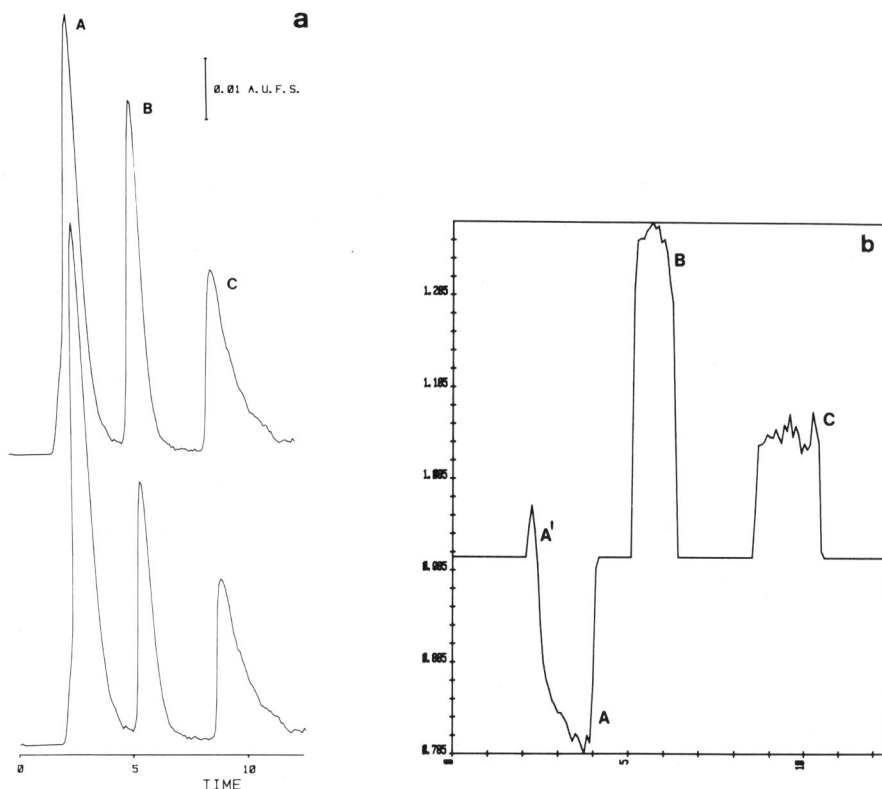

Fig. 7. a: Chromatogram of a mixture of 4 compounds obtained by DAD at 230 nm *(top)* and 240 nm *(bottom)*. b: The resulting ratio plot A_{230}/A_{240}. (Peak **A** = *N*-hydroxytetrahydrothienopyridine.)

and it is pure (i.e. not contaminated with a substance exhibiting an absorption spectrum different from that of the major eluting compound) we see a strong, almost vertical deflection of the baseline (either negative or positive) until the ratio reaches a virtual plateau. This plateau is maintained during the elution of the peak, even when tailing occurs (peak C), and then the ratio falls back to the baseline. However, if an impurity is present (as in peak A), an abnormal ratio signal will be manifest, e.g. an inversion such as shown in Fig. 7b. In general, abnormalities are reflected as deviations of the plateau [5].

The above examples clearly show the potential of HPLC-DAD in DMP. However, some disadvantages and limitations should also be mentioned. Firstly, the limited memory capacity for storing spectral data of the instrument itself (although this can be overcome by introducing additional memory capacity via tapes or discs) and the tremendous

amount of data gathered in each run (in DMP usually between 40 and
100 min). Evaluating these data may take hours or even days, particularly if one is inexperienced. Secondly, the plotting of the data,
especially in 3-D chromatograms, is rather time-consuming. Thirdly,
the limited possibilities for displaying data during the actual run.-
It is desirable that, at least, individual spectra plus the trace
at a pre-selected fixed wavelength can be displayed during the run.
For this reason, we used a conventional single-wavelength detector
in series with the HP 8450 DAD in our experimental set-up.

SYSTEMATIC TOXICOLOGICAL ANALYSIS (STA)

STA comprises the logical search for potentially harmful substances, with uncertain concerning their presence and identities.
The samples usually contain a variety of substances amid matrix compounds representing a complex background. Thus, the ability to record
complete absorption spectra is of paramount interest. Moreover,
it is virtually impossible in the screening for unknown substances,
whether with fixed- or variable-wavelength detectors, to find a single
wavelength that is suitable for all substances. Hence there is a
need for detectors capable of rapidly scanning or recording the complete
absorption spectrum of eluting peaks during the run without disturbing
or stopping the flow.

However, as time usually is literally a matter of life or death
in STA, DAD must be capable of yielding data very quickly. As this
cannot be accomplished with the sophisticated HP 8450 DAD, we selected
the HP 1040A fast-scanning DAD. It has ~200 diodes, monitoring wavelengths from 190 to 600 nm with 2 nm band-width. A single 'scan' is
taken in 10 millisec and can be repeated every 40 millisec [see 5].
With each diode array producing 25 data points per sec, a vast amount
of information is gathered by the detector, and must remain comprehen-
sible to the analyst. This is achieved by the HP-85 desk-top computer, which serves as the operator's terminal, and master computer.
The HP-85 was equippped with input/output, plotter/printer, mass
storage and advanced programming ROM's, 16 kB additional memory, and
an HP-IB IEEE-488 interface. Additional equipment included an HP 7470A
graphics plotter and an HP 82901M dual $5\frac{1}{4}$ inch flexible disc drive.
All software was supplied by Hewlett-Packard.

The HPLC system selected to evaluate the detector was that recommended by Daldrup et al. [6] and was used without further optimization.
It consisted of a 250x4 mm i.d. column of 7 μm Nucleosil C-18 (Machery-
Nagel, Dueren, FRG) and, as mobile-phase mixture, 200 ml of acetonitrile and 340 ml of a pH 2.3 buffer made by mixing 6.66 g KH_2PO_4 and
4.8 g H_3PO_4 (85%) and making up to 1 l with distilled water. Operation was at 25° with ~1 ml/min flow rate; injections were made with a
20 μl loop.

In this system, up to a maximum of 8 parallel signals can be monitored and set by the operator. All are definable as to wavelength and
band-width, which may vary from 4 to 100 nm and can be displayed,
along with one wavelength, on the CRT monitor during the run. The
same or another signal can be designated as the pilot signal, which is
routed through the peak detector that controls acquisition according
to peak status so as to take, display or store scans; 10 scans can be
stored in the local memory. The last chromatographic run, as displayed
on the CRT, or any spectra generated, can be copied by the thermal line-
printer of the HP-85. In addition, the system has two analog outputs
for signal transmission to external integrators, recorders or data
systems.

Though quite useful for various other analytical purposes, it
should be noted that for adequate utilization in STA the basic system
needs to be expanded with the dual disc drive and graphics plotter.
The HP 82901M adds ~50 kB to the memory, enabling multi-signal acquisition and storage, high-density spectral storage and post-analysis data
reduction. Through BASIC language programming the stored data from
an analysis can be treated according to individual needs and answers
can be obtained rapidly. Figs. 8-11 exemplify the potential of the
system as well as ways of presenting the data.

Fig. 8 represents the chromatogram of a mixture of 6 drug standards
monitored in parallel at 8 wavelengths with different band-widths.
The print-outs are normalized so that the differences in response can
be seen. The peak at ~3 min contains both caffeine and strychnine.
Although 8 signals have been monitored, only 6 can be plotted at
once. Evidently, as expected, the lower wavelengths produce the
highest responses. However, as interferences from biological matrices
usually have strong absorbances at the lower wavelengths too, it
can be advantageous to use other signals, e.g. C (254 nm; 4 nm band-
width) or D (260 nm; 80 nm). Generally, a wider band is more suitable
for screening purposes; yet signal F (320 nm; 20 nm band-width) would
be suitable if one were interested in substances that absorb in that
particular region.

Because of the scaling, the appearances of the peaks in Fig. 8
look somewhat unusual; but this can be circumvented by the plotting
applied in Fig. 9. For the same run as in Fig. 8, the data are now
plotted in one diagram, with different types of plot line for the 6
signals (and colours, as a further distinction in the original).

In Fig. 10 the same run is depicted as iso-absorption plots
(contour plots), offering a rough insight into the absorption spectrum of an eluting peak although the plotting is quite time-consuming
and the interpretation requires experience. Another way to plot
the data and visualize the absorption spectra is the 3-D mode
as shown in Fig. 11.

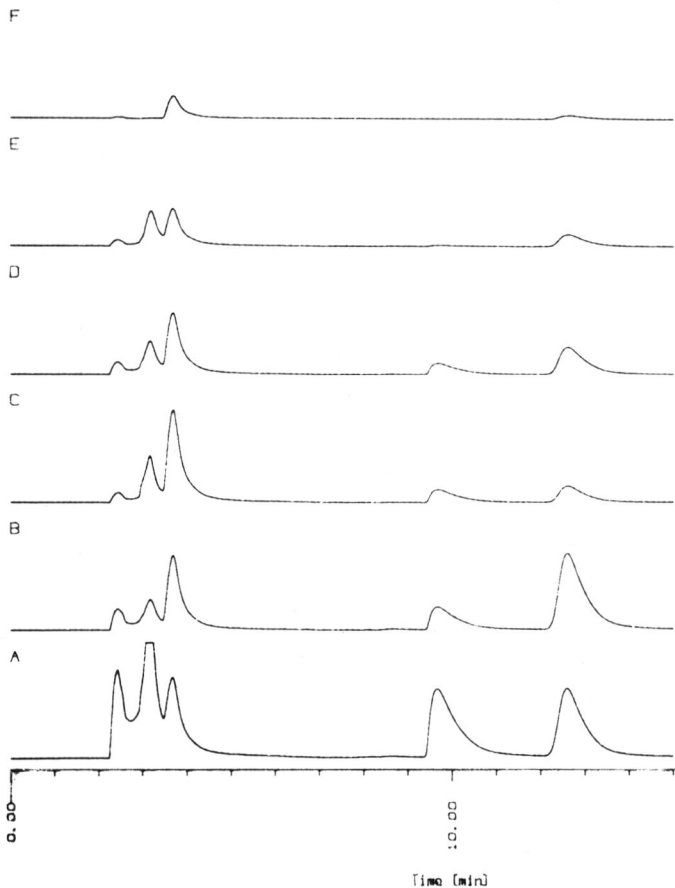

Fig. 8. Separation on a C-18 column of a mixture of 6 drug standards: codeine (retention time 2.4 min), strychnine (3.1), caffeine (3.2), chlordiazepoxide (3.7), amitriptyline (9.6) and methaqualone (12.5). Entries 1-6 at top right (7 & 8 inapplicable; see text) connote each monitoring wavelength and band-width (nm).

Fig. 10, *opposite.* As for Fig. 8, but with diphenhydramine additionally (retention time 5.7 min). Signals plotted as iso-absorbance (contour) lines. Absorbances increase from outside to inside, viz. 50-100-200-300-400-500-600-800 mAU respectively.
Acknowledgement for Figs. 8-15: they are due to appear in an American Chemical Society Symposium volume (lect. by author, Miami, April 1985).

Fig. 9. As for
Fig. 8 (same
print-out at
top), but now with
all absorption
signals plotted
in a single
diagram, distin-
guished by type
of line as in
the key (and, in
the printed-out
copy, by colour).

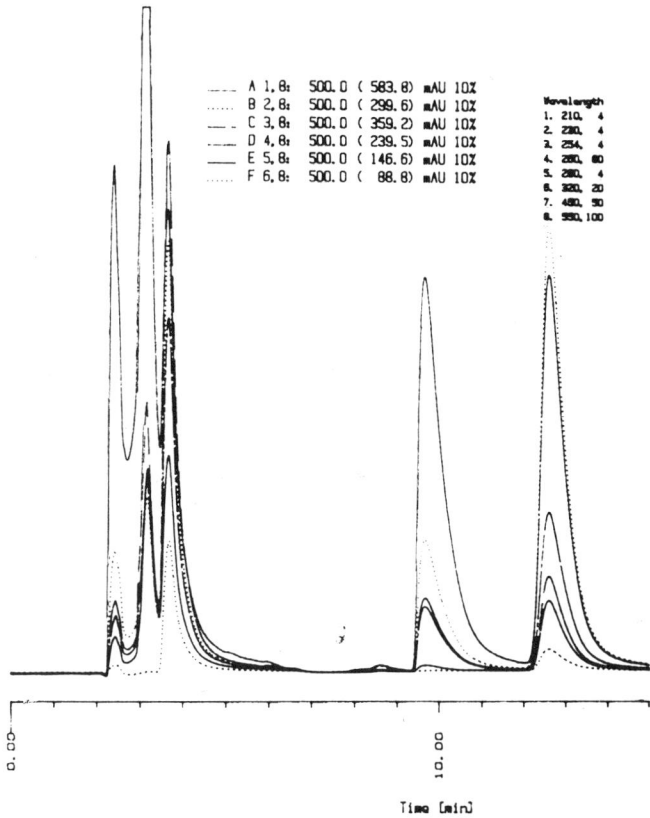

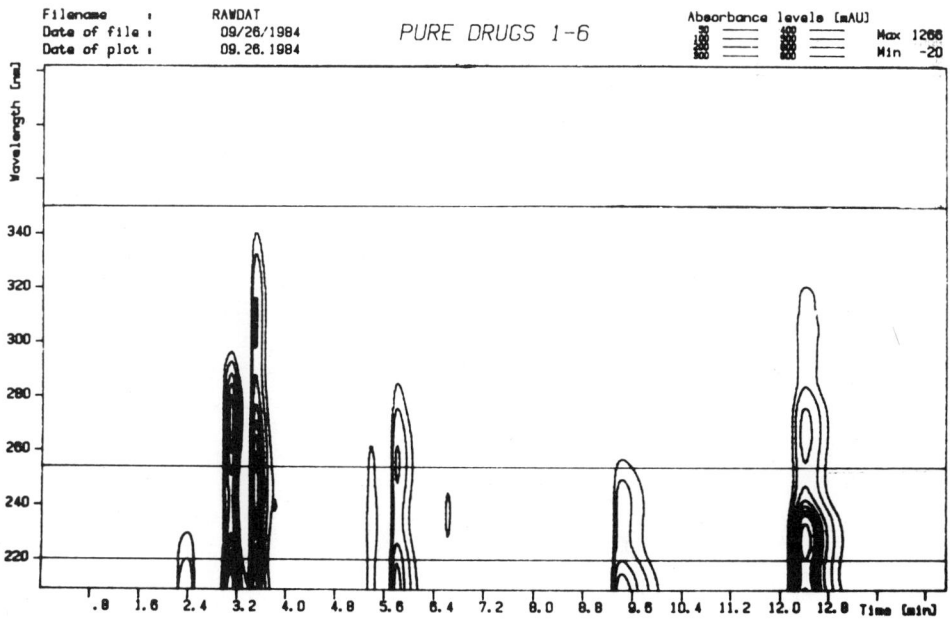

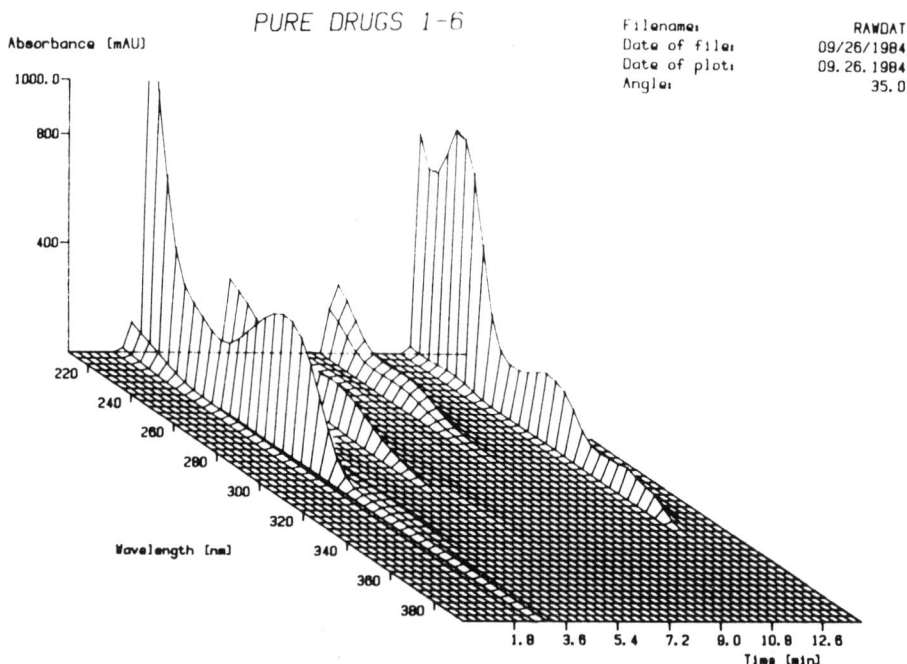

PURE DRUGS 1-6

Absorbance [mAU]

1000.0

800

400

220
240
260
280
300
320
Wavelength [nm]   340
360
380

Filename: RAWDAT
Date of file: 09/26/1984
Date of plot: 09.26.1984
Angle: 35.0

1.8   3.6   5.4   7.2   9.0 10.8 12.6
                              Time [min]

Fig. 11. As for Fig. 10 but with a 3-D mode for plotting the signals: absorbance *versus* wavelength *versus* time.

Fig. 12, *opposite.* HPLC of a mixture (9:1 by wt.) of caffeine and strychnine; retentimes so similar (3.25 & 3.15 min resp.) that only one peak is seen. *At top:* selected spectra taken at various positions in the run, with or without correction as indicated by 'Reference'; small-scale plot.

For general screening purposes in STA we found the plotting of Fig. 12 quite useful. Besides giving the chromatographic profile of the run at a selected wavelength and band-width, it also depicts small-scale absorption spectra over a given range at a given position in the run. Thereby one can get immediate information about the absorption properties of a given peak, with or without corrections for background absorption.

As stated earlier, DAD can help assess the purity of a peak. If there may be more than one component, obtaining individual spectra for identification may be achievable (Figs. 12 & 13) without having

---

Fig. 13, *opposite.* The spectra of Fig. 12: larger-scale plots, at peak apex (3.2215 min) without correction, ———; at 3.1550 min (where strychnine would elute), ----; at 3.2215 min, corrected by subtracting the 3.1550 min spectrum and now showing caffeine characteristics, ·······; and at 3.1550 min, corrected by subtracting the 3.2215 min spectrum and now showing strychnine characteristics, —·—·—. (Cf. Fig. 12 'Sample' values, min.)

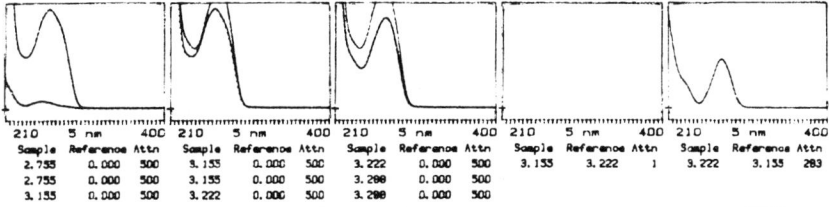

File: RAWDAT   PURE DRUGS   CAFF. +STRYCHN.
Date: 10/08/1984   origin   sample id.

analysis   TEST
inj. vol.   20
mobile ph. DALDRUP
    ''   MECN+BUFFER
    ''   340ML, 'pH=2.97
    ''   RPC18
stat. ph.   RPC18
column   NUCLEOSIL
run no.   1
inj.Time: 12:32
Attn (mAU): 373.7 (320.3)
ZeroL: 10%
Signal: D: 4, 8 Set

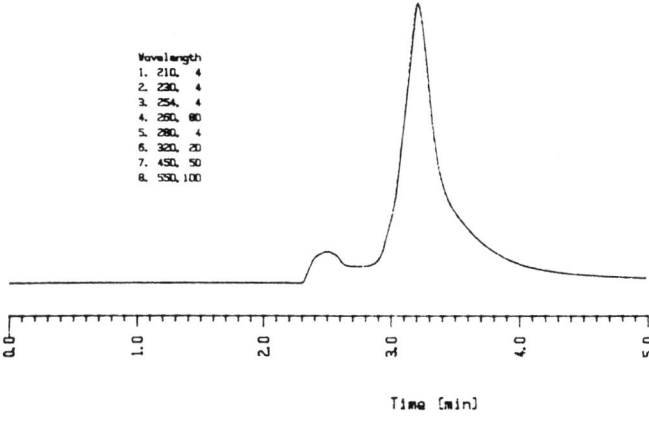

Time [min]

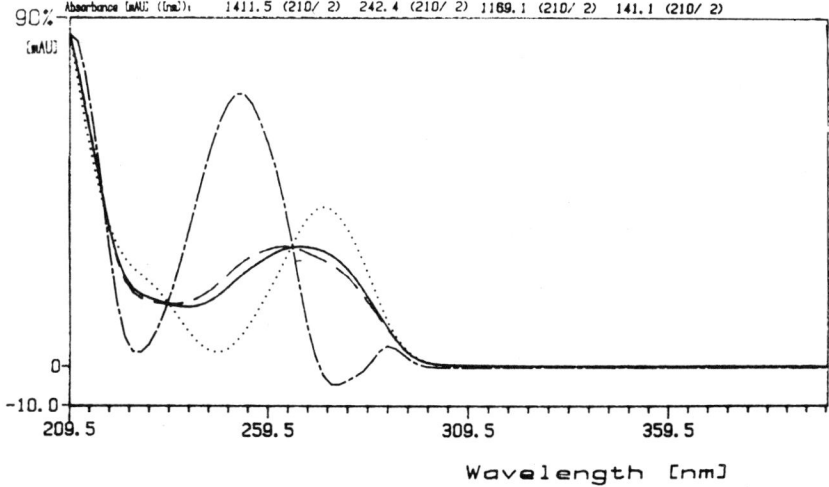

File:	RAWDAT	RAWDAT	RAWDAT	RAWDAT
Date:	10/08/1984	10/08/1984	10/08/1984	10/08/1984
Spectrum [min]:	3.2215	3.2215	3.1550	3.1550
Reference [min]:	no	3.1550	no	3.2882
Attn [mAU]:	1646.7	282.8	1363.9	184.6
Absorbance [mAU (nm)]:	1411.5 (210/ 2)	242.4 (210/ 2)	1169.1 (210/ 2)	141.1 (210/ 2)

Wavelength [nm]

to re-run with different HPLC systems to obtain complete separation. The small-scale spectra in Fig. 12, taken during the elution of the caffeine/strychnine main peak between 3.0 and 3.5 min (the small peak at 2.5 min represents codeine), are not very informative except that the right-hand spectrum obtained by correcting the spectrum at 3.222 min by subtracting that at 3.155 min yields a 'good' caffeine spectrum. Therefore, in Fig. 13 the spectra were plotted on a larger scale. That for the 3.2215 min peak apex (solid line) shows a maximum at 270 nm. The spectrum at 3.1550 min, where one would expect strychnine to elute, has a maximum at 265 nm. Yet by spectral subtraction (3.2215 minus 3.1550 min) one gets an excellent spectrum for caffeine with a maximum at 273 nm and a shoulder at ~225-235 nm. Furthermore, when we deduct 3.2215 from the 3.1550 spectrum and apply a -/+ conversion we can clearly observe the strychnine maximum at 253 nm; but due to the excess of caffeine the shoulder at ~270-290 nm can no longer be observed.

Subtraction of background is also a very important capability of DAD, as in Fig. 14 where plasma amitriptyline elutes at 9.8 min: its uncorrected spectrum (top centre) is totally uncharacteristic for the drug, apparently due to continuous background absorption. When the spectrum at the 9.792 min peak apex was corrected for background, by subtracting either the front at 9.582 min or the rear at 10.098 min, the resulting spectra (Fig. 15) very closely matched that of amitriptyline, with a maximum at 240 nm and a minimum at 230 nm.

From the foregoing examples it can be concluded that the HP 1040 DAD is a very powerful detector and is particularly useful for STA. The instrument is fast and sensitive, and can provide a vast amount of relevant data, in respect of retention behaviour as well as of the absorption spectra of eluting drugs. The resulting identification power based on these two parameters thus becomes comparable to that of a GS-MS or LC-MS combination, but is obtained at a much lower cost. Moreover, it is especially notable that the DAD can produce information on the absorption spectra of drugs at concentrations that are at least 3 orders of magnitude lower than in classical UV-VIS spectrophotometry.

Fig. 15, *opposite.* Enlarged plot of the absorption spectra in Fig. 14 to show impact of continuous background absorption. Spectra: peak apex at 9.792 min, uncorrected, —— ; 9.7915 min corrected for the 9.5615 spectrum, ·······; 9.7915 spectrum corrected for the 10.9802 min spectrum, ----. Both corrected spectra are characteristic for amitriptyline with a maximum at 240 nm and a minimum at 230 nm.

File: *RAWDAT*
Date: 10/12/1984

CP-18
origin

1. 1. 1. 5.
sample id.

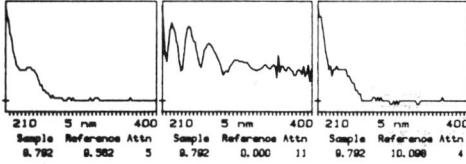

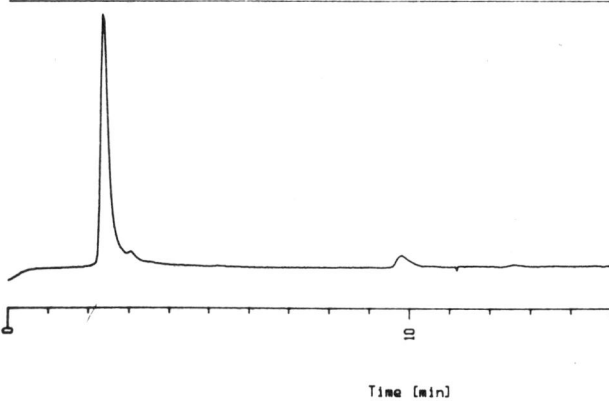

210 5 nm 400   210 5 nm 400   210 5 nm 400
Sample Reference Attn   Sample Reference Attn   Sample Reference Attn
8.792 8.562   5   9.792 0.000 11   9.792 10.098   4

analysis *TEST*
inj. vol. *20*
mobile ph. *DALDRUP*
   ''   *MECN 200+BUFFER*
stat. ph. *RPC18*
column   *NUCLEOSIL*
run no.   *1*
Inj. Time: *10: 43*
Attn [mAU]: *20. 9 (17. 9)*
ZeroX: *10%*
Signal: *D: 4, 8 Set*

Wavelength:
1 . 210,   4
2 . 230,   4
3 . 254,   4
4 . 280, 80
5 . 280,   4
6 . 320, 20
7 . 450, 50
8 . 550, 100

Time [min]

Fig. 14. HPLC of a plasma containing ~1 µg/ml of amitriptyline. The plasma was extracted with chloroform at pH 9.5.

File:	*RAWDAT*	*RAWDAT*	*RAWDAT*
Date:	10/12/1984	10/12/1984	10/12/1984
Spectrum [min]:	9. 7915	9. 7915	9. 7915
Reference [min]:	no	9. 5615	10. 9802
Attn [mAU]:	11. 3	5. 3	5. 4
Absorbance [mAU] ([nm]):	9. 6 (210/ 2)	4. 5 (210/ 2)	4. 6 (210/ 2)

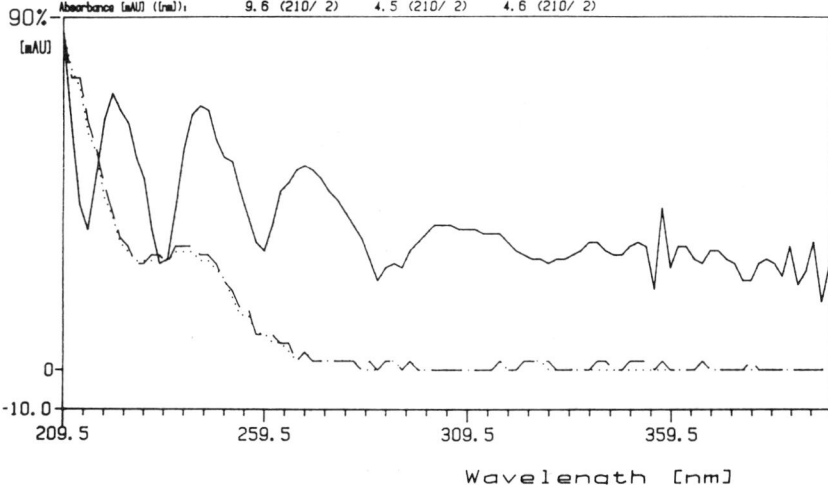

90%
[mAU]

0

-10.0

209. 5   259. 5   309. 5   359. 5

Wavelength [nm]

Acknowledgements

Participants in the experimental work described in this article were M. Bogusz, B.F.H. Drenth, J.P. Franke, T.K. Gerding, R.T. Ghijsen, M. Klys, F. Overzet, A. Burak and H. van der Voet.

References

1. Overzet, F., Ghijsen, R.T., Drenth, B.F.H. & de Zeeuw, R.A. (1982) *J. Chromatog. 240*, 190-195.
2. Overzet, F., Rurak, A., van der Voet, H., Drenth, B.F.H., Ghijsen, R.T. & de Zeeuw, R.A. (1983) *J. Chromatog. 267*, 329-345.
3. Overzet, F. & de Zeeuw, R.A. (1984) *J. Pharm. Biomed. Anal. 1*, 3-17.
4. Ghijsen, R.T., Drenth, B.F.H., Overzet, F. & de Zeeuw, R.A. (1982) *J. High Resolu. Chromatog. Chromatog. Comm. 5*, 192-198.
5. Drouwen, A.C.J.H. (1985) *Ph.D. Thesis*, Delft, The Netherlands, pp. 71-86.
6. Daldrup, T., Susanto, F. Michalke, P. (1981) *Z. Anal. Chem. 308*, 413-427.

#D-5

A ROTATING FILTER DISC ALTERNATIVE TO
PHOTODIODE ARRAY DETECTION SYSTEMS

Peter C. White

Metropolitan Police Forensic Science Laboratory
109 Lambeth Road, London SE1 4LP

With traditional single-wavelength monitoring, solute dis-crimination depends totally on retention-time data. With two detec-tors coupled in series, absorbance ratios are also obtainable; thereby compounds for which the UV profiles appear very similar have been successfully distinguished. Since, however, reproducibility problems can arise with dual detector systems, we developed our own multi-wave-length detector. At the outset, photodiode arrays were not available commercially, and a detector based upon a rotating filter disc was conceived. The disc can hold up to 4 interference filters (UV or visible), and is rotated at a constant speed (2 rev/sec). The absorbance data from the 4 wavelengths are stored on a computer and then processed very quickly, with no operator involvement, to produce a summary of absorbances, absorbance ratios and retention-time data at the end of a chromatographic run.

Consideration is given below to the design of the detector for operation in the UV or visible mode, to performance and cost, and to applications of absorbance ratioing for discriminative purposes as exemplified by the analysis of drugs including barbiturates and dyes. The design is compared with that of multi-wavelength detectors based on photodiode arrays.

A relatively fast and inexpensive analytical technique was required in our Laboratory several years ago for the positive identi-fication of barbiturates. HPLC was found to offer the best discrimi-nation if absorbance ratios and retention-time data were compared. The approach required two UV detectors to be coupled in series, one monitoring continuously at 254 nm and the other at 220 or 240 nm. Using relative retention-time data and two absorbance ratios ($A_{220/254}$ and $A_{240/254}$), the long-term reproducibility of the system was very accept-able and discrimination of 27 out of 29 barbiturates was obtained [1].

This study showed the value of an absorbance-ratio approach for identification purposes, even with a large number of compounds which exhibit similar UV profiles. The limitation of the original approach is that if extended to monitor 3 or more wavelengths it becomes inefficient in terms of sample size, analysis time, space and cost. Furthermore, loss of chromatographic performance and poorer reproducibility will be experienced and hence a loss in discriminatory power.

By developing a single detector which could monitor up to 4 wavelengths simultaneously, two major advantages of multi-wavelength detection could be achieved:
(i) identification could be rendered more definite, based on retention times plus up to 3 absorbance ratios;
(ii) absorbance ratios across a peak could be used to check peak homogeneity, i.e. to confirm that an eluted peak is not a composite of two or more unresolved compounds.
This article concerns the development, performance and applications of such a detector, and comparison with linear diode array (LDA) detectors which are now commercially available. The design and operating principles are described only in outline, since full details have been published elsewhere [2, 3].

THE ROTATING FILTER DISC MULTIWAVELENGTH DETECTOR

Detector design.- The basic optical arrangement is similar to that of a single-beam fixed wavelength detector (Fig. 1; some details in legend). The ^{2}H light is focussed onto a narrow band-pass interference filter, then through a flow-cell mounted in front of a photomultiplier. The disc, housing a filter in each quadrant, is fixed to a stepping motor which produces a constant rotation speed of 2 cycles/sec (cps). With each complete revolution of the disc a signal associated with each of the 4 filters is detected.

Signal monitoring.- When each filter rotates into the light path, one of the 4 metal flags attached to the disc rim triggers an optical light sensor. An additional flag is attached to the disc with its own light sensor and serves as a reference point for the start of each rotation, thus ensuring that the sequence of filter readings is synchronized. Retention time data are also determined with the assistance of this flag.

The separation and storage of signals for each filter is achieved using a microcomputer [PET (Commodore) 4032 with dual $5\frac{1}{4}$ disc drive 8050, Tracor printer 4022 and, as programming language, Basic-Pseudo compiled using PETSPEED (Oxford Computer Systems)]. During analysis it allows signals to be recalled, and hence the absorbance readings for any 2 of the 4 wavelengths can be selected and outputed to a dual-channel recorder to produce chromatograms in the normal manner. An additional option, which can also be in operation during an analysis, is for one channel to plot an absorbance ratio for two selected wavelengths.

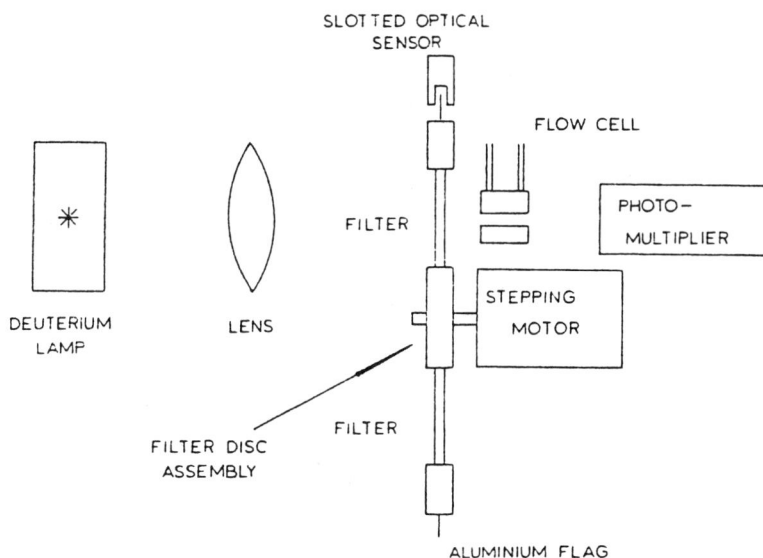

Fig. 1. A schematic diagram of the detector. The filters (25 mm diam.; disc diam. 125 mm) had $\frac{1}{2}$-bandwidths of 20 nm (217 nm) or 12-14 (240, 254, 265; 400, 500, 550, 600 nm). Normally the 2-pen recorder (not shown) received 217 and 240 nm signals. The VIS range of filters was used for (e.g.) dyes, with the same lamp as for UV. *Figs. 1-4 are from ref. [2], courtesy of Elsevier.*

Processing results.- Following an analytical run, which can be terminated either manually or after a pre-selected time, absorbance values for peaks above a pre-determined threshold are calculated together with their retention times. If a reference wavelength has been selected, absorbance ratios will be calculated and these, together with absorbance values and retention times, are presented in a tabulated form on the printer. The processing time depends on the run time and the number of peaks. Generally, for runs of ~25 min duration the data can be printed within 2 min of completing the analysis. Since this whole process can be carried out automatically, operator involvement is minimal.

Detector performance

The chromatograms in Fig. 2 (conditions in Table 1) are from the analysis of a mixture of methylenedioxyamphetamine (MDA) and nortriptyline monitored at 4 wavelengths. The additional information seen from the dramatic changes in relative peak heights confirms the value of multi-wavelength detection. Each analyte was detectable down to 1 ng at 254 nm against a noise level of 1×10^{-4} AU (absorbance units). If the filter disc was not rotated and the 254 nm filter was

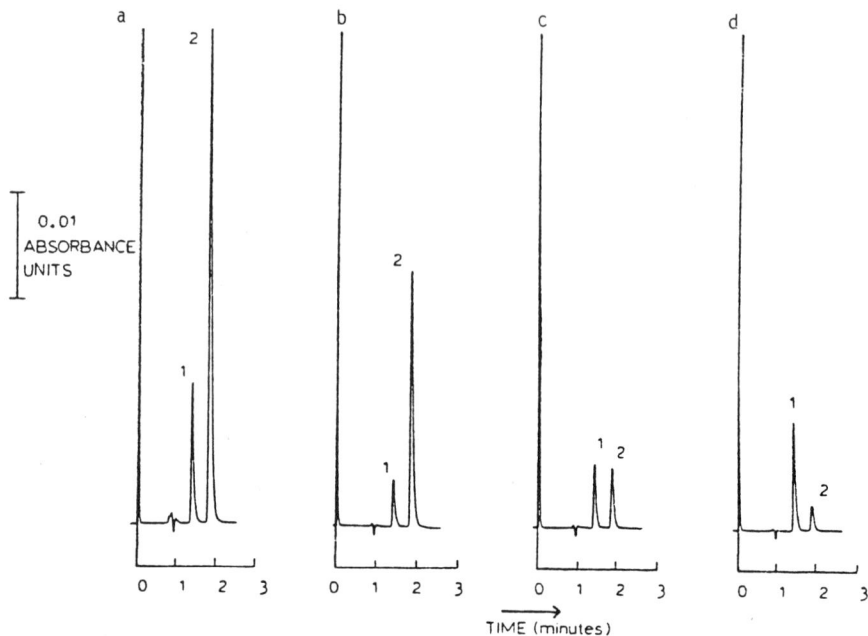

Fig. 2. Chromatograms of a mixture of MDA (1) and nortriptyline (2) monitored simultaneously at (a) 217, (b) 254, (c) 268 and (d) 279 nm.

static in the light path, a slight decrease in noise levels was recorded (Fig. 3). The performance of this detector is, then, very similar to that of a traditional, single-wavelength instrument.

Analytical reproducibilities.- For a mixture of 6 barbiturates analyzed 14 times during 4 weeks, the following average C.V.'s were obtained: for relative retention time, 0.63; for absorbance ratios: 217/254, 1.55; 240/254, 1.08; 265/254, 7.98. Precision was lowest for 265/254 because at 265 nm the test compounds had very low absorbances, just above 1×10^{-4} A.U., i.e. the noise level of the detector. Compared with two detectors in series, in the earlier study [1],

Table 1. Types of HPLC column (typically 125 × o.d. 6 mm) and mobile phase for different applications (details in refs. cited in text).

	MDA/ nortriptyline	Alprenolol/ timolol	Ball-point ink dyes	'Disperse' fibre dyes
Column	Syloid 74 silica	Spherisorb silica S5W	Hypersil ODS	Hypersil ODS
Mobile phase	0.01 M NH$_4$ClO$_4$ in methanol, pH 6.7 (NaOH)	as on left	Acetonitrile/THF/ water + citric acid & hexane sulphonic acid, pH 4.0 (NH$_4$OH)	Acetonitrile/ water + citric acid, pH 3.2

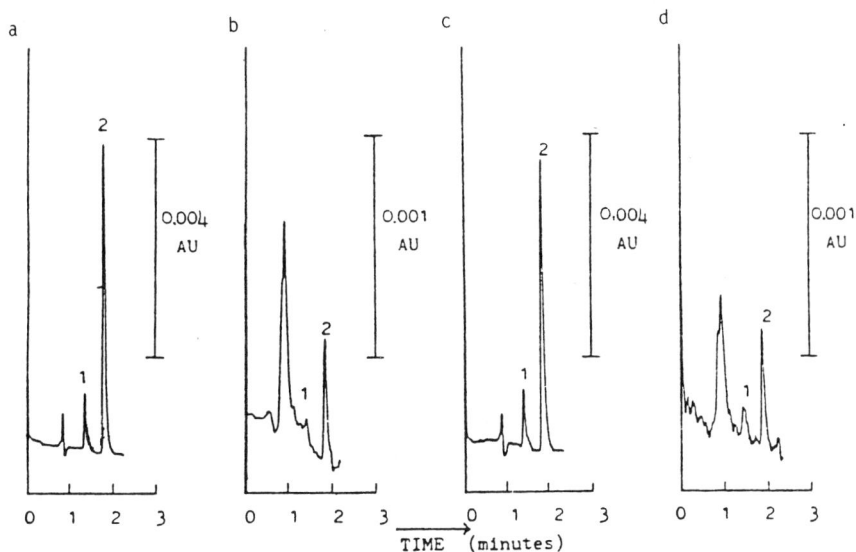

Fig. 3. Chromatograms relevant to detection limits, for MDA (1) and nortriptyline (2) at 254 nm. Stationary disc: **a**, 10 ng injected; **b**, 1 ng. Rotating disc: **c**, 10 ng injected; **d**, 1 ng.

the detector gave more precise absorbance-ratio values. With this enhanced reproducibility greater discrimination could be achieved, and all 29 barbiturates that were analyzed in the earlier study were positively identified with the multi-wavelength detector [4].

Spectra in relation to pH.- For identification purposes it is important to note that if the solutes being examined produce spectra that vary with pH, measurement with a pH meter does not suffice when the eluent is made up: the components of the buffer solution must be weighed out, to give accurate control of pH. If this precaution is not observed, poor reproducibility of the absorbance ratios will be obtained, thereby reducing solute discrimination. The following values for butobarbitone exemplify pH dependence:
- eluent pH: 8.2   8.4   8.6   8.8
   217/254 absorbance ratio: 4.24   4.10   3.41   2.36
   240/254 absorbance ratio: 3.15   3.38   3.28   3.29.

Linearity in relation to concentration.- Detector linearity was maintained over a range of 0-5 µg on-column (absorbance range 0-0.5 AU) at all wavelengths. Performance was similar when the detector was operated in the visible mode for analysis of dyes [5].

Checking peak homogeneity.- Fig. 4 exemplifies the above-mentioned operational mode whereby the homogeneity of an eluted peak can be tested easily and rapidly (provided that any co-eluted compound

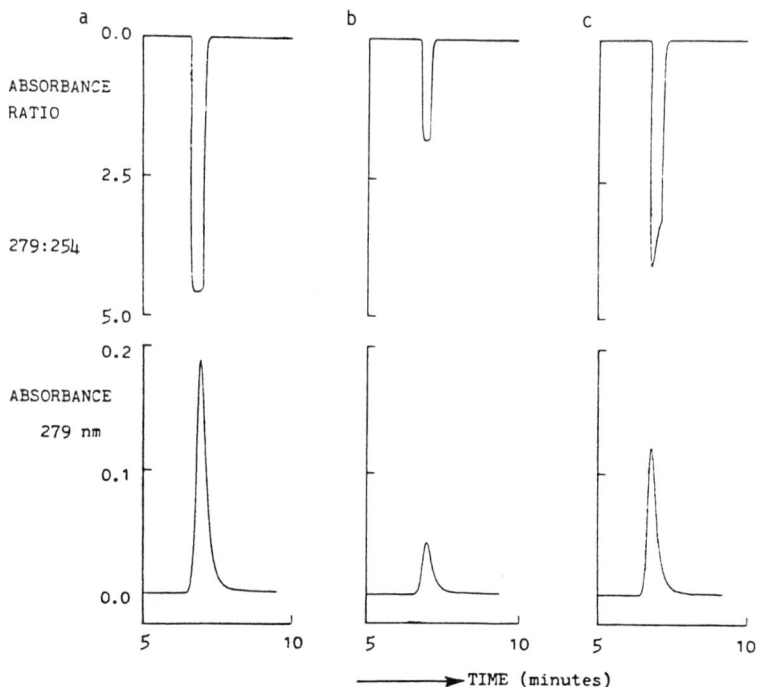

Fig. 4. An example of peak absorbance ratios monitored during the analysis of (**a**) 2 μg timolol, (**b**) 2 μg alprenolol, and (**c**) 1 μg timolol + 1 μg alprenolol. HPLC conditions as in Table 1.

does not have a near-identical absorption spectrum). Timolol and alprenolol co-elute, and when chromatographed separately produce absorbance ratio plots that approximate to a square wave. When a mixture is chromatographed, with monitoring at 279 nm there appears to be a single peak; but a 279/254 plot indicates a continuous change in value as the peak elutes, manifesting the ease of checking peak homogeneity.

APPLICATIONS

The detector has been operated in the UV mode for the identification of barbiturates without any failures in blind trials [4]. During this work, possible interferences from co-formulated drugs were studied (Table 2). Although there are some close similarities in retention times, evidently there are considerable differences in the absorbance ratio values. These values were also quite dissimilar to those obtained for the barbiturates, and clearly indicate that monitoring just 4 wavelengths enables solutes to be positively identified. It is also evident that multi-wavelength detection offers the analyst a relatively inexpensive technique for screening purposes.

Table 2. Relative retention time (RRT) data and absorbance ratios for non-barbiturate drugs that accompany barbiturates in formulations. RRT's relate to heptabarbitone (4.8 min). *From ref. [2], courtesy of Elsevier.*

Drug	RRT	217/254	240/254	265/254
Paracetamol	0.24	0.81	1.00	0.40
Theophylline	0.25	1.58	0.82	1.83
Theobromine	0.25	1.43	0.83	1.69
Orciprenaline	0.26	>10.0	1.39	2.49
Caffeine	0.32	1.68	0.86	1.80
Phenacetin	0.65	0.74	0.98	0.39
Bromvaletone	0.67	6.58	1.27	0.28
Chlormezanone	0.68	>10.0	4.47	0.54
Ephedrine	0.77	>10.0	0.72	0.47
Hyoscine	0.81	>10.0	1.28	0.46
Mephensin	0.83	7.45	0.78	2.26
Phenytoin	1.29	7.20	1.64	0.21
Carbromal	1.31	5.60	1.24	0.33
Mepenzolate bromide	3.83	*Very broad peak*		
Ergotamine, Thenyldiamine, Reserpine –		*not detected*		

Further studies have shown that a solute can be identified by just one value that reflects both the chromatographic and the spectroscopic properties of a compound, thus making comparison or identification much simpler. This is achieved by taking the relative retention time and absorbance ratio values and then either multiplying the values together or dividing one value by another.

More recent studies have concentrated on the analysis of dyes by operating in the visible mode, with 400, 500, 550 and 600 nm filters in the disc [5]. A wide range of dyes originating from inks, fibres and food colourants has been analyzed, and multi-wavelength detection was found to offer several advantages over single-wavelength monitoring. Thus, dye extracts from two ball-pen inks that appeared similar when monitored at 600 nm exhibited quite dissimilar absorbance ratios for both components (Fig. 5), establishing that the inks originated from different sources [5]. This approach can be very useful in identifying and determining common ink dyes. In an example we have published [6], the extracts of two blue ball-pen inks each gave 3 chromatographic peaks. There was the complication that retention times differed slightly between the two runs, because of a change in ambient temperature. However, there was identity in absorbance characteristics between each peak in the second extract and the corresponding peak in the first extract. Of the 3 peaks, two were identified as methyl violet, and the third was confirmed as victoria blue B from its absorbance ratios [6].

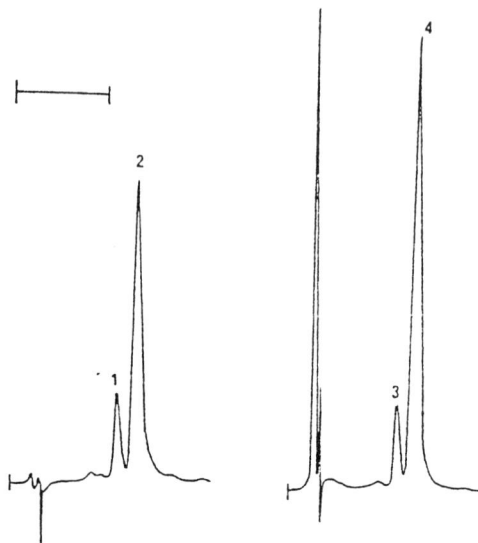

Fig. 5. Chromatograms, monitored at 600 nm, of dye extracts from two inks (time bar = 5 min), and absorbance ratios for the respective peaks. Despite the apparent similarity in the 600 nm traces, the ratios differ between peaks that had apparently corresponded, showing that the inks had not originated from a common source.
From ref. [5], courtesy of Elsevier.

Peak	t_R (min)	400/550	500/550	600/550
1	5.85	0.04	0.26	0.86
2	6.87	0.00	0.21	1.09
3	5.82	0.02	0.28	1.04
4	6.67	0.00	0.18	1.25

Even with single-component dyes, a problem may arise with the rotating filter disc detector operated in the visible mode. Dyes tend to absorb over a relatively narrow range of the visible spectrum, and occasionally it is impossible to obtain more than one absorbance ratio. This could give rise to discrimination difficulties, although this has not been experienced with the range of dyes that we have analyzed [5, 6].

COMPARISON WITH LINEAR DIODE ARRAY DETECTORS

Multi-wavelength detectors are now commercially available, mostly based upon a design that employs linear diode arrays (LDA's) [7]. (The preceding art. by R.A. de Zeeuw is pertinent - *Ed.*) We have evaluated several of these instruments and found the HP 1040A (Hewlett Packard, Palo Alto, CA) most suited to our work, mainly because samples could be monitored at 8 selected wavelengths that covered both the UV and the visible range. For dye analysis, the ability to monitor any selected range of wavelengths is clearly advantageous, as illustrated in Fig. 6 for dyes extracted from two different fibres.

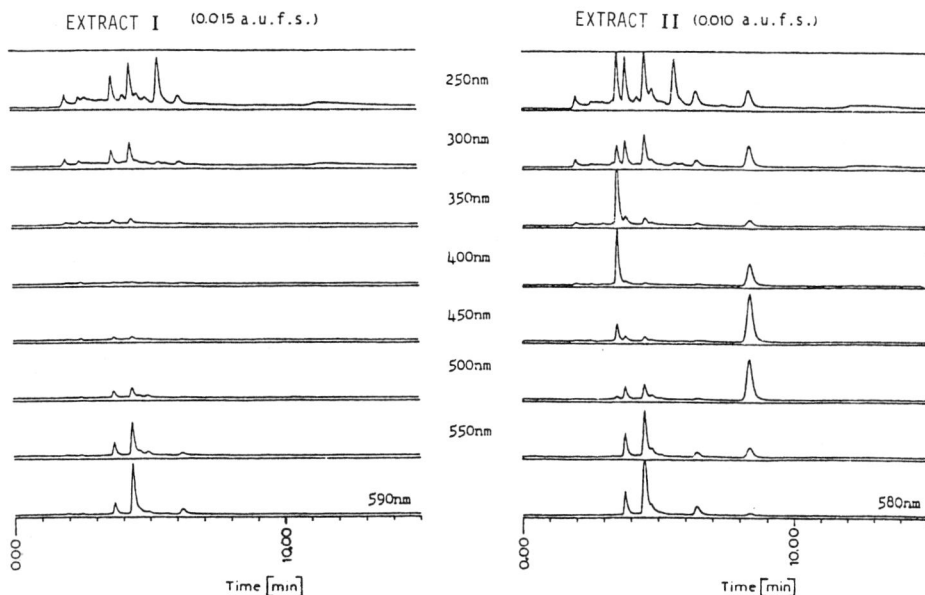

EXTRACT I (0.015 a.u.f.s.) EXTRACT II (0.010 a.u.f.s.)

250nm, 300nm, 350nm, 400nm, 450nm, 500nm, 550nm, 590nm / 580nm

Time [min]

Fig. 6. Chromatograms of dyes from two different fibres each 5 mm long (*left:* extract I; *right:* extract II), in conjunction with multi-wavelength monitoring by use of a HP 1040A detector, illustrating the additional information that can be gained by monitoring at wavelengths besides those related to the absorption maxima of the dye extracts. *From ref. [6], courtesy of Elsevier.*

If the separation of the components in these dye extracts had been monitored only at ~600 nm, the conclusion might have been that the dyes were similar and that the fibres originated from a common source. However, with the LDA detector's ability to monitor up to 8 wavelengths over 190-600 nm it can be seen that extracts I and II do not match; II has additional components.

In a comparative study of detectors for monitoring 'disperse' dyes extracted from fibres, sensitivity was an important consideration. With the LDA detector, detection limits of 200 and 150 pg were obtained with multi- and single-component dyes respectively [6]. These limits were very similar to those obtained with our instrument and only marginally above those for a single-wavelength detector. At these levels, the LDA detector did not give good spectra for the peaks.

A major disadvantage with the HP 1040A detector, and indeed the majority of commercial multi-wavelength instruments, is that with the software currently available the production of a series of absorbance ratios needs much operator time to manipulate the data. Instead of our approach based on absorbance ratios for solute identification and and discrimination, manufacturers have adopted much more time-consuming and less conclusive approaches, e.g. generating and comparing spectra, derivative spectroscopy, and 3-D chromatograms.   De Zeeuw, in the preceding article, also alludes to the time taken for obtaining values, manipulating the data, and printing/plotting.

The cost of producing our instrument is ~$\frac{1}{5}$th that of buying a LDA detector; the price difference is attibutable mainly to the cost of developing very sophisticated software.

CONCLUDING COMMENTS

Evidently our UV/visible multi-wavelength detector based on the principle of a rotating disc housing 4 narrow-bandpass filters performs well in terms of sensitivity and reproducibility when compared with ordinary single-wavelength detectors.   Absorbance ratios can be gained very quickly with virtually no operator involvement, and solutes can thereby be positively identified.   With visible-mode operation some loss in discrimination might be experienced due to the wide spacing of monitoring wavelengths. LDA detectors can improve this situation, but rapid identification of solutes by the absorbance-ratio approach cannot be accomplished at the present time.

Acknowledgements

I thank T. Catterick, J.R. Russell and B.B. Wheals for their valuable contributions to achieve these results.

References

1. White, P.C. (1980) *J. Chromatog. 200*, 271-276.
2. Catterick, T. (1983) *J. Chromatog. 259*, 59-67.
3. Russell, J.R. (1983) *J. Chromatog. 280*, 370-375.
4. White, P.C. & Catterick, T. (1983) *J. Chromatog. 280*, 376-381.
5. White, P.C. & Wheals, B.B. (1984) *J. Chromatog. 303*, 211-216.
6. Wheals, B.B., White, P.C. & Paterson, M.D. (1985) *J. Chromatog. 350*, 205-215.
7. George, S.A. & Maute, A. (1982) *Chromatographia 5*, 419-425.

#NC(D)

NOTES and COMMENTS relating to

APPROACHES TO ANALYTE DETECTION, IDENTIFICATION AND MEASUREMENT

Comments related to particular contributions

#D-1, D-3 & D-4, p. 403
#NC(D)-3 to -5, p. 404

Forum presentations:
  by F.A.A. Dallas on linear analyzer for TLC radiolabel, p. 407;
  by H. de Bree & co-workers on zone refining, p. 408

#NC(D)-1

A Note on

METABOLIC STUDY OF TWO UNLABELLED DRUGS
USING HPLC WITH UV-VIS DIODE ARRAY DETECTION

M.P. van Berkel, B.J. de Jong, H. de Bree,
E. Koorn and W.R. Vincent

Duphar Research Laboratories
P.O. Box 2, 1380 AA Weesp, The Netherlands

UV-VIS detection in HPLC has become very attractive for drug metabolism studies since the introduction of diode array spectrophotometers
[cf. R.A. de Zeeuw, this vol., D-4.-*Ed.*].   From the UV spectra of
the chromatographic peaks, the metabolites can be recognized. The main
advantage of this approach is reduced dependence upon radio-labelled
compounds, since the chromophore acts as a native label.   HPLC with
diode array detection was used to obtain insight into the metabolic
degradation of two potential drugs.

COMPOUND 1

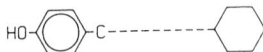

The *in vitro* experiments showed that compound 1 had a very high
affinity for a particular receptor. However, *in vivo* the drug revealed
pharmacological activity for only a very short time, suggesting a
rapid metabolic deactivation.   We therefore studied the metabolism
of this drug in two *in vitro* systems (liver perfusion and microsome
incubation) to elucidate the site of metabolic attack and to obviate
that attack by appropriate synthesis.

Liver perfusion.– The bile duct, portal vein and posterior vena
cava of a male rat (Sprague Dawley, ~300 g) were cannulated under
ether anaesthesia.   The liver was rapidly removed, placed in a heated
cabinet (37°) and perfused via the portal vein in a recirculating
system.   The perfusion medium (described by Meyer [1]) consisted
of diluted rat blood and was supplemented by compound 1 (10 mg/100 ml).

Samples of the perfusate and the bile were taken every 15 min
during 2-3 h; the volume of the bile was determined gravimetrically.

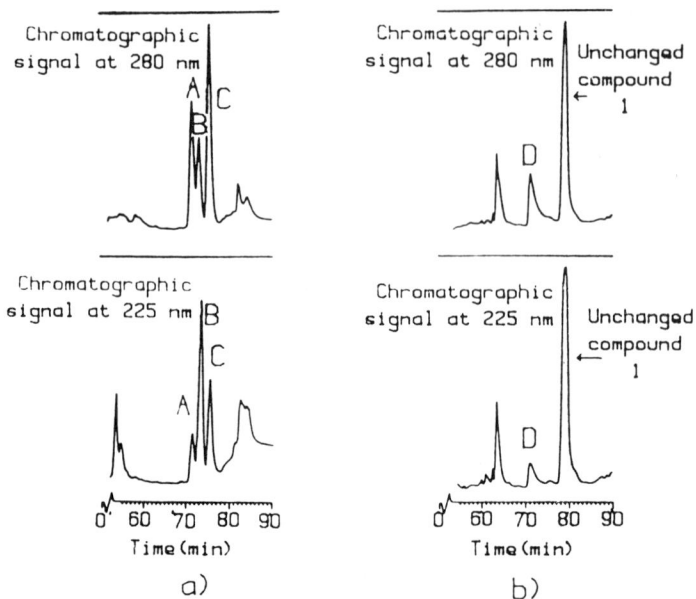

Fig. 1. RP-HPLC metabolite patterns: a) 2 ml bile after liver per-fusion for 30 min; b) 20 ml liver microsomal preparation (see text). Zorbax C-8 column, 500×9 mm i.d., with a precolumn [3]; total sample loaded. Elution with water-to-methanol gradient.

The perfusate was analyzed after centrifugation for 10 min at 3000 rpm, whereas bile was analyzed directly, by HPLC (Fig. 1, legend) with UV-VIS diode array detection (Hewlett Packard model 1040A detector).

Microsome incubation.- Compound 1 was incubated with 10,000 g supernatant from a rat liver homogenate. The incubation mixture [2] contained 75 µg/ml of the drug; incubation was at 37°, followed by centrifugation and filtration of the supernatant for HPLC.

RESULTS AND DISCUSSION

The perfusate analysis showed only a decrease of the parent drug, which had disappeared completely within 60 min. The metabolite pattern of the bile (Fig. 1a) showed three peaks (A, B & C) with reten-tion times between 70 and 80 min. From their spectra we concluded that they might have originated from compound 1. The other peaks in the chromatogram represented endogenous compounds. Components A-C were isolated and shown, by ^{1}H NMR and MS, to have the structures shown in Fig. 2 (left part).

In the microsomal incubation experiment we expected metabolite(s) having a (vulnerable) catechol function, and hence used an acidic eluent for determining the pattern (Fig. 1b).

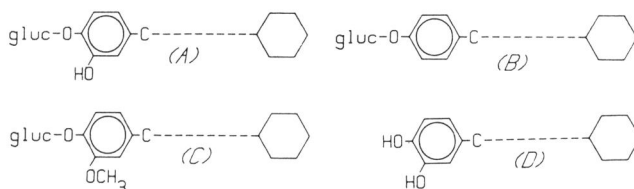

Fig. 2. Structures established for components shown in Fig. 1.

By comparing the spectra of peak D with compound 1 we observed shifts - bathochromic at 225 and 280 nm and hyperchromic at 280 nm. We therefore postulated the presence of a catechol function in peak D, as verified by isolation and identification: the structure is shown in the right portion of Fig. 2.

COMPOUND 2

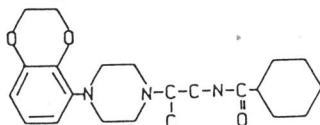

The *in vivo* experiments with the antihypertensive compound 2 revealed a different pharmacological profile in the two species investigated; the duration of activity in the rat was much shorter than in the rabbit. This difference could be explained by either a metabolic deactivation in the rat or an activation in the rabbit. The *in vitro* metabolism of compound 2 was therefore investigated by incubating it, as for compound 1, with liver microsomes, both rabbit and rat. After 35 min at 37°, metabolite patterns were examined by HPLC with the same conditions as for compound 1.

RESULTS AND DISCUSSION

The difference between the incubations with microsomes from rabbit (Fig. 3a) and rat (Fig. 3b) was mainly quantitative, the conversion appearing much slower for rat than for rabbit microsomes. From the full spectra (not illustrated) of the peaks eluting between 35 and 60 min we concluded that they might have originated from compound 2. The other peaks represent endogenous compounds, being present in the blank also. We isolated the components representing the peaks between 43 and 50 min, and identified them by ^{1}H NMR and MS. The proposed structures are as shown in Fig. 4. The greater extent of metabolism with rabbit liver accords with the metabolic-activation explanation of the species difference in response.

COMMENT ON USEFULNESS OF THE DIODE-ARRAY DETECTION MODE

Simultaneous acquisition of light-intensity data at wavelengths spanning the range 190-600 nm allows recognition of the chromophore-containing metabolites, based on the UV-spectra of the HPLC peaks; thereby the need for radiolabelled compounds in metabolism studies is reduced. However, parent-drug bioconversion may cause batho-/hypsochromic shifts.

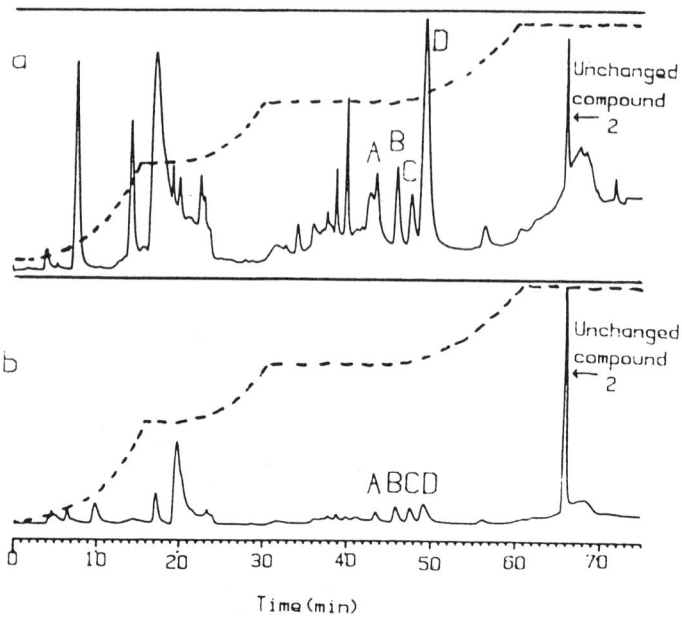

Fig. 3. RP-HPLC metabolic pattern after incubating compound 2 with liver microsomes: a) rabbit, b) rat. Interrupted line denotes the methanol gradient.

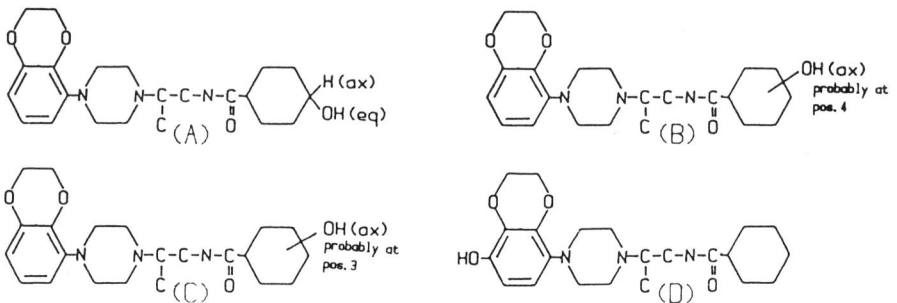

Fig. 4. Proposed structures for components shown in Fig. 3.

References

1. Meyer, D.K.F., Keulemans, K. & Mulder, J. (1981) *Meths. Enzymol. 77*, 81-94.
2. Mazel, P. (1972) in *Fundamentals of Drug Metabolism and Drug Disposition* (La Du, B.N., Mandel, H.G. & Way, W.L., eds.), Williams & Wilkins, Baltimore, pp. 527-536.
3. Ruijten, H.M., Van Amsterdam, P.H. & De Bree, H. (1984) *J. Chromatog. 314*, 183-191.

#NC(D)-2

A Note on

DETERMINATION OF THE GLUCURONIDE(S) OF THE
ANTINEOPLASTIC AGENT ETOPOSIDE

J.J.M. Holthuis, W.J. van Oort and A. Hulshoff

Department of Analytical Pharmacy
State University of Utrecht
Pharmaceutical Laboratory, Catharijnesingel 60
3511 GH Utrecht, The Netherlands

Etoposide (VP 16-213; I in Fig. 1) is used clinically as an antineoplastic agent. Its analysis, pharmacokinetics and mode of action receive increasing attention [1, 2], but little has been paid to the isolation and identification of its metabolites. Colombo et al. [3] reported the presence of two different glucuronides in rat bile after its intravenous administration; but no other information has been published concerning the glucuronidation of this drug in humans. Our present aim was to identify possible glucuronides of etoposide in the urine of cancer patients after intravenous administration.

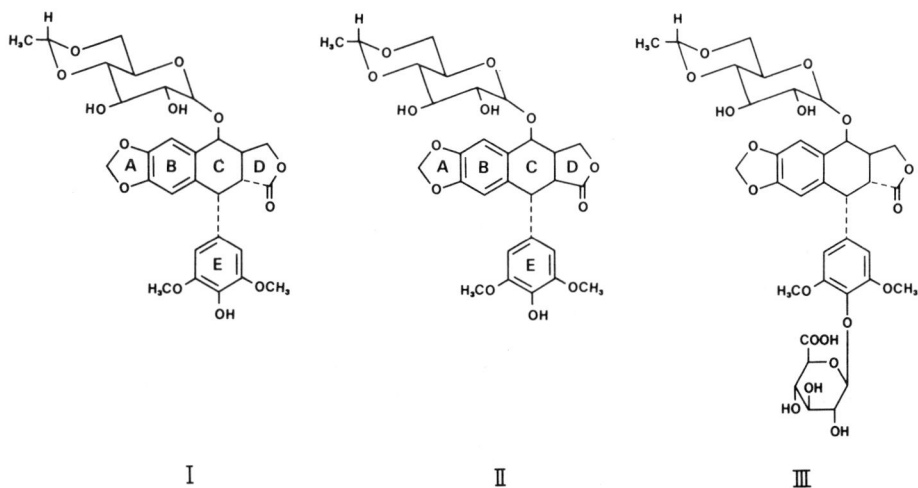

I   II   III

Fig. 1. Formulae of etoposide (**I**), cis etoposide (**II**) and etoposide glucuronide (**III**).

Fig. 2. HPLC of an extract from 50 µl of a patient's urine: glucuronide of etoposide (I) and of cis etoposide (II).
Waters Assoc. pump (6000A), injector (U6K) and column: µBondapak phenyl (10 µm), 300×4.6 mm i.d.
Mobile phase: methanol/ water/acetic acid, 25:73:2 by wt.; 1.0 ml/min. Detection at 280 nm (Kratos Spectraflow detector).
The patient's etoposide dosage was 1.2 g i.v.; urine sample only 0–6 h.

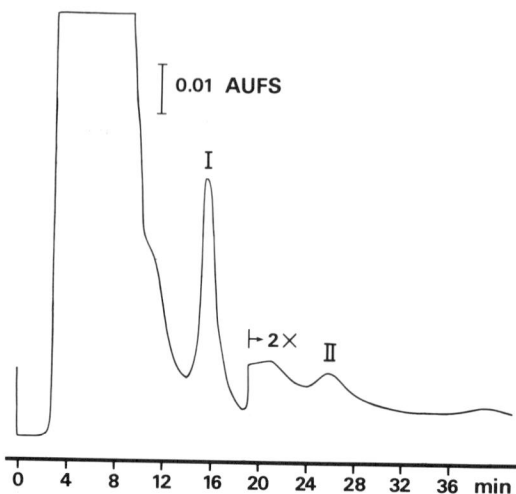

EXPERIMENTAL

Chemicals.– Sodium acetate, acetic acid, 1,2-dichloroethane (DCE) and methanol, all reagent grade, were from E. Merck. Etoposide was furnished by Bristol Myers Nederland B.V. The 1,4-saccharolactone and β-glucuronidase from either bovine liver (BL; 2.8×10^6 U/g) or *Helix pomatia* (HP; 92×10^3 U/ml) were from the Sigma Chemical Co. The enzyme solutions were prepared by dissolution in acetate buffer pH 5.0 (0.2 mM) to a concentration of 2000 Fishman units/ml.

Mass spectrometry.– For electron-impact examination (EI–MS) the sample was introduced by DI probe into the ion source (250°) of a Kratos MS–80; the settings were 70 eV for electron energy and 100 µA for ionizing current. For fast atom bombardment (giving positive ions; FAB–MS) the instrument was a VG–ZAB–ZF equipped with a saddle field FAB gun. The energy of the argon beam was 1 mA and 7 kV, and the acceleration voltage 8kV. To 100 µl of the matrix (glycerol containing 1% acetic acid and 10% NaCl, w/w) 0.5 mg samples were added.

Isolation and identification of etoposide glucuronide(s).– A sample (1.0 ml) of patient's urine was extracted twice with 6 ml DCE. The organic phases, containing the unchanged etoposide, were discarded, and the aqueous phase was freeze-dried. The residue was extracted with 10 ml of methanol. After filtration through paper the filtrate was evaporated down to 1.0 ml; this solution was centrifuged for 5 min at 5000 **g**, and 50 µl aliquots of the supernatant were chromatographed (Fig. 2), with collection of 0.5–1 ml eluate fractions for 25 min. The chromatograms were scrutinized for peaks lacking in blank urine and attributable to etoposide administration. Fractions possibly containing glucuronides were dried down under N_2 at room temperature. (The 'phenyl' column gave particularly good separations.)

Part of the residue was incubated for 14 h at 37° with β-glucuronidase BL, then extracted twice with DCE. The extract was investigated by EI-MS, and also analyzed by HPLC with electrochemical (EC)
detection [2] at +500 mV *vs.* Ag/AgCl. Other portions of the residue
were investigated by FAB-MS, both directly and after diazomethane
treatment aimed to furnish the methyl ester of any glucuronides
present. The diazomethane (in ether) was added to the residue dissolved in 100 μl methanol, and after 2 min at room temperature the
solvent was evaporated under reduced pressure; the residue was methylated again according to the same procedure.

RESULTS

Fig. 2 shows a chromatogram for a 5000 **g** methanol supernatant,
prepared as described above. When the fraction containing peak I
was incubated with β-glucuronidase BL and the subsequent DCE extract
was analyzed by HPLC with EC and UV detection, a compound was obtained
with the same chromatographic and (examined off-line) EC properties
as etoposide. The EI-MS spectrum of this aglycone was identical
to that of etoposide (Fig. 3A); the specific fragments were m/z
588 (M^+), 400 (M-glucopyranosyl+H^+) and 382 [(M-glucopyranosyl-OH)$^+$].

When the fraction containing peak II was incubated, a compound
with the same properties as cis etoposide (Fig. 1, II) was obtained;
but the amount was insufficient for MS identification. The compounds of peaks I and II, without enzymatic incubation, proved to
be electrochemically inactive when the HPLC system (Fig. 2) was
combined with an EC detector [2] at a potential of +750 mV *vs.* Ag/AgCl.

Peak I, probably an intact glucuronide of etoposide, was analyzed by FAB-MS. The highest mass fragment was at m/z 747 (M+H^+-H_2O)
with a low intensity. The most intense ion was at m/z 658 (Fig. 3B).
The mass spectrum with FAB for the methylated product of peak I
(Fig. 3C) showed the highest mass at m/z 801; the most intense ion
was at m/z 612, and there was also an ion at m/z 658. The rest
of this spectrum is almost identical to that of the underivatized
glucuronide. The presence of $BaCl_2$ during the incubation of the pre-
extracted urine with β-glucuronidase HP had no influence on the
hydrolysis. Control incubations of urine in acetate buffer pH 5.0
or 5 mM H_2SO_4 in the absence of enzyme yielded no free etoposide.

DISCUSSION

For the identification of glucuronides, generally it is highly
preferable to analyze them intact, because procedures based on enzymatic or chemical hydrolysis are insufficiently selective and because
the optimum incubation conditions for different glucuronides vary
greatly [4, 5] (see arts. in Vol. 12, this series, especially p. 268
– *Ed.*). The nature of the linkage between the parent compound and
glucuronic acid can commonly be elucidated by derivatization and EI-MS.

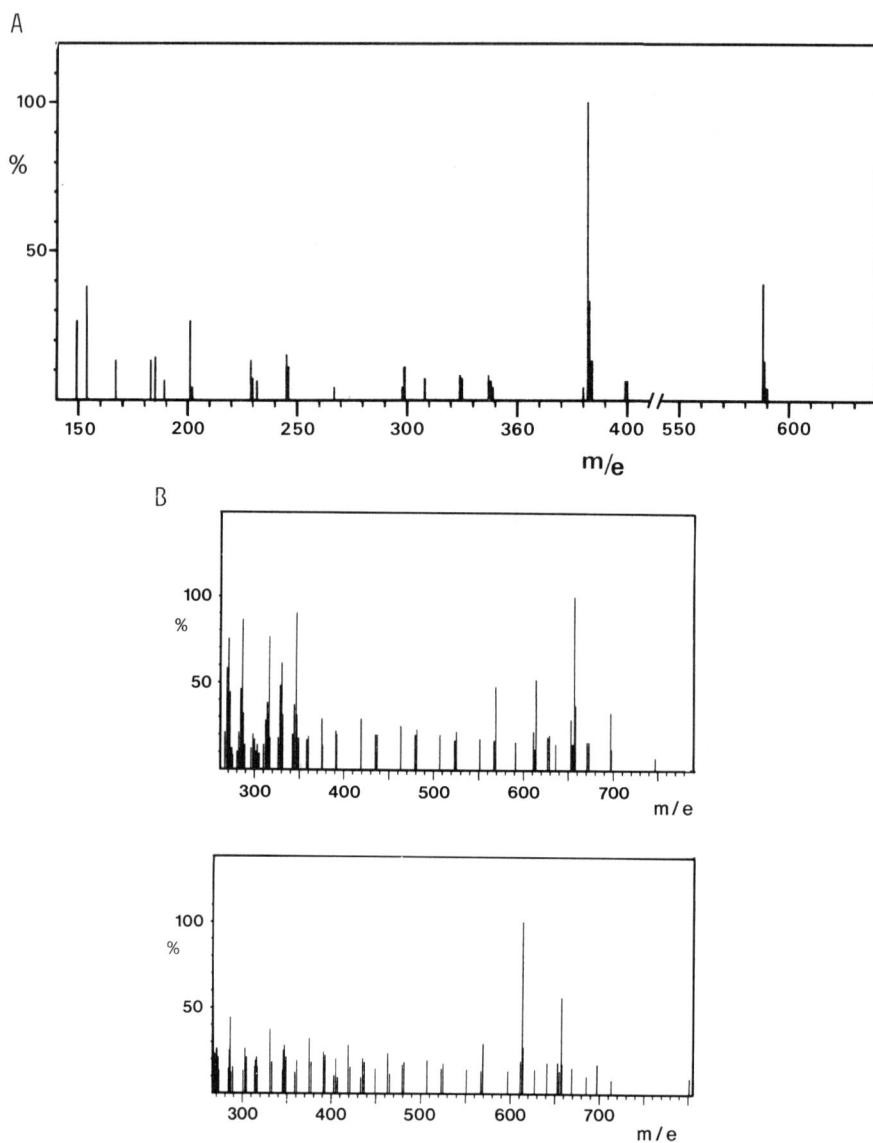

Fig. 3. Mass spectra. [In text, 'm/e' is rendered as 'm/z'.]
A: The EI spectrum of etoposide.
B: The FAB spectrum of etoposide glucuronide (peak I, Fig. 2).
C: The FAB spectrum of the methyl ester of etoposide glucuronide.

Thereby it is possible to distinguish between linkages to aliphatic or aromatic hydroxyl groups because of different fragmentation patterns [5]. In the case of etoposide glucuronide, however, it was not possible to obtain a good EI-MS spectrum, even after methylation of the carboxylic group and silylation of the remaining hydroxyl groups with BSTFA. When etoposide glucuronide (M_r 764) was investigated by FAB-MS, the formation of the following mass fragments was anticipated: 764 (M^+) and 787 ($M+Na^+$). However, the highest mass found was 747, with a low intensity, corresponding to ($M+H^+-H_2O$). Normally the abundance of molecular ion is greatly increased in FAB-MS. After methylation of the carboxylic group of the glucuronide moiety (M_r of the product = 778) with diazomethane the largest ion was found at m/z (m/e) 801 corresponding to ($M+Na^+$) (Fig. 3C). Surprisingly, the ion corresponding to etoposide (at m/z 588) is not present in FAB mass spectra of the glucuronide (methyl ester) of etoposide. The aglycone peak has proved to be the most intense ion in the FAB-mass spectra of ether-glucuronidated phenols [6]. These ions are normally produced through the loss of the dehydrated glucuronic acid moiety ($M+H^+-176$) or its methyl ester ($M+H^+-190$).

The interpretation of most of the FAB-mass spectrum of etoposide glucuronide is probably hampered by the formation of artefactual matrix ions. However, the identity of this glucuronide is firmly established. The liberation of etoposide upon incubation of the pre-extracted urine with β-glucuronidase HP was completely inhibited by 1,4-saccharolactone. The β-glucuronidase HP preparation also possesses sulphatase activity. However, as no etoposide is produced with the inhibitor present, evidently etoposide is not excreted as a sulphate. When etoposide glucuronide was subjected to HPLC with EC detection, no signal was observed, strongly indicating that the glucuronic acid is attached to the phenolic group in ring E (Fig. 1, III).

Peak II in Fig. 2 may represent the glucuronide of cis etoposide (cf. Fig. 1, II); but its identity has not yet been established by MS.

References

1. Holthuis, J.J.M. (1985) *PhD. Thesis*, University of Utrecht.
2. Holthuis, J.J.M., Römkens, F.M.G.M., Pinedo, H.M. & van Oort, W.J. (1983) *J. Pharm. Biomed. Anal. 1*, 89-97.
3. Colombo, T., D'Incalci, M., Donelli, M.G., Bartosek, I., Benfenati, E., Farina, P. & Guaitani, A. (1985) *Xenobiotica 15*, 343-350.
4. Fenselau, C. & Johnson, L.P. (1980) *Drug Metab. Dispos. 8*, 274-283.
5. Billets, S., Lietman, P.S. & Feneslau, C. (1973) *J. Med. Chem.. 16*, 30-33.
6. Fenselau, C., Yelle, L., Stogniew, M., Liberato, D. Lehman, J. Feng, P. & Colvin, M. (1983) *Int. J. Mass Spectrom. Ion Phys. 46*, 411-414.

#NC(D)-3

A Note on

RECENT DEVELOPMENTS IN POST-COLUMN REACTORS FOR HPLC

U.A.Th. Brinkman[*]

Department of Analytical Chemistry
Free University
De Boelelaan 1083, 1081 HV Amsterdam, The Netherlands

In the past decade, HPLC has been shown to be a very versatile, highly efficient and rapid method of analysis. Detection, however is still a relatively weak point in HPLC. This is a major drawback, because trace analysis requires the use of highly sensitive and selective detection principles. Besides on-line trace enrichment, derivatization has emerged in recent years as a powerful tool – applied either pre-column or post-column – to obtain the necessary sensitivity and selectivity in the determination of trace constituents in biological or other complex matrices.

Earlier studies from our laboratory were published in Vol. 7 (R.W. Frei) and Vol. 14 (U.A.Th. Brinkman & R.W. Frei) of this series. The present sketch deals exclusively with on-line post-column derivatization (or reaction detection), which is somewhat more sophisticated than pre-column detection and can be more easily adapted to automation. The latter is a distinct advantage when one has to deal with large series of samples.

REACTION DETECTION

On-line post-column detectors for HPLC utilize a variety of chemical and physicochemical principles to convert the analyte of interest into a suitable end-product. Detection is generally carried out with a selective detector, e.g. a fluorescence spectrophotometer. A few relevant examples are discussed below.

Chemical derivatization is often carried out with fluorescamine or *o*-phthalaldehyde (OPA). With OPA, primary amines are converted into highly fluorescent products, and detection limits are often as low as 10 pg. OPA is especially recommended because it possesses no native fluorescence (low background; no removal of excess reagent

[*] *may be contacted for a list of references*

required) and because a reaction time of ~20 sec often suffices (small contribution to extra-column band broadening; no air or solvent segmentation required).

Ion-pair formation with fluorigenic counter-ions such as substituted naphthalene and anthracene sulphonic acids has been used for a variety of interesting compounds (pheniramines, secoverine; see Vol. 14 of this series). An alternative is the use of acridine at low pH values, i.e. of acridine-H^+, for the determination of sulphonic acids. The general position of these systems - and, indeed, of all systems involving the use of a reagent which is itself fluorigenic, or else electroactive - is that the excess of reagent must be removed via on-line extraction of the reaction product into a suitable organic solvent. This seriously complicates the system because an additional pump, tee-piece and phase separator are required. Nevertheless, good results are obtainable, and relative S.D.'s of 2-3% are typically found for the analysis of 'real samples' such as body fluids.

POST-COLUMN OPERATIONS, AND THE WHEREWITHAL TO PERFORM THEM

On-line post-column **extraction**, not in conjunction with ion-pair formation, has been used successfully in HPLC-mass spectrometry (LC-MS) and (cf. a Note that follows) in HPLC with electron-capture detection. In both cases, the extraction step is included to separate the analytes of interest (substituted phenoxyacetic acids, pentachlorophenol in urine; low-pH extraction to suppress analyte ionization) from interfering polar compounds which remain in the aqueous phase.

Recently, **miniaturization** of tee-pieces, extraction coils and phase separators has been attempted. First results are highly promising and narrow-bore HPLC (1 mm i.d. analytical columns) can now be combined with on-line post-column reaction/extraction detectors without significant loss of chromatographic resolution.

Consideration is given in Vol. 14 to the **solid-phase reactor**, a short (3-6 cm) s.s. column packed with reagents, e.g. finely divided Zn or Cu, reagents immobilized on inert glass beads (reductants, oxidants, enzymes) or catalysts such as cation- or anion-exchange resins. Such resin-packed reactor columns are especially popular because many derivatization reactions are based on a pH effect. One can now discard older systems utilizing aggressive aqueous solutions such as 1-5 M NaOH or H_2SO_4, and replace them by a solid-phase reactor that can easily and continuously be operated at up to 100°. Thus, we have studied the conversion of non-reducing carbohydrates, guanidines and *N*-methylcarbamates, derivatizing one of the products on-line in a second reactor. With a urease reactor we have determined urea and ammonia in mixtures and in body fluids, with reactor columns of i.d. 4-6 mm or only 1 mm. To determine thiram and disulfiram we are using a Cu reactor, in which Cu-containing complexes are formed which can easily be monitored by absorption measurements in the visible range.

#NC(D)-4

A Note on

HPLC WITH ON-LINE ELECTRON-CAPTURE DETECTION

U.A.Th. Brinkman[*]

Department of Analytical Chemistry
Free University
De Boelelaan 1083, 1081 HV Amsterdam, The Netherlands

In recent years, HPLC has emerged as an analytical technique that is equivalent in performance to GC. Today, HPLC and GC are seen as supplementary rather than competitive, each having its specific advantages and drawbacks, and each having its preferred fields of application. A drawback of HPLC is the lack of detectors that can match the sensitivity of GC detectors. In order to improve this situation, the on-line use of the electron-capture detector (ECD) in HPLC has repeatedly been advocated.

The present sketch summarizes the work that has been carried out in our laboratory in the past decade. Virtually all these HPLC-ECD studies have been carried out using a ^{63}Ni ECD from Pye Unicam Ltd. (Cambridge, U.K.). The evaporation interface inserted between the outlet of the HPLC column and the inlet of the ECD is usually a coiled stainless-steel capillary of, typically, 50-75 cm length and of i.d. 0.25-0.50 mm, mounted in a stainless-steel block to achieve efficient heat transfer, and kept at a temperature of 250-300°.

NORMAL-PHASE HPLC-ECD

Early work on HPLC-ECD dealt almost exclusively with adsorption chromatography on silica, using hexane or iso-octane as eluent. Such systems can be used conveniently and continuously at eluent flow-rates of 0.5-0.8 ml/min, provided that the organic solvent is purified by a 1-2 h treatment with a dispersion of sodium in high-b.p. paraffin and subsequent distillation. More recently it has been shown that hexane can be replaced by toluene, which is more polar (but has the same low background as hexane), thus extending the range of application of NP-HPLC-ECD. Such systems can be miniaturized rather easily, and with a Brownlee Micropump a gradient elution system can even be set up.

[*] *may be contacted for a list of references and reprints of certain papers*

Another approach to extend the range of applicability of HPLC-ECD is the addition of a suitable polar modifier to the alkane used as eluent. Best results are obtained with dioxan, and in several recent applications hexane containing 10-15% (v/v) of dioxan has been utilized. A further possibility is the derivatization of the analytes of interest with electron capture-sensitive reagents so as to decrease their polarity, while simultaneously increasing the sensitivity towards the ECD.

REVERSED-PHASE HPLC-ECD

With RP-HPLC-ECD, on-line coupling is feasible, either directly – provided that miniaturized systems are used – or after post-column extraction of the analytes into, e.g., hexane or toluene. In the direct mode, methanol/water and dioxan/water mixtures containing up to at least 50-70% of water can be used at flow rates of ~50 μl/min. Pure water can be used at a flow-rate of ~25 μl/min. The presence of small amounts of acid in the eluent can be tolerated. In the extraction mode, conventional-scale HPLC equipment and normal flow-rates of ~1 ml/min can be employed.

ANALYTICAL ASPECTS AND APPLICATION

On-line NP- and RP-HPLC-ECD have been carried out for many analytes (~50). For favourable compounds, the detection limits in the conventional NP mode are 5-10 pg (but <1 pg in a miniaturized system), and much the same values are recorded for direct, i.e. miniaturized, RP-HPLC-ECD. The detection limits in terms of concentration are, self-evidently, distinctly worse in the latter case (smaller injection volume!). In all cases, plots of response against concentration are linear over at least 2-3 orders of magnitude.

Applications to 'real samples' have included the determination of chloroxuron in strawberries, phenylurea herbicides in surface water, pentachlorophenol in urine, liver and wood samples, polychlorinated biphenyls in various environmental samples, and of vitamin K, chloroanilines, organochlorine pesticides and low-mol. wt. halogenated aliphatic hydrocarbons.

#NC(D)-5

A Note on

LIQUID CHROMATOGRAPHY - MASS SPECTROMETRY (LC-MS)

L.E. Martin, M.S. Lant and Janet Oxford

Glaxo Group Research Ltd.
Ware, Herts. SG12 0DJ, U.K.

Three systems for the on-line coupling of HPLC to a mass spectrometer (MS) are commercially available. (1) In the system with a moving belt interface, the eluent is deposited in droplets or sprayed onto a moving polyimide belt, and the solvent is evaporated before the belt reaches the MS ion source [1]; MS operation can be in the electron-impact (EI) or chemical ionization (CI) mode. Thermolabile compounds, e.g. ranitidine and its *N*-oxide, decomposed at the high temperatures required to evaporate mobile phases containing large amounts of water [1]. The other systems now to be considered entail (2) direct liquid introduction (DLI) or (3) a thermospray (TSP) interface. For all three, volatile buffers are normally employed.

In the DLI system [2] the mobile phase flows through a low dead volume water-cooled stainless steel (s.s.) probe into the MS. A s.s. diaphragm with a 5 μm orifice is fitted into the probe tip. A proportion of the solvent passes through the orifice and enters a quadrapole MS source as a stream of fine droplets. The solvent is evaporated in the source, and the vapour acts as a CI reagent gas. The system can be used with mobile phases containing up to 80% water. However, if more than ~40 μl/min enters the MS an adequate vacuum cannot be maintained, and the operating conditions of the MS are affected. The sensitivity has been improved by using columns of only 2 mm diam. and reduced flow-rates (150-300 μl/min). The use of micro-columns with 20-60 μl/min flow would further improve the sensitivity, but they have a limited capacity and are unlikely to be used routinely. Further disadvantages are that the DLI system can be used only in the CI mode, and that its routine use for quantitative analysis is limited due to blockage of the orifice by the deposition of dissolved silica from the column packing.

The DLI system is, however, suitable for studying thermolabile molecules. The $[M+H]^+$ ion of m/z 315 was the base peak in the mass spectrum of ranitidine and was used for its quantitative analysis [3];

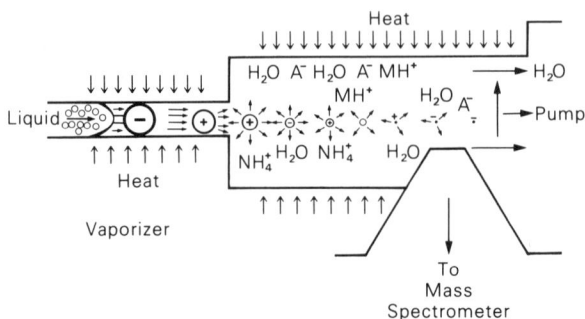

Fig. 1. Schematic representation of thermospray (TSP) ionization. M represents the molecular ion of the analyte, and A the anion. (The arrow ↑ near right indicates passage of analyte + buffer to purge.)

deutero-ranitidine was used as an internal standard (i.s.). The mass spectrum of ranitidine-*N*-oxide showed that some fragmentation of the molecule had occurred: the ion of m/z 315 was the base peak, and the pseudo-molecular ion $[M+H]^+$, m/z 331, of ranitidine-*N*-oxide was ~25% of the intensity of the base peak [4].

About two years ago the TSP interface became commercially available. This method of sample introduction and ionization was pioneered by M.L. Vestal and co-workers in Houston [5]. The eluent from the chromatograph (0.8-2 ml/min) is passed through a 100 µm diam. s.s. tube which protrudes into a region of reduced pressure (~1 torr) and is heated up to 400° by passing an electric current through it, producing a supersonic vapour jet with entrained particles or droplets.

In the presence of polar analyte molecules and a polar mobile phase containing volatile buffers, viz. ammonium acetate or formate, or trifluoroacetic acid, ions of the analyte M are formed without any external ionization (Fig. 1). The ions are sampled by either a quadrupole or magnetic-sector MS [5]. Some analytes, e.g. non-polar molecules, are not ionized under these conditions; to ionize such compounds a thoriated-iridium filament has been installed in the TSP system.

ANALYSES IN OUR LABORATORY WITH THE TSP INTERFACE

We have used a Hewlett-Packard quadrupole MS (5987A) and liquid chromatograph with the TSP interface (Vestec Corpn., Houston, TX), to assay ranitidine, its *N*-oxide, and beclomethasone-17,21-dipropionate (BDP; an anti-inflammatory steroid).

The column, 100 × i.d. 4.6 mm, was packed with 5 μm Hypersil-ODS. The mobile phase was 0.1 M ammonium acetate/acetonitrile (60:40 v/v) and the flow-rate was 1 ml/min.

The mass spectrum for ranitidine was similar to that obtained using DLI. That for the *N*-oxide showed that ~90% of the ion current was due to fragment ions. The base peak was m/z 315, and the intensity of the [M+H]$^+$ ion was 18% of the base peak; the extent of fragmentation was similar irrespective of whether the DLI or TSP technique was used [4].

BDP was used to compare the 'filament on' and 'filament off' modes of TSP operation. The MS was operated in both the positive- and the negative-ion mode. When the filament is on, the MS is operating in the CI mode. Fig. 2 compares the mass spectra obtained in each mode fron 36 ng BDP injected on-column. The 'filament off' and 'filament on' spectra (positive-ion mode) were very similar, the base peak being the [M+H]$^+$ ion of BDP.

In the negative-ion mode, with the filament off the base peak was the [M]$^-$ (m/z 520) plus [CH$_3$COO]$^-$ adduct (m/z 579); with the filament on, the base peak due to [M]$^-$ was seen, also an [M−15]$^-$ ion at m/z 505 due to loss of a methyl group, and the adduct ion at m/z 579 (Fig. 2). The limit of sensitivity was determined by injecting solutions of BDP onto the column and measuring in the SIM mode the intensity of the [M+H]$^+$ ion or the [M]$^-$ ion. The 'filament on' nega- tive-ion mode was 10 times as sensitive as 'filament off', and 20 times as sensitive as 'filament on' in the positive mode. The limit of detection for the [M]$^-$ m/z 520 ion was 150 pg on-column. The signal- to-noise ratio was 3 at this sensitivity.

The TSP interface has proved reliable over six months. If volatile buffers are used there is no blockage of the vapouriser. Where the use of ammonium acetate would interfere with the chromatography, the buffer may be added post-column through a T-piece. A wide range of mobile phases ranging from water to 100% tetrahydrofuran, hexane and dichloromethane can be used. For the non-polar solvents the TSP should be operated with the filament on. The system is reliable enough to be automated using an AASP or column-switching system [3].

References

1. Martin, L.E., Oxford, J. & Tanner, R.J. (1982) *J. Chromatog. 251*, 215-224.
2. Melera, A. (1980) *Adv. Mass Spectrom. 8B*, 1597-1615.
3. Martin, L.E. (1986) *J. Pharm. Biomed. Anal.*, in press.
4. Lant, M.S., Martin, L.E. & Oxford, J. (1985) *J. Chromatog. 323*, 143-152.
5. Vestal, M.L. (1984) *Science 226*, 275-281.

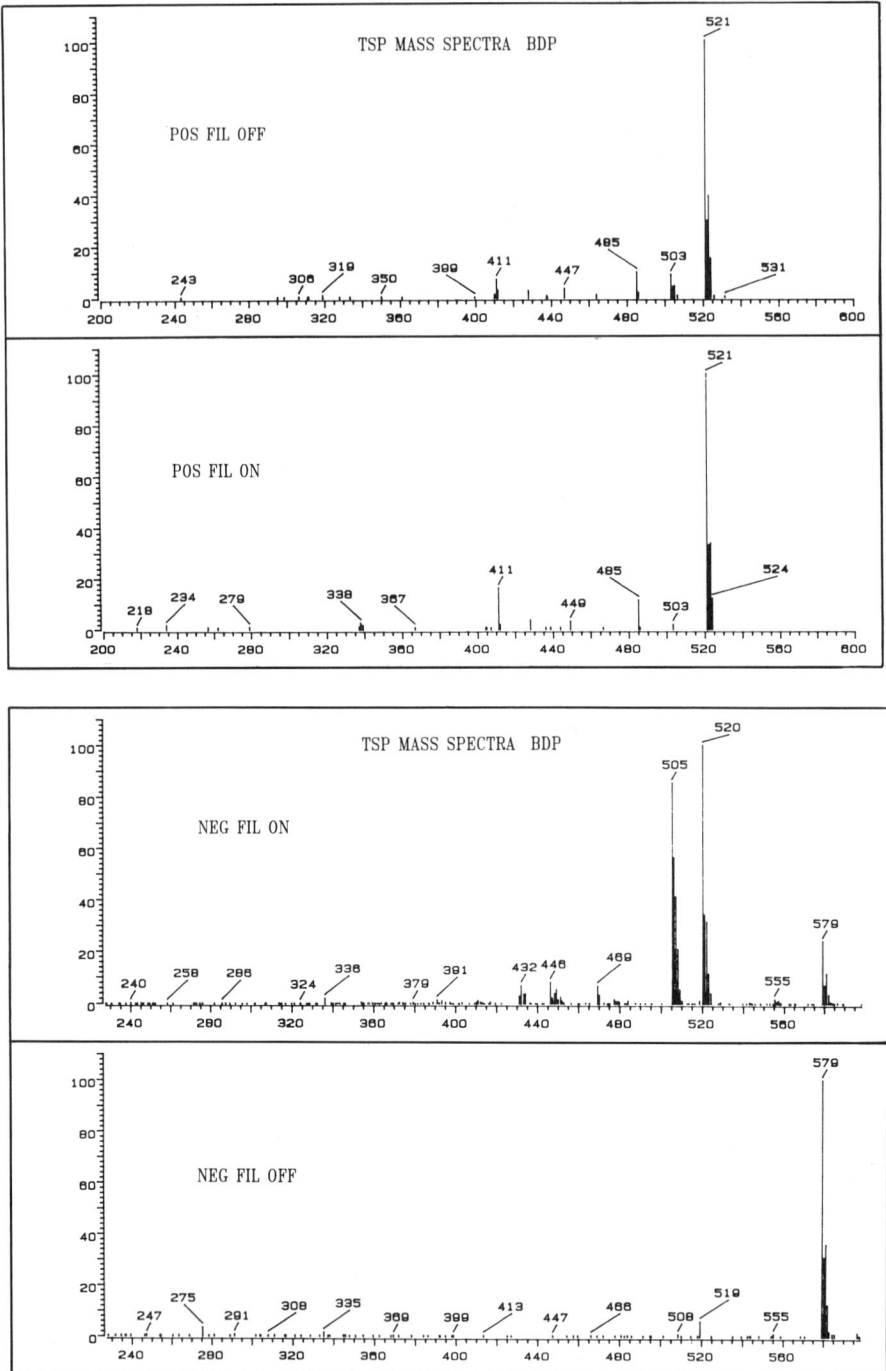

Fig. 2.   Mass spectrum of BDP under different ionization conditions.

Comments on material in #D

Comment on #**D-1**, J.K. Nicholson - ^{1}H NMR FOR METABOLITE DETECTION

Remark by D. Dell.- As a variation on the choice of proton NMR for metabolic studies, there is a published example of the use of ^{19}F NMR, where metabolites of 5-fluorouracil were being investigated; the pattern was notably 'clean', because there are no endogenous fluorine-containing compounds that would interfere.

Comments on #**D-3**, P.C. White - MULTI-WAVELENGTH DETECTOR

Question by P.G. Ashton.- Your system is able to distinguish between 29 different barbiturates; but in forensic toxicology we need to identify only a few barbiturates and their metabolites amongst the endogenous material present: is your system capable of doing this? **Reply.-** This has yet to be investigated. **Reply to query by A. Electricwala**, relating to comparison of two ball-point inks: in comparing two absorbance-ratio values, the S.D. is important for the discrimination.

Comments on #**D-4**, A. Hulshoff & al.- FLUOROPHORE-LABELLED GLUCURONIDES

R. Schmid asked how the derivatization procedure compared, in respect of sensitivity and sample handling, with other carboxyl derivatization procedures. **Reply.-** The publication text (above) is pertinent. Our method is selective and sensitive, and mild reaction conditions suffice - which applies also to other published procedures. **Answers to further questions.-** Comparing the fluorescence labels with those in the literature, no marked difference is apparent; the dansyl nucleus behaves badly in water-rich media, and also differences in detection limits can be caused by factors besides the fluorescent properties of the derivatives. A query about nitro-phenol-type glucuronides (indeed investigated) led to mention of two problems: the derivative is so polar that one may get interfering peaks from reagents and derivatized endogenous compounds, and the fluorescence signal of the derivative may be very low, possibly due to an inner filter effect insofar as the excitation wavelength is near that of the nitrophenol nucleus. **Question by K-H. Lehr.-** Did you try to determine the glucuronides of phenolphthalein or nitrophenol by means of your method? **Reply.-** With nitrophenol there are two problems: the fluorescence response of the derivatives is low, and the peak is close to or under the reagent-blank peak.

Comments on #**NC(D)-3,-4,** U. A. Th. Brinkman – POST–COLUMN REACTORS; ECD
       & #**NC(D)-5,** L.E. Martin – LC-MS

D. Dell asked about the reliability of the solid phase used
for derivatization: had it been used for, and survived, the analysis
of hundreds of plasma samples? **Reply.-** The system, further developed
and tested by Kratos, indeed performs well in sustained use, e.g.
the hydrolysis of amides to amino acids for OPA derivatization,
and thiram assay is another example; the pre-columns are in use
in company laboratories, even 3 in sequence. **Response to R.D. McDowall,**
who sought a recapitulation of the benefit to sensitivity from
use of microbore columns.- They give lower detection limits because
of the lower dispersion volumes, ~20-fold lower for 1 mm compared
with 4.6 mm; however, the injection volumes have to be lower, which
can be an actual advantage if only a limited amount of sample is
available, but in terms of analyte concentration in the sample
there is no gain from microbore operation. **Practical tip from
H. de Bree,** for purifying methanol, provided that its water content
is <5%: an effective procedure is to treat with sodium, ~1 g/1
of methanol; leave to react until H_2 evolution ceases, then distil 80%
off for use.

M. Uhlein asked whether assay problems had been encountered
where LC-MS direct coupling was the only way to solve them. **L.E.
Martin's answer.-** An example is the steroid BCD [see foregoing
'Note'], for which the dose in man (i.v., oral or by inhalation)
is typically 100 μg. **Question from U.A.Th. Brinkman.-** Have you
any experience of introducing pure organics such as hexane into
the TSP system? **Reply.-** No, but a 1985 paper by D.A. Garteiz &
M.L. Vestal describes the analysis of hydrocarbons in hexane extracts
using the filament-on mode. **Replies to questions by K.K. Midha.-**
Concerning the ability of the system to detect an on-column load
of 5 ng, for ranitidine in urine (100 μl injected) this means that
50 ng/ml is detectable. Use of the TSP with a magnetic-sector
rather than a quadrupole MS has not been tried by us; but M.L. Vestal
reckons this is feasible, and Kratos advertize a TSP interface
for the MS 25. **Answer to R. Schmid,** who asked if the MS ion source
had to be modified: the interface contains the ion source, which
is fitted with heaters, thermocouples and vapour exhaust manifold.

Citations contributed by Senior Editor

Special techniques in GC

In a further contribution to the problem of **derivatizing tertiary amines** for GC [1], an optimized two-phase procedure has been
developed, using ethyl chloroformate, for assaying **pentazocine** in
plasma; detection was by **MS** (SIM), coupled to the capillary column.

GC—MS (conventional column) was employed in an assay procedure for **diclofenac**, extracted by benzene from acidified plasma [2], and in a procedure for assay of plasma or urine for **captopril** and metabolic 'conjugates' (the disulphide dimer, and *S*-methylated drug and its sulphone) [3].

Using a bench-top instrument if CI is not needed as a gentler alternative to EI, **GC—MS** enables **enantiomer investigation** with the aid of stable isotopes [4]. Thus, for **warfarin** (whose enantiomers differ in activity) values for its enantiomers, in plasma from dosed volunteers, were individually obtained by GC-MS after adminis-tration of a 'racemate' comprising [^{12}C(*R*)]- and [^{13}C(*S*)]-warfarin; this neat approach (EI-MS; SIM) has elucidated the pharmacokinetics of warfarin enantiomers [authors concerned included R.A. O'Reilly & W.F. Trager, as cited]. GC-MS enabled the pharmacokinetics to be investigated, in the same subject, for **procainamide** and its ***N***-acetyl metabolite, by co-injecting ^{12}C-drug and ^{13}C-metabolite [5].

HPLC, e.g. with EC detection [cf. **NC(C)**:- UV or intrinsic fluorescence]

An example of **pre-column fluorophore generation** is the analysis of serum for **bestatin**, a drug potentially effective in cancer and other diseases [6]: the drug and the *p*-hydroxy drug were converted by periodate oxidation to the aldehydes, which by a further reaction yielded fluorescent products. For detection by **UV in the absence of intrinsic absorption**, RP-HPLC may be performed with a ion-pairing UV-absorbing agent in the mobile phase, as investigated with Na naph-thalene-2-sulphonate; its retention should be similar to that of the analyte [7].

Analytes that can be determined in plasma with the **EC detection mode** include **timolol** [8], **salbutamol** [9] and **noradrenaline** along with a **glycol** metabolite (3,4-dihydroxyphenylethylene glycol) [10]. The reductive rather than oxidative mode of EC detection was used for **misonidazole** and its desmethyl metabolite [11]. Both modes – and, in some laboratories, use of the traditional dropping mercury electrode – feature in a reviewers' tabulation (with HPLC condit-ions) of **various drugs** amenable to EC detection [12]. For **melphalan** and **chlorambucil** in plasma, the **UV, fluorescence and EC** detection modes have been carefully compared, in the pharmacokinetic context [13]: with the UV mode, baseline noise (caused mainly by pump pulsa-tions) was minimal and sensitivity was greatest. **EC circuitry** can readily be assembled, saving outlay on instrument purchase [14]. The analytical usefulness of HPLC-UV with **photodiode array for urapidil** has been demonstrated [15] (cf. **trimethoprim** and **sulfamethoxazole** [16]).

Comparisons between analytical approaches, including RIA

For **nimodipine** in plasma, accurate assay was achievable by either GC-ECD or HPLC-UV, for demethylated metabolites also; assays on CSF were performed by GC-ECD after 'clean-up' by TLC or HPLC [17]. GC-ECD and HPLC also correlated well for **butofilol** in plasma; one solvent-extraction step sufficed for HPLC, whereas GC entailed multi-stage clean-up and derivatization [18].[⊗]

GC-MS checking of a **propranolol** RIA with 'specific' Ab's showed the need to remove an interfering conjugate by pre-extraction [19]. For **adriamycin** in plasma and urine, RIA showed lower specificity than HPLC (fluorescence detection; initial solid-phase extraction) [20]. Non-chromatographic approaches were compared with HPLC preceded by deproteinization (phenol/TCA) and followed by fluorescent derivatization, to determine **tobramycin** in serum [21]. Taking account of cost as well as speed, HPLC in comparison with three immunoassays took the lead; but a microbiological assay was easiest to perform, albeit slow. A comparison between microbiological assay and HPLC has also been reported for **imipenem** [22]; RP-HPLC was used for deproteinized plasma, and anion-exchange HPLC for urine. In the assay of patients' urine for **EGF-URO**[gastrone], RIA correlated poorly with RRA [23]; possible reasons are discussed.

Enzymatic and TLC approaches

Besides HPLC and RIA, enzyme inhibition (angiotensin-converting enzyme) was used for assaying **enalapril** and a metabolite in plasma, following extraction onto XAD-4 and elution by methanol [24]; the study also dealt with urine and liver, and was aided by TLC. Based on published methods for assaying **2'-deoxycoformycin** in biological fluids through inhibition of adenosine deaminase, an enzymatic kinetic method was developed, taking enzyme inactivation into account [25]. TLC with fluorescence measurement was used for determining **maprotiline** in urine and plasma after solvent extraction and derivatization by 7-chloro-4-nitrobenzofurazan [26].

[⊗]Likewise for **nomifensine** HPLC was simpler, and more selective[27].

References

1. Hartvig, P., Fagerlund, C. & Bondesson, U. (1984) *J. Pharm. Biomed. Anal. 2*, 509-517.
2. Kadowaki, H., Schlino, M. & Uemara, I. (1984) *J. Chromatog. 308*, 329-333.
3. Drummer, O.H., Jarrot, B., & Louis, W.J. (1984) *J. Chromatog. 305*, 83-93.
4. Toon, S., & Davidson, E.M. (1986) *Lab. Pract.*, January, 52-55.
5. Butcher, J.S., Strong, J.M., Lucas, S.V., Lee, W.K. & Atkinson, Jr., A.J. (1977) *Clin. Pharmacol. Ther. 22*, 447-457.
6. Ishida, J., Yamaguchi, M., Kay, M., Ohkura, Y. & Nakamura, M. (1984) *J. Chromatog. 305*, 381-389.
7. Hackzell, L., Rydberg, T. & Schill, G. (1983) *J. Chromatog. 282*, 179-191.
8. Gregg, M.R. & Jack, D.B. (1984) *J. Chromatog. 305*, 244-249.

9. Tan, Y.K. & Soldin, S.J. (1984) *J. Chromatog. 311*, 311-317.
10. Howes, L.G., Miller, S. & Reid, J.L. (1985) *J. Chromatog. 338*, 401-403.
11. Meering, P.G., Baumann, R.A., Zijp, J.J. & Maes, R.A.A. (1984) *J. Chromatog. 310*, 159-166.
12. Smyth, M.R. & Egan, A.M. (1986) *Anal. Proc. 23*, 87-89.
13. Adair, C.G., Burns, D.T. & Harriott, M. (1986) *Anal. Proc. 23*, 30-33.
14. Russell, J.R. (1986) *Lab. Pract.*, January, 99-101.
15. Zech, K., Huber, R. & Elgass, H. (1983) *J. Chromatog. 282*, 161-167.
16. Weber, A., Opheim, K.E., Siber, G.R., Ericson, J.F. & Smith, A.L. (1983) *J. Chromatog.278*, 337-345.
17. Krol, G.J., Noe, A.J. & Yeh, S.C. (1984) *J. Chromatog. 305*, 105-118.
18. Jeanniot,J.P., Houin, G. & Ledudal, P. (1983) *J. Chromatog. 278*, 301-309.
19. Eller, T.D., Knapp, D.R. & Walle, T. (1983) *Anal. Chem. 55*, 1572-1576.
20. Rahmani, R., Gil, P., Martin, M., Durand, A., Barbet, J. & Cano, J-P. (1983) *J. Pharm. Biomed. Anal. 1*, 301-309.
21. Stobberingh, E.E., Houben, A.W. & Van Bove, C.P.A. (1982) *J. Clin. Microbiol. 15*, 795-801.
22. Gravallese, D.A., Musson, D.G., Pauliokonis, L.T. & Bayne, W.F. (1984) *J. Chromatog. 310*, 71-84.
23. Nexφ, E., Lamberg, S.I. & Hollenberg, M.D. (1981) *Scand. J. Clin. Lab. Invest. 41*, 577-582.
24. Toco, D.J., de Luna, F.A., Duncan, A.E.W., Vasssil, T.C. & Ulm, E.H. (1982) *Drug Metab. Dispos. 10*, 15-19.
25. Staubus, A.E., Weinrib, A.B. & Malspeis, L. (1984) *Biochem. Pharmacol. 33*, 1633-1637.
26. Prinoth, M. & Mutschler, E. (1984) *J. Chromatog. 305*, 508-511.
27. Lindberg, R.L.P., Salonen, J.S. & Iisalo, E.I. (1983) *J. Chromatog. 276*, 85-92.

Use of a linear analyzer for radiolabel measurement on TLC plates

  - from a Forum Abstract by F.A.A. Dallas (Glaxo Ltd., Ware)

     Past approaches for radioactivity on chromatographic surfaces included elution analysis, zonal analysis, autoradiography, radioscanning, beta cameras, spark chambers and various types of proportional counters. Our drug-metabolism group has been using a modern position-sensitive proportional counter (Lab Logic Ltd.). It can be used at various voltages, and discriminators allow a restricted band of energy values to be detected. Up to 40 tracks may be set up at one time, and new tracks may be added as original tracks are completed. The instrument has a high throughput, requires minimum operator time, and has high sensitivity, moderate resolution and a low cost-per-sample. The major disadvantage is that to improve resolution one must decrease sensitivity. Even when sensitivity is not a problem, generally the radio-TLC chromatograms are assessed in tandem with autoradiograms of the TLC plates.

Trace enrichment from urine by zone refining

- from a Forum Abstract (relevant to sect. #C) by
  H.M. Ruijten, H.P. van Berkel & H. de Bree (Duphar, Weesp)

If HPLC is performed for an analyte in 1-5 l of sample, concentration is conveniently achieved by cone-shaped pre-columns which were described in Vol. 14, this series. However, if a much larger volume has to be processed or the analytes have a definite limited k' in the concentrating medium, a less time-consuming pre-treatment to remove the bulk of water can be used, based on the zone-refining principle. In a specially designed glass vessel, with a temperature gradient from +4° at the centre to -10° at the wall enables most of the water to be frozen out in nearly pure form. Thereby the urine volume can be reduced to ~10% containing 70-99% of the solutes.

Further citations by Senior Editor, relevant to sects. #C & #D

Problems in the HPLC determination of **thiols** and **disulphides** in biological fluids have been reviewed [28]. To minimize thiol losses caused by binding to proteins and to autoxidation to disulphides, samples are collected into EDTA and quickly acidified to remove protein and inhibit disulphide formation; any storage (at -20°) should be brief. A mobile phase at pH 1-2 containing EDTA to reduce chelative losses onto stainless-steel surfaces allowed **RP-HPLC** separation for captopril and thiomalate. (Cysteine and GSH were also studied; for D-penicillamine a cation-exchange column worked well.) Following runs with thiomalate, it appeared as a 'ghost' peak when samples lacking the drug were run: evidently thiols can bind to ODS-silica, displaceable by other thiols or a high concentration of organic modifier. A method for pre-derivatizing thiols would help. **EC detection** can be performed with Au or Pt (not Au/Hg amalgam) electrodes; but no EC system has yet proved satisfactory for disulphides (which are not difficult to chromatograph). Cf. #C-1 in Vol. 14.

Radioenzymatic assay of urinary **histamine** was found to greatly underestimate its level, as shown by GC-MS after derivatization [29]. Apparently urine contains an inhibitor for the histamine N-methyltransferase on which the assay relies.

28. Perrett, D. & Rudge, S.R. (1985) J. Pharm. Biomed. Anal. 3, 3-27
    (& Perrett, D., Chromatog. Soc. Bull. 21 (March 1986), 14-15).
29. Roberts, L.J., Aulsebrook, K.A. & Oates, J.A. (1985) J. Chromatog.
    338, 41-49.

Analyte Index

Key overleaf to the 10-category **chemical classification** (collation based on some analytically relevant features). Use of a compound as a internal standard is **not** indexed, nor all tabulated data (e.g. R_T's).
Hyphen '-' as in '17-' connotes *et seq.*, i.e. treatment in depth.

Prefixes to some page entries, *besides* ch = *chiral distinction:*

$\#$ Superscript, e.g. ^{1}, signifies that the study included **metabolite(s)** of the listed compound (**see over**).
$\#$ Subscript $_r$ signifies that 'real' **samples** (animal or human) were assayed, usually including blood or plasma. This may also be the case for some entries lacking the prefix $_r$; but mostly these concern pure compounds, or non-biological samples (see 'Environmental' entry in General Index).
$\#$ See IIa heading for p, denoting that a **precursor** was studied.

Any **index search of earlier vols.** (listed opposite title p.) can be confined to Vols. 12 (index **cumulative**) & 14; same 10 categories but fuller indication of sample type. The present prefix system is a stylistic innovation.

··

CATEGORY I (no amino group, nor cyclic N except maybe imide)

#Ia: acid *(other than conjugate),* or *ester (criterion: OVERLEAF)*

Bile acids: ^2_r318
Carboxylic acids, besides particular entries: 262; ch: 264-, 317
Cephalosporins: **see** IIa (even if of Ia type)
Dichloroacetic acid: $_r$109

Eicosanoids (**& see** Leuko..., Prost..., Thromb...): $_r$117-, $_r$126
Etodolac: ch: $_r$250
Ibuprofen, ch: $_r$244, $_r$250-
Isosorbide dinitrate: ^1_r310
Isoxepac: 341
Leukotrienes, e.g. LTB$_4$: $_r$117-, 119, $_r$130

Mandelic acid, ch: 261-, 278-
α–Methylarylacetic acids, e.g. Benoxaprofen, Fenoprofen, Naproxen (**& see** Ibuprofen; also Indoprofen, in IIIa), ch: 244, 250, 252
Nimodipine: ^1_r405
Nitroglycerin: Iz entry
Prostaglandins, e.g. PGE$_2$: $_r$117, $_r$129, $_r$130
Thiomalate: $_r$408
Thromboxanes, e.g. TXB$_2$: $_r$117-, $_r$130
Tropic acids, ch: 249-, 259-, 262

═══════

#Iy: not acid *(unless conjugate)* or ester, & no halo, N or P

Benzo(a)pyrene: **see** Polynuclear
Estrogens: **see** Oestrogens
Etiocholanolone: ^{2}348-
Etoposide: $_r$348, ^2_r389-

ASSIGNMENT 'CATECHISM'   *(See previous p. for other guidance)*

\# **Metabolites** are not separately listed; the parent molecule's entry is preceded by a superscript: *Phase I* metabolite(s),[1] or, if including *N*-desalkyl, [1] (i.e. **bold**); *Phase II (conjugates)*, [2].

\# **Parent molecules as indexed** bear generic names, where applicable, as listed (with formulae) in the *Merck Index*. Note, however, that some analytes fall under a group title (or a title cross-referenced therein). Examples: **Steroids**; **Phenylethylamine** (notional parent molecule for, e.g. noradrenaline), for which the listings (IIb' & IIb") indicate how to look up metabolites such as HMPG. **Peptides/ Proteins** entry in IIa gives guidance on retrieval.

\# **Assignment as 'acidic'** (to Ia, IIa or IIIa) applies where the pKa is <6; this excludes phenols, and **conjugates are excluded** since only the parent molecule is listed (prefixed [2]; see above). Also 'acidic' (notional) are **esters** yielding an acidic group in the main moiety if hydrolysed (as may happen *in vivo*).

\# **Cyclic *N*** is never treated as 'amino'; it is 'imide' (possible category: Ic) if -CO-N-CO-, but otherwise *may* be basic.

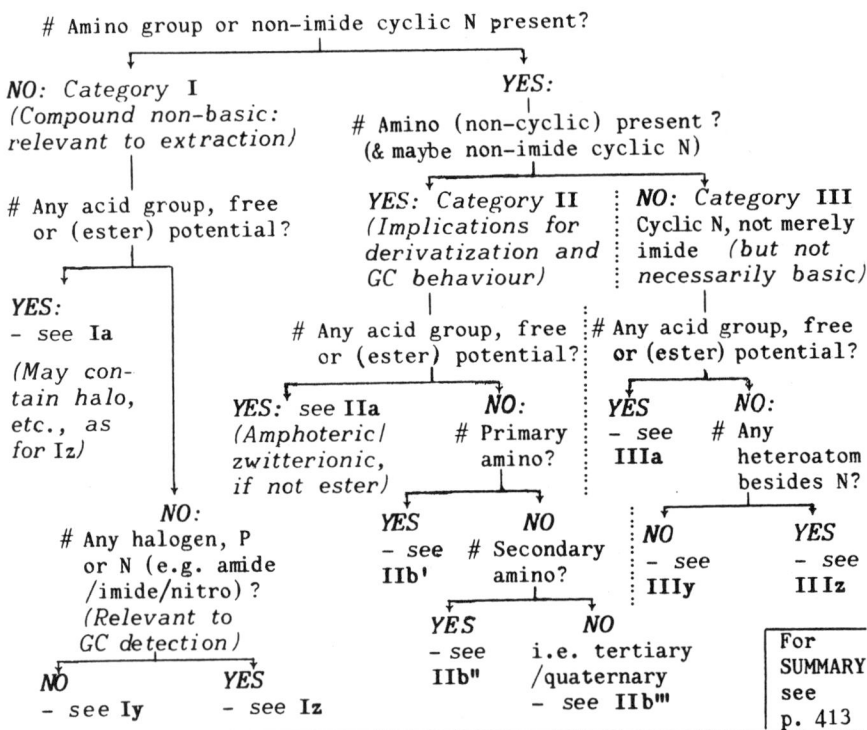

\# Amino group or non-imide cyclic N present?

NO: Category **I**
(Compound non-basic: relevant to extraction)

\# Any acid group, free or (ester) potential?

YES:
- see **Ia**
(May contain halo, etc., as for Iz)

NO:
\# Any halogen, P or N (e.g. amide /imide/nitro) ? *(Relevant to GC detection)*

NO - see **Iy**   *YES* - see **Iz**

YES:
\# Amino (non-cyclic) present ? (& maybe non-imide cyclic N)

YES: Category **II** *(Implications for derivatization and GC behaviour)*

\# Any acid group, free or (ester) potential?

YES: see **IIa** *(Amphoteric/ zwitterionic, if not ester)*

NO: \# Primary amino?

YES - see **IIb'**

NO \# Secondary amino?

YES - see **IIb"**

NO i.e. tertiary /quaternary - see **IIb"'**

NO: Category **III** Cyclic N, not merely imide *(but not necessarily basic)*

\# Any acid group, free or (ester) potential?

YES - see **IIIa**

NO: \# Any heteroatom besides N?

NO - see **IIIy**   *YES* - see **IIIz**

For SUMMARY see p. 413

#Iy, *continued*

Glycols, esp. amine-derived: r312, r405

Nabumetone: $\frac{1}{r}$311
Nadolol, ch: r317
Oestrogens: ^{2}348–
Phenprocoumon: r311
Polynuclear aromatic hydrocarbons (PAH's), ch: 250, r251
Steroids (& see other Iy entries; also Bile... in Ia, & Beclo... in Iz): 24, 312, ^{2}348
Thiram: 396
Warfarin, ch: 244, 317, 405

#Iz: as for #Iy, but with halo, P, or N as (e.g.) amide, imide, $-NO_2$

Acetaminophen: see Paracetamol
Barbiturates: 222–, 378; ch: 244, 248, 249
Beclomethasone: r400
Benzamides (& see Sul... below; also 'RIV..' in IIb'): 189–

'BCNU': r311

Ethosuximide, ch: 244, 249
Glutethimide, ch: 244, 249, r252–
Hydantoins, e.g. Mephenytoin (& see Phenytoin), ch: 244, 285, $\frac{1}{r}$316

N-Methylformamide: $\frac{1}{r}$341–
Nitroglycerin (cf. Isosorb... in Ia): 110

Paracetamol (Acetaminophen): $^{12}_{r}$325–, 379
Phenytoin: 379
2-Pyrrolid(in)one: r113–, 126
Succinimides, ch: 244, 248, 249
Sulpiride/Sultopride: r191–

CATEGORY II (amino, not in a ring)

#IIa: acid *other than conjugate* or ester *(main moiety = acid)*

For **Peptides** & **Proteins**:
– look for 'family name' (e.g. Growth factors), not merely entries for individual components (e.g. EGF);
– p as prefix signifies precursor(s) studied; thus pGastrin covers (pre)progastrin;
– analytes with amino acid(s) attached, e.g. LTE, may not be in IIa; all eicosanoids are in Ia

N-Acetyl derivs.: see parent compound, e.g. Muramic
ACTH: p55, 70, r99–
Amino acids (esp. endogenous; & see Cysteine): 37, 129, r326; ch: 316, 317
Aminobenzoic acid, ch: 264
Ampicillin: $\frac{1}{r}$333
Angiotensins: 39, r130; ch: 317
α-Atrial natriuretic peptide (ANP): 69
Azeonam: r312
Baclofen: r216

C-peptide: r127
Calcitonin/CGRP: 24, 72
Captopril: r216, r408
S-Carboxymethylcysteine, ch: 285
Cephalosporins (listed here even if really Ia type): 306, r312
– Ceftriaxone: r311
Chlorambucil: r405
Cholecystokinin: 37, p_r76
Cortinarins: $\frac{1}{r}$13–
Creatine/Creatinine: r326
Cysteine (not in conjugate; cf. r324): r130, r408
– N-acetyl: 110, r130; ch: 285–

Diclofenac: r405

#IIa, *continued*

Dipyrone: $_r$311
Dynorphin (**& see** Opioid): 121,
127, p129, 155
EGF: **see** Growth
Eicosanoids: see IIa heading
Enalapril: $\frac{1}{r}$406
Endorphins (**& see** Opioid): 55,
$_r$60-, 70-, $_r$128, p129
Enkephalins (**& see** Opioid):
$_r$128, p129
- Leu-: 39, 121
- Met-: 39, p55, $_r$129
[Flucloxacillin: in IIIa, though
most penicillins are in IIa]
GABA: $_r$113, 126
Gastrin: p$_r$76-, 125
Glucagon: $_r$68
Glutathione: 110, $_r$408
Growth factors, e.g. EGF: 17-,
$_r$34, 70, $_r$406
- IGF-I: $_r$130
Growth hormone (GH): 127
Imipenem: $_r$406
Insulin: $_r$68
Kinins: see Cholecys..., Tachy...
Leukotrienes: **see** IIa heading
β-Lipotropin: 55, $_r$60-

Melphalan: $_r$216
Methyldopa: ch: 317
MSH: 55
Muramic acids (free or peptido-
glycan): $_r$4-, $\frac{1}{r}$6
Neurokinins (Neuromedins): $_r$46-
Neurotensin: 37, 39, 70
Opioid peptides (& see Dyn...,
Endor..., Enkeph..., β-Lipo...,
POMC): 37, p129, $_r$130
Oxytocin: 37, 39, $_r$127

Peptides/Proteins: see IIa
heading, & General Index
Peptidoglycans: 3-, $_r$8-
POMC: 55, 62
Somatomedins: $_r$89-
Substance P: p$_r$46-
Tachykinins: see Neuro..., Subs...
Tensins: see Angio..., Neuro...
Thyroxine/Iodothyronines, ch: $_r$317

TSH: $_r$102
Vasoactive intestinal peptide
(VIP), & PHM, PHI: 70, p$_r$76-,
84, $_r$127
Vasopressin, esp. AVP: $_r$37-,
39-, $_r$127

═══════════

#IIb': primary amino; *no* acid
    (unless conjugate) or ester

'A643C' (an acetamide deriva-
tive): $_r$216
Adriamycin: **see** Doxo...
Amphetamines: 233, 375; ch: 233,
249, 251, 317
Dapsone: 299
Doxorubicin (Adriamycin):
$_r$406
4'-Epi-doxorubicin: $\frac{1}{r}$311
Histamine: $_r$408
Metoclopramide: 189-
Nomifensine: $\frac{1}{r}^2$211, $_r$406
Nucleobases (Ade, Cyt, Gua): 306
Phenylethylamines (if not
IIb"; **& see** Amphet...), ch: 316
Polyamines: $_r$129
Procain(amid)e: 233, $\frac{1}{r}$405
Pyrimethamine: 299
'RIV 2093' (an aminobenzamide):
$_r$192
Tobramycin: $_r$406
Tocainide, ch: $_r$316
Trimethoprim: $_r$405

───────────

#IIb": secondary amino, not in a
    ring; otherwise as for IIb'

Acebutolol, ch: $\frac{1}{r}$283
Albuterol: **see** Salbutamol
Bupranolol: $\frac{1}{r}$311
Bupropion: $\frac{1}{r}$151-
Chlordiazepoxide: $_r$141-, 233,
366
Chloroquine: $\frac{1}{r}$309
Desimipramine (cf. Imipramine
entries prefixed ^{1} in IIb'''):
$_r$134-, $\frac{1}{r}$149-
Fenfluramine: $_r$167; ch: $\frac{1}{r}$273
Maprotiline: $_r$406

#IIb", *continued*

Methaqualone: 233, 366
Oxmetidine: $^1_r^2$313

Phenylethylamines, *N*–alkylated
(cf. IIb'):
- Ephedrines: 233, 379; ch: $_r$165,
  249, 317
- Noradrenaline: $_r$405
Propranolol: 406; ch: $_r$250–,
$_r$316
Salbutamol: $_r$405, 314
Timolol: $_r$405

#IIb''': tert. amino or quaternary
  ammonium, not in a ring; otherwise as for IIb'

Adinazolam: $_r$203
Amitriptyline (**& see** Nortript...,
  = metabolite): 366, 370, 375
Butoprozine: ^1_r356–
Chlorpromazine: ^1_r133–, $_r$160–,
^1_r164–, 167
Clomipramine: ^1_r217
Dibenzazepines: see Clomipramine,
  Imipramine; also (IIb") Chlordiaz-
  epoxide, Desipramine, & (IIIy)
  Carbamazepine;
  cf. Tricyclics entry below

Dicyclomine: $_r$310
Dimethylpropion: ch: ^{1}317
Diphenhydramine: 366
Disopyramide, ch: ^{1}254–
Doxepin: $_r$167

Flurazepam: ^1_r216
Glycopyrronium: $_r$310
Imipramine (cf. Desimipramine,
  IIb"): $_r$134–, ^1_r149–

Nortriptyline: 377
Oxyphenonium, ch: 260

Pentazocine: $_r$404
Prifinium: $_r$311
Ranitidine: ^1_r399

Tricyclics, including Dibenzaz-
epines (above; **& see** Amitriptyline,
Imipramine): $_r$149–, $_r$165, $_r$217
Verapamil: ^1_r311

CATEGORY III (cyclic N, not
merely imide; *no* amino)

#IIIa: acid *(other than conjugate)*
  or ester *(main moiety = acid)*
Cocaine: 233
Fl(ucl)oxacillin: ^1_r333
Indoprofen, ch: $_r$317
Temocillin, ch: 317
Zomepirac: $_r$216

#IIIy: only N-hetero (nor merely
  imide); *no* amino, & not acid or
  (main moiety) potential acid

Benzodiazepines/Benzodiazepinones
(**& see** Chlordiazepoxide in
IIb", Flurazepam in IIb'''):
$_r$133–, $^1_r^2$141–, 232; ch: ^{2}145,
316
- triazolo/imidazolo type:
  142, $_r$216
  including: *see over*

SUMMARY OF CATEGORIES

	I	II	III
Amino?	no	✓	no
Non–imide hetero-N?	no	maybe	✓
Acid or potential acid (not conjugate)?	✓ = Ia	✓= IIa	✓= IIIa
– no! (and not an ester)	Halo, P or N?	Primary amino?	Hetero atom besides N?
	– no: **Iy**	✓ = IIb'	
	– ✓ = **Iz**	If no:	– no = IIIy,
		2^y= IIb"	✓= IIIz
		3^y or 4^y = IIb'''	

Only **parent compound** listed; prefix
^{1} if Phase I metabolites studied [or
^{1} (**bold**) if dealkylated amino], & ^{2} if
Phase II (conjugate); prefix $_r$ = 'real'
(biological) sample. *Full Key: p. 410*
Chiral distinction denoted ch .

#IIIy, *continued*
Benzodiazepines, *continued*
  including:
- Adinazolam: $_l$201–
- Alprazolam: $_l$143, $_r$216
- Triazolam: $_l$143
- **other types:** 142
  including:
- Diazepam: $_r$144, ^{1}233; ch: 249
- Lorazepam, ch: 249
- Midazolam: $_l$216
- Nitrazepam: $_r$134, $_r$144,
  $_r$216, 233
- Oxazepam: 233

2'-Deoxycoformycin: $_r$406
2'-Deoxynucleosides: 306
5'-Deoxy-5-fluoro-[or -6-aza-]-
  uridine: $_l$303–
Diclofensine: $_l$213
Diethylcarbamazine: $_r$310
5-Fluorouracil: 303–
Haloperidol: $_r$138
Metronidazole: $_r$311, $_r$313,
  333
Misonidazole: $_r$405

Naloxone: 129, $_r$216

Omeprazole: $_l$311
Oxpentifylline: $_l$216–
Physostigmine (Eserine): $_r$181–
Sulfamethoxazole: $_r$405
Tinidazole: $_r$311
Toloxatone: $_l$216
Trazodone: $_l$154–

Reminder: **KEY** *on p. 409 and, for classification (based on* **parent** *compound's structure), on p. 410.*

#IIIz: heteroatom besides N;
  otherwise as for #IIIy

Codeine: 233, 266, 366
'DU 29373': $_r$297
Morphines: 233
Oltipraz (a pyrazine): $_r$310
Phenothiazines (**& see** Chlorproma-
zine, IIb''''): $_l$134–, $_l$159–, ^{1}210
  including:
- Mesoridazine: $_r$173–
- Sulphoridazine: $_l$207–
- Thioridazine: ^{2}134, $_l$161,
  $_l$164, $_l$207
- Trimeprazine: $_r$164, 167
  and the following, *all* $_r$160–
  (*esp.* $_r$162):
- Butaperazine (also $_r$134),
  Fluphenazine, Perazine,
  Perphenazine (also $_r$167),
  Pipotiazine, Prochlorperazine
  (also $_r$165, $_r$167), Promazine,
  Promethazine, Thioperazine,
  Trifluoperazine (also 138),
  Trifluphenazine

Piperazine-type analgesic,
ch: $_r$317
'SK&F 94120': ^1_r239–
Strychnine: 366, 368

Thioxanthenes, esp. *cis(Z)*-
isomers: $_r$173–
  including:
- Chlorprothixene: 176–
- Clopenthixol/Zuclopenthixol:
  $_l$174–
- Flupentixol: $_r$177–
- Thiothixene: $_r$216

General Index

This Index deals mainly with features studied and with approaches and points of technique, indexed similarly to previous 'A' vols. (listed opposite title p.) so as to facilitate back-searching. The preceding Analyte Index deals with compounds investigated; exceptionally, a few types are also listed below according to their nature, e.g. 'Antineoplastics', 'Benzophenones...'.

In a page entry such as '17-', the '-' means '*et seq.*', i.e. coverage in depth.

Accuracy of analyses: **see** Assay ...comparisons, Automated

Adjuvants: **see** Antisera...raising, & Peptidoglycans

Adsorbents in sample preparation (**& see** Bonded, Cartridges, Solid-): 42, 236
- XAD-4: 406; XAD-2: 350

Adsorptive losses (**& see** GC, HPLC, Vessels): 56, 160
- minimization by solvent additive: 153, 175

Affinity separations (**& see** Protein A): 7, 9

Albumins (incl. ovalbumin), esp. separation: 24
Antibodies (Ab's; **& see** Antisera, Cross-, Immunoglob...):
- circulating (measurement, diagnostic role): 9
- monoclonal (MAb's): e.g. 98, 165

Anticholinergics: 254, 260

Antidepressants/Antipsychotics: sect. #B (see Contents list, viii)

Antigenicity: **see** Immunogenicity

Antineoplastics: 303, 311, 312, 389, 405

Antisera (**& see** Cross-, Immuno...):
- raising/assessing: 47, 78, 90, 99, 118, 166, 178
- specificity enhancement: 46-

Arachidonic acid: 117

Assay approaches, esp. comparisons for accuracy etc. (**& see** Bio..., Enzymes, Immunoassays, RRA): e.g. 38, 96, 134-, 145, 160, 167, 173-, 405-, 408

Automated methods (**& see** Robot..):
- GC: 291, 309, 312, 401
- sample preparation/HPLC: 236, 297-, 309-

Bacteria: **see** Cell...wall, Infect...

Benzophenones as 'derivatives': 143, 145, 216

Bile analytes: 318, 359-, 385

Bioassays (not immuno; cf. Enzymes): 88, 117, 121
- microbiological: 406

Biogenic amines: **see** IIa in Analyte Index (Histamine, Phenylethylamine)

Blood analytes: **see** Erythro..., Sample collection (& in Analyte Index, where prefix r commonly connotes assay in plasma)

Bonded-phase materials (**& see** GC, Ion-exchange):
- for HPLC (**& see** HIC; cf. HPLC packings), besides C-18 (e.g. C-2, CN): 21, 129, 136, 177, 216, 254
- for sample preparation (**& see** Cartridges): e.g. 185, 202
  - comparison with solvent extraction: 312
  - types other than C-18: 185, 202, 217, 236

Brain analytes: 38-, 47, 156, 162, 216

Calibration-curve determination /features: e.g. 39, 154, 156, 194

Cancer/Tumour studies (cf. Anti-neo-), Analytes in tumours/metastases: 50, 84

Carboxylic acids: **see** Conjugates, Deriv...; & Analyte Index, Ia

Cartridges for sample preparation (**& see** Bonded-): e.g. 114, 127, 185, 202, 236-, 297, 309, 318
- apparatus for (**& see** Automated): 185, 312

Cell features/studies (**& see** Immunomic..., Liver, Metab..., Processing):
- type differences, peptides: 84
- wall components, bacteria: 3, 6

Cerebrospinal fluid: **see** CSF

Chiral differentiation (**& see** Enantiomers, & Analyte Index p. nos. preceded by ch; cf. Diastereo..., Stereo...):
- derivatization, esp. to form diastereoisomers (& problems): 245, 274, 316, 317
- GC with a CSP: 285-, 316
- HPLC with a CSP: 145-, 245-, 316
  - cavity CSP, esp. cyclodextrins (Inclusion chromatography): 246-, 261-

- HPLC with a CSP, *continued*
  - ligand-exchange/metal complex: 246-
  - protein type, e.g. α-glycoprotein (AGP): 214, 246, 248, 254, 315
- HPLC with a chiral/ion-pair eluent: 261-, 317
  - cyclodextrins: 261, 317
- TLC: 237-, 317

Chromatography: **see** Affinity, Assay...comparisons, Exclusion, GC, HIC, HPLC, Ion-, TLC

Conjugates ('Phase II'; cf. superscript [2] in Analyte Index; **& see** Glucuronides):
- extractability: 318, 348-, 360
- NMR investigation: 326-

Conjugation to confer immunogenicity (**& see** Iodin...): e.g. 47, 58-, 76, 78, 86, 118, 178

Contaminants (analytical): **see** Cartridges, Interfer..., Plasticizers, Solvent

Cross-reactivity (**& see** Assay ...comparisons, Metabolites, Peptides, RIA, RRA): e.g.: 165, 167-, 180

CSF analytes: 57-, 128, 406

Cyclodextrins (**& see** Chiral): 279

Data handling/interpretation (**& see** Multi-): e.g. 356-, 364, 374-

Denaturation (cf. Protein precip...), esp. inadvertent (**& see** Peptides): 21, 25-, 29

Derivatization, pre-chromatographic (**& see** Benzophenones, Chiral):
- for GC: e.g. 291, 309, 317
  - for ECD: e.g. 113, 143, 316
  - obviation in capillary GC: 143; **& see** GC
  - tertiary amines: 313
- for HPLC (**& see** Electro...), esp. for fluorimetry: e.g. 113,

Derivatization sub-entry, *ctd.*
145, 214, 249, 403, 405
- carboxylic acids: 152, 344-,
354-
- oxazolid-ine/-one formation:
249, 317
- for TLC: 5, 406

Derivatization, post-column:
see Fluor...

Diastereoisomers (for formation,
see Chiral...deriv...), esp.
separation: 245
- by GC: 250, 274-, 316
- by HPLC: 145, 283, 317

Disulphides: 405, 408

Dyes (ink, fabrics): 379

Eicosanoids (**& see** Analyte Index,
Ia): 117

Electrochemical (EC) assay:
- derivatization for: 37
- DPP: 144
- HPLC detection: e.g. 37-,
136, 145, 164, 391, 405, 408
- baseline/noise problems:
124, 310
- modes/electrode types/settings:
39-, 123-, 408
- dual-channel: 38-, 182-

Electrophoresis: 7

ELISA applicability: 10, 98

Eluents (esp. composition; **& see**
Cartridges, Ion-pair, Resol...):
- optimization/modifiers: e.g.
23-, 123, 154, 299, 313, 314,
348
- used with CSP's: e.g. 262-,
316
- peptide/protein separation:
e.g. 19-, 24-, 114
- pH & salt influences: e.g.
23, 26, 31, 262-
- with volatile buffers: 60,
128, 401

Emulsions (in extraction), &
obviation: 153, 156, 214, 236

Enantiomers, differential aspects:
& see Chiral; cf. Diastereo...,
Stereo...

Endogenous analytes [some name-
listed (e.g. Growth, Prosta...),
in Analyte Index too]: e.g.
109-, 113-, 325-, 396

Endorphins/Enkephalins (**& see**
Analyte Index, IIa): e.g. 55-,
121

Environmental samples: 4, 398

Enzymes:
- as tools (**& see** Glucuronidase,
Lysozyme, Proteases): 7, 10,
129
- for analyte measurement
(**& see** ELISA): 406
- 'indicator' reactions, e.g.
with NAD: 6
- chromatography: 24, 29
- detriment to analyte (**& see**
Proteases): 183-

Erythrocytes, drug levels/shifts:
151, 160, 161, 184, 192, 194

Evaporations: **see** Solvent

Exclusion chromatography (Gel
'filtration'/'permeation'):
32-, 66, 79, 127, 130
- with ion-exchange too: 7, 31
- with lipophilic groups: 30,
33, 318

Extraction of analytes: **see**
Conjugates, Sample, Solvent,
Tissues

Fluorimetric methods (**& see**
Derivatization):
- in HPLC (without pre-column
reaction): 145, 395
- in TLC: 5, 174-, 406
- sensitivity attainment: 349,
403

Forensic/toxicological (esp.
drug) analytes: 221-, 233,
264, 373-
- biological specimens (SPA): 239

Freezing (**& see** Storage, Zone),
esp. effects (**& see** Storage):
239
- tenacious binding: 203

GC (Gas chromatography; commonly
capillary mode; **& see** Automated,
Derivatization): e.g. 135, 289-,
312
- adsorptiveness ('activity'),
  & obviation: 217, 222, 229,
  289
- analyte degradation/injection
  strategies/obviating derivatization: 142-, 162, 289, 310,
  312
  - solids injector: 143
- assessment, e.g. with Grob
  mixtures: 226, 289
- detection modes other than
  FID (**& see** MS): 273, 287
  - AFID (NPD): e.g. 136, 144,
    162, 215, 287
  - ECD: e.g. 143, 162
- stationary phases incl. SCOT
  /WCOT columns: 143, 177, 216,
  221, 289, 309
  - with barbiturate moiety: 222-

Gel chromatography/'filtration':
see Exclusion

Glucuronides (examined intact;
& see Conjugates): 350
- HPLC: 145, 389-
  - derivatized: 355-
- NMR study: 326
- types/hydrolysis: 212, 214,
  343, 344, 390
  - *N*-/labile: 211

Glutathione (GSH; cf. Conjugates),
esp. drug influences: 111, 342

Glycoproteins: 30, 103, 123,
151
- AGP (**& see** Chiral): 248-,
  253

Growth factors (GF's; **& see**
Analyte Index, IIa): e.g. 17-,
24-, 33-, 88

Growth hormone: 24, 31
- somatomedin as index: 87-

HIC (Hydrophobic interaction
chromatography): 30-, 127

HPLC (**& see** next entry, & Assay,
Automated, Chiral, Sample):
- column size etc., & microbore
  /capillary choice: 177, 200,
  217, 396, 404
  - losses onto surface: 56,
    408
- detection (**& see** Derivatization, Electrochemical, Fluo...,
  MS, Multi-..., RIA): e.g.
  145, 405
  - ECD: 397
  - post-column reactors, incl.
    solid-phase: 395, 404
  - serial detectors: 358, 374
- equilibrium/flow-rate influence
  /ghost peaks (**& see** Peaks):
  20, 28, 156, 408
- pre-column/coupled columns
  /switching: 129, 203-, 254,
  312, 314, 348, 408
  - plasma loaded 'raw': e.g.
    311
- pump problems: 29
- radial compression 'columns':
  e.g. 38, 40, 124
- retentions/identifications
  (**& see** MS, Multi-): e.g.
  356, 359
- strategies/optimization/gradi-
  ent use (**& see** Eluents, Peptides):
  e.g. 27, 300, 355, 360, 386
- temp. choice/influence (incl.
  CSP's): 30, 190, 264, 314

HPLC packings (**& see** Chiral, HIC,
Ion-): 264
- alumina: 313
- CSP's: **& see** Chiral
- comparisons/supposed equiva-
  lences: 21, 49, 313
- 'FPLC': 130
- mixed-mode/ion-exchange also:
  18, 27, 30, 313, 348

HPLC packings, *continued*
- NP (usually silica): e.g.
  154, 175, 182, 313
- pre-treatment/exposed groups):
  19, 24, 202, 260, 264, 313
- resin-based, e.g. XAD (**& see**
  HIC, Ion-): 311
- RP: **see** Bonded

Hydrophobicity (**& see** HIC):
e.g. 134
- molecular regions, esp.
  peptides: 18, 21

Identification approaches: **see**
HPLC...retentions, Forensic,
Metabolites,
MS, NMR, Multi-

Immunoassays (**& see** Antisera,
Cross-, Ligand, Peptides, RIA),
esp. mode comparisons: e.g.
90-, 103
- immunometric (IMA's): 95, 126
  - 2-site: 97-
- non-isotopic (**& see** ELISA):
  97, 102
- sample dilution/pre-treatment
  (**& see** RIA): 11, 89-

Immunogenicity (**& see** Conjugation):
- peptide sequences: e.g. 9-,
  46-, 78, 83-, 91, 99-, 118,
  165
- peptidoglycans: 8-

Immunoglobulins (Ig's): 8, 9,
123

Immunomicroscopy: 76, 84 (histo-
chem.); 129 (e.m.)

Inclusion chromatography: **see**
Chiral

Infections, manifestation: 5, 9-

Insulin/Insulin-like activity
(**& see** Processing): 68, 87-

Interferences, esp. chromatographic (**& see** Contam...): e.g.
42, 50, 182, 192, 313

Iodination for Ab generation:
56, 65-, 125, 126
- product heterogeneity/remedies:
  66, 125
  - storage of product: 72

Ion-exchange approaches (**& see**
Exclusion, HPLC pack...):
- chromatography (IEC): 66,
  125
  - HPLC: e.g. 30-, 66-, 127,
    303-, 314, 348
- sample preparation: 312, 314

Ion-pair approaches:
- conferring fluorescence/UV
  detectability: 396, 405
- extraction: 311, 314, 350
- HPLC (**& see** Eluents): e.g.
  314
  - 'bulky ion-pair': 303-
  - for peptides/proteins: 3-, 25-,
    28, 33, 123

Isotope derivative assay (cf.
Radioenz...): 134

Kidney analytes: 15

Kinins: **see** Analyte Index, IIa

Lability problems (**& see** Storage):
- analytes (**& see** GC...degradation,
  Glucuronides, Metabolites,
  N-Oxides, Sulph...): e.g.
  114, 183, 211
  - circumvention (**& see** Sample
    collection): 114, 136, 161,
    184, 322
- reagents, e.g. racemization:
  72, 245, 283

Ligand assays (**& see** Immuno...,
RIA, RRA), esp. comparisons:
e.g. 89, 97, 147, 406

Lipophilicity: **see** Hydrophobicity

Liver (**& see** Gluta...), esp.
analytes/drug transformation:
129
- *in vitro* studies (incl. perfusion): 385

Liver, *continued*
- microsomes: 250, 386
- stereoselectivity: 250

Losses: **see** Adsorptive, Denat...,
Erythrocytes, Proteases, Vessels

Lysozyme:
- chromatography: 24, 46
- fission by: 4

Mass spectrometry: **see** MS

Metabolites (cf. [1] [1] & [2] entries,
explained on p. 409, in the
Analyte Index; & Conjugates,
Cross-reactivity, Glucuronides,
Identification, Liver, NMR,
N-Oxides, Stereo..., Sulph...):
e.g. 135, 142, 164, 359, 385
- profiling (DMP)/pathways:
  e.g. 216, 333, 338, 356-

Methionine oxidation: **see**
Sulph...

Modifiers: **see** Eluents

Monoclonal antibodies (MAb's):
see Antibodies

MS (Mass Spectrometry, esp. for
assay; usually electron-impact
(EI):
- chemical ionization (CI):
  138, 144, 390-
  - negative-ion: 113, 215,
    401
- fast atom bombardment (FAB):
  8, 128, 390
- GC-MS: 119, 138, 144, 163,
  287, 404, 405
- HPLC-MS (LC-MS): 128, 399
  - thermospray (TSP): 128,
    400-, 402
- identifications (e.g. by molecular ions): 14, 209, 251

Multi-wavelength HPLC detection
(**& see** Wave...): 355-, 373
- photodiode array (PDA) detectors: 355-, 380, 387, 405
- rotating-disc detector: 373-

Muramic acids: 4-

Mushroom toxins: 13-

Neuropeptides (generally **see**
type names, esp. in Analyte
Index, IIa): e.g. 37-, 55-, 70-

NMR (esp. proton) for
identification/assay: 317, 319-,
337-, 386, 403
- 'COSY' (2-D): 322, 326
- endogenous analytes: 323-

Nomenclature: e.g. vi, 46, 88,
312

Nuclear magnetic resonance: **see**
NMR

Opioids (**see** Analyte Index,
IIa): 37-, 55-, 70-, 128

N-Oxides: 135, 160, 167, 215,
400

Pain, & peptides role: 55-,
124

Peak quality/problems in HPLC
(cf. TLC), e.g. split peaks
(**& see** HPLC...equil...): 30,
80, 114, 123, 264, 300, 313, 408

Peptides (**& see** Conjugation,
Precursor, Proteases; also name
entries, incl. Analyte Index,
IIa):
- artefactual changes: e.g.
  80, 122
- authentic/purity (**& see**
  Iodin...): 56, 82
- cross-reactivities: e.g. 46-,
  85, 100
- cryptic regions (flanking
  sequences): 76-, 125
- cyclic: 13-
- establishing amino acid composition: 83
- HPLC (**& see** Proteins): e.g.
  17-, 49-, 59-, 81, 121
- immunoassay approaches/problems
  (**& see** Immuno..., Iodination):
  numerous allusions in Sect. A
- MS: 128

Peptides, *continued*
- sequence homologies/excisions
  (**& see** Immunogenicity, Precursors): e.g. 46, 55, 76

Peptidoglycans, incl. isolation
& assay: 3-
- disease changes: 11
- metabolism/adjuvant use: 4, 6-
- structure studies: 4, 6

Pharmacokinetic studies, esp.
analytical feasibility: e.g.
144, 163-, 196-, 405
- enantiomers: 405

Photodiode array detectors:
see Multi-wavelength

Pituitary analytes, e.g. GF's:
17-, 37-

Plasticizers, interfering in
analyses: 151, 160, 238

Polarography: **see** Electro...DPP

Precision assessment: e.g. 102

Precursors/processing (cellular;
& see Cell) of peptides (**& see**
Analyte Index IIa entries preceded by *p*): 30, 46, 55, 76-,
83-, 121
- POMC: 55, 67

Prostaglandins (**& see** Ia in
Analyte Index): 117

Proteases:
- analyte detriment/suppression
  (**& see** Peptides): 24, 71, 121
- *in vivo* actions (**& see** Precursors): 80
- use to split peptides: 4, 79

Protein A, use of: 10, 99

Protein binding, esp. drugs
/analytical relevance (cf. Chiral):
151, 203, 215, 248, 313, 408
- carriers: 88-
  - use for assay (CPBA): 90

Protein precipitation/removal,
esp. plasma (cf. Interferences):
e.g. 203, 214, 312, 313

Proteins (**& see** Antibodies,
Denaturation, Enzymes, Glyco...):
- separation, esp. HPLC (**& see**
  Peptides): e.g. 18, 21-, 30, 127

Radioisotope use/features relevant
to isotope choice   (**& see** Iodination, RIA, RRA): e.g. 70, 97,
118

Radioenzymatic assay: 408

Radioreceptor assay: **see** RRA

Receptors (cf. RRA): 71, 73, 129
- assay: 67
  - interferences: 89

Resolution/Retention: **see**
Eluents, GC, HPLC, Peak

RIA (radioimmunoassay; **& see**
Assay, Cross-, Immuno...,
Peptides):
- for drugs: e.g. 164-, 177
- for peptides: e.g. 9-, 68-, 90,
  96
- geometrical isomer distinction:
  167
- interferences/dilution, solvent
  extraction, or other pre-
  treatment: 11, 47, 126, 179
  - HPLC: e.g. 34, 37-, 49-,
    128, 130, 406
- ligand homogeneity: 65-
- separation of ligand (e.g.
  with PEG)/solid-phase systems
  /'SPRIA': e.g. 10, 48, 119
- sequence-specific: e.g. 47, 90,
  167

Robotics in analysis: 291, 293-,
310, 312

RRA (receptor binding assay;
& see Immuno..., Ligand): e.g.
70-, 89, 145-, 216, 406
- cross-reactivity & possible
  advantage: e.g. 146-
- interferences/prior extraction
  or HPLC: 146
- receptor preparation: 146, 215

Salt effects: **see** Eluents; some
Solvent extr... entries also apply

Sample collection/storage (blood, etc.; & see Eryth..., Lability, Plasticizers): 50, 57, 151, 156, 160, 184, 191, 408

Sample preparation: see Adsorb.., Automated, Bonded, GC...pretreatment, HPLC...sample, Protein, RIA, Solid-, Solvent, Tissue, TLC

Sensitivity/Detection limit (& see Assay, Immuno...): e.g. vi, 38, 90, 97, 145, 154

Sequences: see Immunogenicity, Peptides, RIA

Sex differences: 16-

Size-exclusion chromatography: see Exclusion

Sleep factors: 4, 7-

Solid-phase (liquid-solid) processing (& see Adsorbents, Bonded, Cartridges, RIA): e.g. 5, 201-, 206, 207, 348

Solvent extraction (& see Adsorptive, Emulsions, Ion-pair, RIA): e.g. 153, 156, 182, 191, 236, 313, 350
- evaporation step: 153, 204
- of impurities (washing): e.g. 212, 187, 350
- pH influence/selective: 133, 136, 153, 161
- purification of solvent: 182, 404
- shaking: 154

Somatomedins, & clinical relevance: 88-

Species differences, e.g. in metabolites: 16, 275
- peptides: 81

Stereoisomers: see Chiral, Diastereo...

Stereoselectivity (cellular /pharmacological; cf. Liver): e.g. 244, 248, 250, 253, 260, 274-

Storage, survival of analytes (cf. Iodin..., Lability): 151, 160-

Sulphoxides/Sulphones (cf. Disulphides): 15, 161, 311, 313, 405
- formed in vitro: 47, 49, 51, 67-, 73
  - minimization: 51, 57, 161
- ring-S: 136, 161-, 207-
- separation (peptides): 49

Tachykinins (& see Analyte Index, IIa): 46

Therapeutic monitoring: e.g. 134, 149, 169

Tissues (besides Index entries), esp. analyte comparisons: 85, 88
- extraction: 5, 40, 51, 76, 80, 153, 156, 216
- regional differences (e.g. brain; cf. Cell): 122, 146

TLC (& see Chiral, Fluori...): 5, 130, 190, 208, 212, 251
- HPTLC: 174
- for sample-preparation: 7, 406
- radio-scanning: 407
- spot troubles, e.g. duality: 278, 280

Toxins: see Mushroom

Trace enrichment (& see HPLC... pre-.. , Zone): 408

Tumours: see Cancer

UV detection in HPLC: see Multi-, Wave... , Ion-pair

Vessels (& see Adsorptive, Plasticizers) & choice/treatment (e.g. silanization): 58, 153, 156

Wavelength ratios (& see Multi-), usefulness: 356-, 376-, 387

Zone refining: 408